Application of Artificial Intelligence to Advance Individualized Diagnosis and Treatment in Emergency and Critical Care Medicine

Application of Artificial Intelligence to Advance Individualized Diagnosis and Treatment in Emergency and Critical Care Medicine

Editor

Zhongheng Zhang

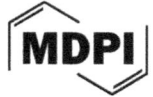

Basel • Beijing • Wuhan • Barcelona • Belgrade • Novi Sad • Cluj • Manchester

Editor
Zhongheng Zhang
Department of Emergency
Medicine, Sir Run Run Shaw
Hospital, Zhejiang University
School of Medicine
Hangzhou
China

Editorial Office
MDPI
St. Alban-Anlage 66
4052 Basel, Switzerland

This is a reprint of articles from the Special Issue published online in the open access journal *Diagnostics* (ISSN 2075-4418) (available at: https://www.mdpi.com/journal/diagnostics/special_issues/AI_Emergency).

For citation purposes, cite each article independently as indicated on the article page online and as indicated below:

Lastname, A.A.; Lastname, B.B. Article Title. *Journal Name* **Year**, *Volume Number*, Page Range.

ISBN 978-3-7258-0909-7 (Hbk)
ISBN 978-3-7258-0910-3 (PDF)
doi.org/10.3390/books978-3-7258-0910-3

Cover image courtesy of Zhongheng Zhang

© 2024 by the authors. Articles in this book are Open Access and distributed under the Creative Commons Attribution (CC BY) license. The book as a whole is distributed by MDPI under the terms and conditions of the Creative Commons Attribution-NonCommercial-NoDerivs (CC BY-NC-ND) license.

Contents

About the Editor vii

Jie Yang, Bo Zhang, Xiaocong Jiang, Jiajie Huang, Yucai Hong, Hongying Ni and Zhongheng Zhang
Application of Artificial Intelligence to Advance Individualized Diagnosis and Treatment in Emergency and Critical Care Medicine
Reprinted from: *Diagnostics* **2024**, *14*, 687, doi:10.3390/diagnostics14070687 1

Kuan-Chi Tu, Eric nyam tee Tau, Nai-Ching Chen, Ming-Chuan Chang, Tzu-Chieh Yu, Che-Chuan Wang, Chung-Feng Liu, et al.
Machine Learning Algorithm Predicts Mortality Risk in Intensive Care Unit for Patients with Traumatic Brain Injury
Reprinted from: *Diagnostics* **2023**, *13*, 3016, doi:10.3390/diagnostics13183016 6

Chin-Choon Yeh, Yu-San Lin, Chun-Chia Chen and Chung-Feng Liu
Implementing AI Models for Prognostic Predictions in High-Risk Burn Patients
Reprinted from: *Diagnostics* **2023**, *13*, 2984, doi:10.3390/diagnostics13182984 20

Jerome Rambaud, Masoumeh Sajedi, Sally Al Omar, Maryline Chomtom, Michael Sauthier, Simon De Montigny and Philippe Jouvet
Clinical Decision Support System to Detect the Occurrence of Ventilator-Associated Pneumonia in Pediatric Intensive Care
Reprinted from: *Diagnostics* **2023**, *13*, 2983, doi:10.3390/diagnostics13182983 37

Xiaofei Chen, Huaiyu Zhu, Linli Mei, Qi Shu, Xiaoying Cheng, Feixiang Luo, Yisheng Zhao, et al.
Video-Based versus On-Site Neonatal Pain Assessment in Neonatal Intensive Care Units: The Impact of Video-Based Neonatal Pain Assessment in Real-World Scenario on Pain Diagnosis and Its Artificial Intelligence Application
Reprinted from: *Diagnostics* **2023**, *13*, 2661, doi:10.3390/diagnostics13162661 49

Hsin-Hung Liu, Yu-Tseng Wang, Meng-Han Yang, Wei-Shu Kevin Lin and Yen-Jen Oyang
Exploiting Machine Learning Technologies to Study the Compound Effects of Serum Creatinine and Electrolytes on the Risk of Acute Kidney Injury in Intensive Care Units
Reprinted from: *Diagnostics* **2023**, *13*, 2551, doi:10.3390/diagnostics13152551 61

Ozum Tuncyurek, Koray Kadam, Berna Uzun and Dilber Uzun Ozsahin
Applicability of American College of Radiology Appropriateness Criteria Decision-Making Modelfor Acute Appendicitis Diagnosis in Children
Reprinted from: *Diagnostics* **2022**, *12*, 2915, doi:10.3390/diagnostics12122915 73

Khandaker Reajul Islam, Jaya Kumar, Toh Leong Tan, Mamun Bin Ibne Reaz, Tawsifur Rahman, Amith Khandakar, Tariq Abbas, et al.
Prognostic Model of ICU Admission Risk in Patients with COVID-19 Infection Using Machine Learning
Reprinted from: *Diagnostics* **2022**, *12*, 2144, doi:10.3390/diagnostics12092144 85

Xiaoying Cheng, Huaiyu Zhu, Linli Mei, Feixiang Luo, Xiaofei Chen, Yisheng Zhao, Shuohui Chen, et al.
Artificial Intelligence Based Pain Assessment Technology in Clinical Application of Real-World Neonatal Blood Sampling
Reprinted from: *Diagnostics* **2022**, *12*, 1831, doi:10.3390/diagnostics12081831 104

Umran Aygun, Fatma Hilal Yagin, Burak Yagin, Seyma Yasar, Cemil Colak, Ahmet Selim Ozkan and Luca Paolo Ardigò
Assessment of Sepsis Risk at Admission to the Emergency Department: Clinical Interpretable Prediction Model
Reprinted from: *Diagnostics* **2024**, *14*, 457, doi:10.3390/diagnostics14050457 . . . . **116**

Ke Pang, Liang Li, Wen Ouyang, Xing Liu and Yongzhong Tang
Establishment of ICU Mortality Risk Prediction Models with Machine Learning Algorithm Using MIMIC-IV Database
Reprinted from: *Diagnostics* **2022**, *12*, 1068, doi:10.3390/diagnostics12051068 . . . . **130**

About the Editor

Zhongheng Zhang

Zhang Zhongheng is a distinguished medical professional and scholar known for his significant contributions to emergency and critical care medicine. He obtained his Bachelor's, Master's, and Doctoral degrees in Clinical Medicine from Zhejiang University between 2007 and 2021. A member of the Jiusan Society, Zhang's research focuses on sepsis, challenging traditional medical paradigms with precision treatment models. His work identifies sepsis subtypes based on clinical phenotypes and genotypes, offering personalized management strategies. Zhang's innovative use of machine learning predicts volume responsiveness and proposes ideal body weight correction for acute respiratory distress syndrome (ARDS) patients. Currently serving as Chief Physician and Associate Professor at Sir Run Run Shaw Hospital, Zhejiang University, Zhang's research is supported by national grants, including from the National Natural Science Foundation of China. His scholarly contributions have earned him numerous awards and honors, with publications in high-impact international journals and over 6,000 citations in the Web of Science (WoS) database, reflecting his global influence. Zhang's dedication to precision medicine has garnered recognition, including the Zhejiang Medical Science and Technology Award, solidifying his position as a leading figure in healthcare advancement and medical research.

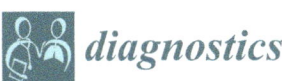

Editorial

Application of Artificial Intelligence to Advance Individualized Diagnosis and Treatment in Emergency and Critical Care Medicine

Jie Yang [1], Bo Zhang [1], Xiaocong Jiang [1], Jiajie Huang [1], Yucai Hong [1], Hongying Ni [2,*] and Zhongheng Zhang [1,*]

1. Department of Emergency Medicine, Sir Run Run Shaw Hospital, Zhejiang University School of Medicine 3#, East Qingchun Road, Hangzhou 310016, China; 22218206@zju.edu.cn (J.Y.); 3414285@zju.edu.cn (B.Z.); jxc506180@163.com (X.J.); 22218207@zju.edu.cn (J.H.); realhealth@zju.edu.cn (Y.H.)
2. Department of Critical Care Medicine, Affiliated Jinhua Hospital, Zhejiang University School of Medicine, No.365 Renmin East Rd, Jinhua 321000, China
* Correspondence: nihongying2@163.com (H.N.); zh_zhang1984@zju.edu.cn (Z.Z.)

Emergency and critical illnesses refer to severe diseases or conditions characterized by rapid changes in health that may endanger life within a short period [1]. With the development of information technology [2], the storage, sharing, and use of medical data have become more convenient. Furthermore, with the rapid development of artificial intelligence technology [3,4], we are at the forefront of a medical information revolution. The emergence of AI has brought new possibilities for the treatment of critically ill patients [5,6]. Through big data analysis and machine learning, we are able to predict the progression of diseases more accurately and adjust treatment plans in a timely manner [7–9]. This trend towards precision medicine has had a profound impact on medical practice [10]. In this context, we have organized a Special Issue to discuss the application of AI in the management of critical illnesses, aiming to achieve greater advancements in future healthcare.

In this Special Issue, researchers from various countries and regions have explored the application of artificial intelligence in critical care, covering aspects such as diagnosis, management, and prognosis. (Figure 1) Several previous studies have explored the realm of diagnosis. Aygun et al. (Contribution 1) aimed to develop an interpretable predictive model based on Explainable Artificial Intelligence (XAI) to forecast sepsis and identify significant biomarkers. Within a cohort of 1572 patients, they utilized biomarkers including age, respiratory rate, blood oxygen saturation, procalcitonin, and positive blood culture to predict sepsis. The results of SHapley Additive exPlanations (SHAP) indicate that factors such as advanced age, increased respiratory rate, and decreased procalcitonin elevate the risk of sepsis. By enhancing transparency in the decision-making process, XAI models enable clinicians to comprehend and trust the predictive capabilities of AI systems [11]. During the diagnostic process, multiple methods are often available to assist physicians in making a diagnosis. Tuncyurek (Contribution 2) conducted an evaluation using artificial intelligence methods to determine the optimal selection of methods. Acute appendicitis stands as one of the most common causes of abdominal pain in the emergency department and is the leading surgical emergency among children under 15, posing a significant risk upon rupture. The selection of radiological methods is paramount for accurate diagnosis, thereby averting unnecessary surgeries. The aim of this study is to evaluate the effectiveness of the American College of Radiology (ACR) Appropriateness Criteria in diagnosing acute appendicitis using multivariable decision criteria. This study's uniqueness lies in its provision of an analytical ranking of results for this intricate decision problem, showcasing the merits and demerits of each alternative in different scenarios, even accounting for the ambiguity of emergency situations concerning the diagnosis of pediatric appendicitis. We applaud the utilization of a novel model to test the ACR qualification criteria, aiming to minimize confusion in the diagnostic process.

Citation: Yang, J.; Zhang, B.; Jiang, X.; Huang, J.; Hong, Y.; Ni, H.; Zhang, Z. Application of Artificial Intelligence to Advance Individualized Diagnosis and Treatment in Emergency and Critical Care Medicine. *Diagnostics* **2024**, *14*, 687. https://doi.org/10.3390/diagnostics14070687

Received: 15 March 2024
Revised: 20 March 2024
Accepted: 21 March 2024
Published: 25 March 2024

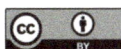

Copyright: © 2024 by the authors. Licensee MDPI, Basel, Switzerland. This article is an open access article distributed under the terms and conditions of the Creative Commons Attribution (CC BY) license (https:// creativecommons.org/licenses/by/ 4.0/).

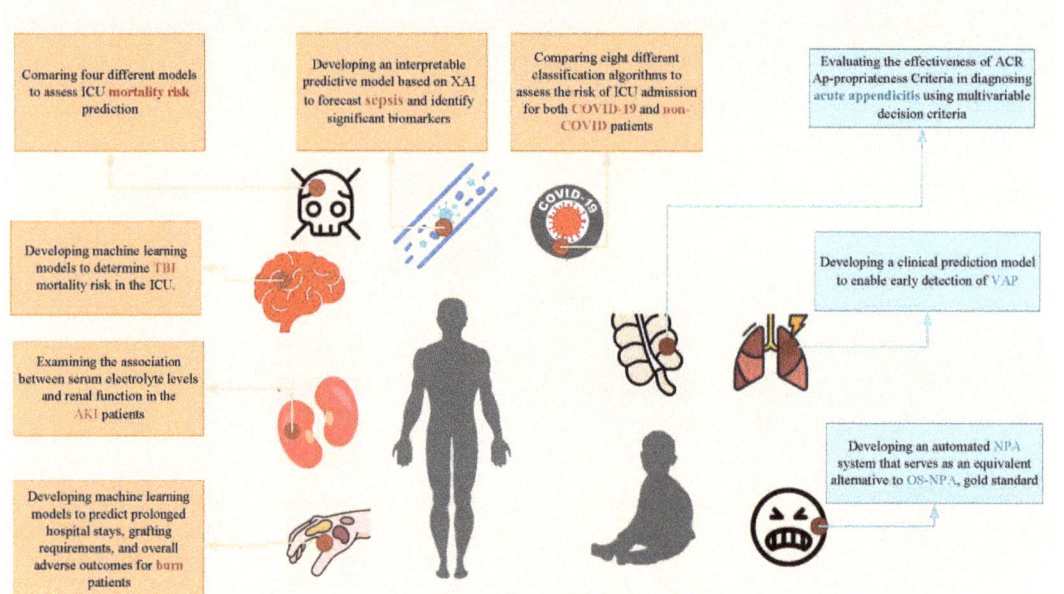

Figure 1. The figure provides a visual summary of the contents covered in the special issue. Through these visual elements, readers can quickly grasp the various topics and related content featured in the issue. XAI: Explainable Artificial Intelligence; TBI: Traumatic Brain Injury; ICU: Intensive Care Unit; AKI: Acute Kidney Injury; COVID-19: Coronavirus Disease 2019; VAP: Ventilator-Associated Pneumonia; NPA: Neonatal Pain Assessment; OS-NPA: on-site Neonatal Pain Assessment; ACR: the American College of Radiology.

Figure 1 provides a visual summary of the contents covered in the Special Issue. Through these visual elements, readers can quickly grasp the various topics and any related content featured in the Issue. XAI: Explainable Artificial Intelligence; TBI: Traumatic Brain Injury; ICU: Intensive Care Unit; AKI: Acute Kidney Injury; COVID-19: Coronavirus Disease 2019; VAP: Ventilator-Associated Pneumonia; NPA: Neonatal Pain Assessment; OS-NPA: On-Site Neonatal Pain Assessment; ACR: The American College of Radiology.

The risk of acute kidney injury (AKI) has long presented a challenge for clinicians in the intensive care unit (ICU) [12,13]. The combined effects of serum creatinine, blood urea nitrogen (BUN), and clinically relevant serum electrolytes have yet to be comprehensively studied. Through a screening of the MIMIC-IV Database, the association between serum electrolyte levels and renal function was examined (Contribution 3), revealing that levels of serum creatinine, chloride, and magnesium emerged as the three primary factors requiring monitoring in this patient cohort. Thus, it is imperative to undertake larger-scale studies based on this research to strengthen and refine the clinical guidelines pertaining to AKI.

Rambaud et al. developed a clinical prediction algorithm using prospective clinical data from 827 pediatric patients stored in a Canadian tertiary pediatric hospital database (Contribution 4). This algorithm aims to enable the early detection of ventilator-associated pneumonia (VAP). Notably, this study demonstrates the most accurate sensitivity achieved by a Clinical Decision Support System (CDSS) to date in identifying VAP. We anticipate the implementation of the results of this algorithm by Jerome Rambaud in the Pediatric Intensive Care Unit (PICU), and we look forward to seeing its outstanding performance in multicenter trials.

Furthermore, artificial intelligence has numerous applications in prognosis. In the fields of traumatic brain injury (TBI) and burn injuries, artificial intelligence (AI) technologies have significantly advanced the predictive accuracy of patient outcomes beyond traditional models. Tu et al. and Yeh et al. conducted retrospective studies in their respective areas, gathering extensive patient data to employ machine learning models in the prediction of mortality and adverse outcomes. The researchers focused on 2260 TBI patients in the ICU, using four machine learning models and 42 features. Their study outperformed traditional tools like APACHE II and SOFA scores in predicting mortality risk (Contribution 5). Similarly, Yeh et al. analyzed data from 348 burn patients, demonstrating AI's ability to predict prolonged hospital stays, grafting needs, and other adverse outcomes more accurately than the commonly used Baux score (Contribution 6). Both studies highlight the role of modern AI in enhancing the stratification and assessment of patients, marking significant progress towards intelligent healthcare in their respective domains. In another study (Contribution 7) utilizing the MIMIC-IV Database, multiple machine learning models were employed to predict patient mortality, with the findings indicating that the XGBoost machine learning method outperformed traditional models through comparative analysis.

Furthermore, artificial intelligence plays a significant role in disease management [14]. Amidst the outbreak of the COVID-19 pandemic, the escalating number of critically ill patients in global intensive care units (ICUs) has placed a strain on ICU resources. The early prediction of ICU demand is crucial for effective resource management and allocation. Islam et al. conducted a retrospective cohort study focusing on data collected from the Pulmonology Department of a state hospital in Moscow (Contribution 8). Various feature selection techniques were investigated, and a stacked machine learning model was proposed. This model was compared with eight different classification algorithms to assess the risk of ICU admission for both COVID-19 and non-COVID patients, as well as for COVID patients separately.

Artificial intelligence also plays an important role in image recognition and assessment in the medical fields. The assessment of neonatal pain (NPA) has not received sufficient attention in clinical practice, leading to widespread instances of undertreatment of pain severity. In clinical NPA, facial expressions are considered the most explicit indicators, upon which various pain assessment scales are designed. Zhu et al. aimed to develop an automated NPA system that meets actual clinical needs (Contributions 9 and 10). To achieve this, a video database capturing the facial expressions of neonates during blood collection procedures in the neonatal ward was established, and an AI-NPA method was developed based on real-world data. The clinical utility of the automated NPA system was validated by recruiting 232 pediatric patients from a tertiary children's hospital in China. According to the OS-NPA results of 232 neonates, the accuracy of the automated NPA system was 88.79%. Although video-based NPA (VB-NPA) protocols facilitate remote or post hoc pain diagnosis by experts, serving as an equivalent alternative to the on-site NPA (OS-NPA) gold standard, VB-NPA may suffer from partial inaccuracies due to information loss in neonatal pain videos captured in real NICU settings. Nonetheless, it remains comparable to OS-NPA. Video-based assessment for neonatal pain evaluation in clinical settings is feasible and allows for the real-time, remote assessment of neonatal pain severity. We anticipate further applications of this technology in neonates with larger-scale data and potential migration to adult pain assessment.

Collectively, these studies illuminate the transformative impact of AI and ML in medical diagnostics and prognostics, heralding a new era of precision medicine that promises enhanced patient outcomes and optimized healthcare delivery [15]. Additionally, in the application of artificial intelligence, there are characteristics of overfitting and poor generalization; some models produce very precise predictions, but this precision may not necessarily translate into clinical benefits [16]. To address these issues of generalization, further validation is needed through randomized controlled trials (RCTs) across multiple centers.

Funding: The study was founded by the China National Key Research and Development Program (NO.: 2022YFC2504503, 2023YFC3603104), the Huadong Medicine Joint Funds of the Zhejiang Provincial Natural Science Foundation of China under Grant No. LHDMD24H150001; National Natural Science Foundation of China (82272180) and the Project of Drug Clinical Evaluate Research of Chinese Pharmaceutical Association NO. CPA-Z06-ZC-2021–004.

Conflicts of Interest: The author declares no conflicts of interest. The funders had no role in the design of the study; in the collection, analyses, or interpretation of data; in the writing of the manuscript, or in the decision to publish the results.

List of Contributions:

1. Aygun, U.; Yagin, F.H.; Yagin, B.; Yasar, S.; Colak, C.; Ozkan, A.S.; Ardigò, L.P. Assessment of Sepsis Risk at Admission to the Emergency Department: Clinical Interpretable Prediction Model. *Diagnostics* **2024**, *14*, 457. https://doi.org/10.3390/diagnostics14050457.
2. Tuncyurek, O.; Kadam, K.; Uzun, B.; Uzun Ozsahin, D. Applicability of American College of Radiology Appropriateness Criteria Decision-Making Model for Acute Appendicitis Diagnosis in Children. *Diagnostics* **2022**, *12*, 2915. https://doi.org/10.3390/diagnostics12122915.
3. Liu, H.-H.; Wang, Y.-T.; Yang, M.-H.; Lin, W.-S.K.; Oyang, Y.-J. Exploiting Machine Learning Technologies to Study the Compound Effects of Serum Creatinine and Electrolytes on the Risk of Acute Kidney Injury in Intensive Care Units. *Diagnostics* **2023**, *13*, 2551. https://doi.org/10.3390/diagnostics13152551.
4. Rambaud, J.; Sajedi, M.; Al Omar, S.; Chomtom, M.; Sauthier, M.; De Montigny, S.; Jouvet, P. Clinical Decision Support System to Detect the Occurrence of Ventilator-Associated Pneumonia in Pediatric Intensive Care. *Diagnostics* **2023**, *13*, 2983. https://doi.org/10.3390/diagnostics13182983.
5. Tu, K.-C.; Tau, E.n.t.; Chen, N.-C.; Chang, M.-C.; Yu, T.-C.; Wang, C.-C.; Liu, C.-F.; Kuo, C.-L. Machine Learning Algorithm Predicts Mortality Risk in Intensive Care Unit for Patients with Traumatic Brain Injury. *Diagnostics* **2023**, *13*, 3016. https://doi.org/10.3390/diagnostics13183016.
6. Yeh, C.-C.; Lin, Y.-S.; Chen, C.-C.; Liu, C.-F. Implementing AI Models for Prognostic Predictions in High-Risk Burn Patients. *Diagnostics* **2023**, *13*, 2984. https://doi.org/10.3390/diagnostics13182984.
7. Pang, K.; Li, L.; Ouyang, W.; Liu, X.; Tang, Y. Establishment of ICU Mortality Risk Prediction Models with Machine Learning Algorithm Using MIMIC-IV Database. *Diagnostics* **2022**, *12*, 1068. https://doi.org/10.3390/diagnostics12051068
8. Islam, K.R.; Kumar, J.; Tan, T.L.; Reaz, M.B.I.; Rahman, T.; Khandakar, A.; Abbas, T.; Hossain, M.S.A.; Zughaier, S.M.; Chowdhury, M.E.H. Prognostic Model of ICU Admission Risk in Patients with COVID-19 Infection Using Machine Learning. *Diagnostics* **2022**, *12*, 2144. https://doi.org/10.3390/diagnostics12092144.
9. Chen, X.; Zhu, H.; Mei, L.; Shu, Q.; Cheng, X.; Luo, F.; Zhao, Y.; Chen, S.; Pan, Y. Video-Based versus On-Site Neonatal Pain Assessment in Neonatal Intensive Care Units: The Impact of Video-Based Neonatal Pain Assessment in Real-World Scenario on Pain Diagnosis and Its Artificial Intelligence Application. *Diagnostics* **2023**, *13*, 2661. https://doi.org/10.3390/diagnostics13162661.
10. Cheng, X.; Zhu, H.; Mei, L.; Luo, F.; Chen, X.; Zhao, Y.; Chen, S.; Pan, Y. Artificial Intelligence Based Pain Assessment Technology in Clinical Application of Real-World Neonatal Blood Sampling. *Diagnostics* **2022**, *12*, 1831. https://doi.org/10.3390/diagnostics12081831.

References

1. Crawford, A.M.; Shiferaw, A.A.; Ntambwe, P.; Milan, A.O.; Khalid, K.; Rubio, R.; Nizeyimana, F.; Ariza, F.; Mohammed, A.D.; Baker, T.; et al. Global critical care: A call to action. *Crit. Care* **2023**, *27*, 28. [CrossRef] [PubMed]
2. Pandit, J.A.; Pawelek, J.B.; Leff, B.; Topol, E.J. The hospital at home in the USA: Current status and future prospects. *NPJ Digit. Med.* **2024**, *7*, 48. [CrossRef] [PubMed]
3. Rampton, V. Artificial intelligence versus clinicians. *BMJ* **2020**, *369*, m1326. [CrossRef] [PubMed]
4. He, X.; Liu, X.; Zuo, F.; Shi, H.; Jing, J. Artificial intelligence-based multi-omics analysis fuels cancer precision medicine. *Semin. Cancer Biol.* **2023**, *88*, 187–200. [CrossRef] [PubMed]
5. Komorowski, M.; Celi, L.A.; Badawi, O.; Gordon, A.C.; Faisal, A.A. The Artificial Intelligence Clinician learns optimal treatment strategies for sepsis in intensive care. *Nat. Med.* **2018**, *24*, 1716–1720. [CrossRef]
6. Devis, L.; Catry, E.; Honore, P.M.; Mansour, A.; Lippi, G.; Mullier, F.; Closset, M. Interventions to improve appropriateness of laboratory testing in the intensive care unit: A narrative review. *Ann. Intensive Care* **2024**, *14*, 9. [CrossRef] [PubMed]

7. Myszczynska, M.A.; Ojamies, P.N.; Lacoste, A.M.B.; Neil, D.; Saffari, A.; Mead, R.; Hautbergue, G.M.; Holbrook, J.D.; Ferraiuolo, L. Applications of machine learning to diagnosis and treatment of neurodegenerative diseases. *Nat. Rev. Neurol.* **2020**, *16*, 440–456. [CrossRef] [PubMed]
8. Ngiam, K.Y.; Khor, I.W. Big data and machine learning algorithms for health-care delivery. *Lancet Oncol.* **2019**, *20*, e262–e273. [CrossRef] [PubMed]
9. Goecks, J.; Jalili, V.; Heiser, L.M.; Gray, J.W. How Machine Learning Will Transform Biomedicine. *Cell* **2020**, *181*, 92–101. [CrossRef] [PubMed]
10. Denny, J.C.; Collins, F.S. Precision medicine in 2030—Seven ways to transform healthcare. *Cell* **2021**, *184*, 1415–1419. [CrossRef] [PubMed]
11. Tjoa, E.; Guan, C. A Survey on Explainable Artificial Intelligence (XAI): Toward Medical XAI. *IEEE Trans. Neural Netw. Learn. Syst.* **2021**, *32*, 4793–4813. [CrossRef] [PubMed]
12. Chronopoulos, A.; Rosner, M.H.; Cruz, D.N.; Ronco, C. Acute kidney injury in elderly intensive care patients: A review. *Intensive Care Med.* **2010**, *36*, 1454–1464. [CrossRef] [PubMed]
13. Kellum, J.A.; Prowle, J.R. Paradigms of acute kidney injury in the intensive care setting. *Nat. Rev. Nephrol.* **2018**, *14*, 217–230. [CrossRef] [PubMed]
14. Komorowski, M. Clinical management of sepsis can be improved by artificial intelligence: Yes. *Intensive Care Med.* **2020**, *46*, 375–377. [CrossRef] [PubMed]
15. Gutierrez, G. Artificial Intelligence in the Intensive Care Unit. *Crit. Care* **2020**, *24*, 101. [CrossRef] [PubMed]
16. Goodman, K.; Zandi, D.; Reis, A.; Vayena, E. Balancing risks and benefits of artificial intelligence in the health sector. *Bull. World Health Organ.* **2020**, *98*, 230. [CrossRef] [PubMed]

Disclaimer/Publisher's Note: The statements, opinions and data contained in all publications are solely those of the individual author(s) and contributor(s) and not of MDPI and/or the editor(s). MDPI and/or the editor(s) disclaim responsibility for any injury to people or property resulting from any ideas, methods, instructions or products referred to in the content.

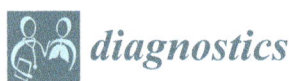

Article

Machine Learning Algorithm Predicts Mortality Risk in Intensive Care Unit for Patients with Traumatic Brain Injury

Kuan-Chi Tu [1], Eric nyam tee Tau [1,*], Nai-Ching Chen [2], Ming-Chuan Chang [2], Tzu-Chieh Yu [2], Che-Chuan Wang [1,3], Chung-Feng Liu [4] and Ching-Lung Kuo [1,3,5,*]

1. Department of Neurosurgery, Chi Mei Medical Center, Tainan 710402, Taiwan; gary12223@hotmail.com (K.-C.T.); wangchechuan@gmail.com (C.-C.W.)
2. Department of Nursing, Chi Mei Medical Center, Tainan 710402, Taiwan; patty11@gmail.com (N.-C.C.); h85068132@yahoo.com.tw (M.-C.C.); fish5777@yahoo.com.tw (T.-C.Y.)
3. Center for General Education, Southern Taiwan University of Science and Technology, Tainan 710402, Taiwan
4. Department of Medical Research, Chi Mei Medical Center, Tainan 710402, Taiwan; chungfengliu@gmail.com
5. School of Medicine, College of Medicine, National Sun Yat-sen University, Kaohsiung 804, Taiwan
* Correspondence: ronaldowen@gmail.com (E.n.t.T.); kuojinnrung@gmail.com (C.-L.K.); Tel.: +886-6-281-2811-57423 (C.-L.K.)

Abstract: Background: Numerous mortality prediction tools are currently available to assist patients with moderate to severe traumatic brain injury (TBI). However, an algorithm that utilizes various machine learning methods and employs diverse combinations of features to identify the most suitable predicting outcomes of brain injury patients in the intensive care unit (ICU) has not yet been well-established. Method: Between January 2016 and December 2021, we retrospectively collected data from the electronic medical records of Chi Mei Medical Center, comprising 2260 TBI patients admitted to the ICU. A total of 42 features were incorporated into the analysis using four different machine learning models, which were then segmented into various feature combinations. The predictive performance was assessed using the area under the curve (AUC) of the receiver operating characteristic (ROC) curve and validated using the Delong test. Result: The AUC for each model under different feature combinations ranged from 0.877 (logistic regression with 14 features) to 0.921 (random forest with 22 features). The Delong test indicated that the predictive performance of the machine learning models is better than that of traditional tools such as APACHE II and SOFA scores. Conclusion: Our machine learning training demonstrated that the predictive accuracy of the LightGBM is better than that of APACHE II and SOFA scores. These features are readily available on the first day of patient admission to the ICU. By integrating this model into the clinical platform, we can offer clinicians an immediate prognosis for the patient, thereby establishing a bridge for educating and communicating with family members.

Keywords: artificial intelligence; machine learning; traumatic brain injury; mortality; intensive care unit; computer-assisted system

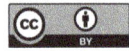

1. Introduction

Traumatic brain injury is a global issue that not only impacts patients' health but also imposes a significant burden on social, economic, and medical resources [1]. The age-adjusted mortality rate in Europe is 11.7 per 100,000 and 17.0 per 100,000 in the US [2,3]. In contrast to Western countries, where TBI is often associated with war, Asia experiences TBI due to falls and road traffic injuries [4]. As low- to middle-income countries undergo industrial transformation leading to increased mechanization and urbanization, the incidence of brain injuries is gradually rising. However, the slow growth of medical resources in these countries results in more severe disabilities compared to developed nations [4].

Survivors of TBI typically face neurological deficits and disabilities. Those with severe TBI receive treatment in the intensive care unit (ICU). Various efforts have been made to predict the prognosis of TBI patients, exploring factors such as Glasgow Coma Scale (GCS), age, pupillary reactivity, injury severity, and clinical condition (e.g., hypoxia, respiratory distress, and hypotension) in numerous studies. The evaluation of brain injury extent and classification using CT scans is also closely linked to mortality [5–8].

A previous retrospective study found variability in the use of a single predictive model across populations [9]. Although studies of IMPACT and CRASH are widely known, they may not be applicable to each individual patient [10]. The SOFA (Sequential Organ Failure Assessment), introduced in 1996, is designed to describe the progression of complications in critically ill patients and an elevated SOFA score is associated with a higher likelihood of mortality [11,12]. APACHE II relies on 12 physiological variables measured within the first 24 h of ICU admission to predict ICU patient outcomes [13]. However, the use of APACHE II and SOFA has only shown marginal improvement in prognostic performance [14]. Therefore, we need to seek more accurate predictive models for prognosis and mortality in ICU settings.

Machine learning (ML) approaches require more input and output data for analysis, but they excel at handling complex interrelationships. Compared to classical linear regression statistics, machine learning processes data directly, resulting in more accurate predictions [15]. However, the "black-box" nature of AI, characterized by its lack of explanation, is still the main reason for the low clinical application. In order to improve the predictive explanation of AI models, Explanatory Artificial Intelligence (XAI) techniques have been introduced, with SHAP (SHapley Additive exPlanations) being the most widely used XAI technique for explaining which clinical features are important for predicting various diseases or patient prognosis. Therefore, it is very important to use XAI to better interpret how each feature contributes to the associated outcome in the AI prediction model [16].

Courville E et al. reported a systematic view and meta-analysis (2013–2020) demonstrating that much of this literature discusses in-hospital mortality and poor prognosis, but lacks a more specific focus on the ICU population to understand the predictive power of AIs in TBI patients [17]. In the last three years, there have been several reports on the prognosis and mortality risk of brain injury using ML techniques. However, some of these studies may not have selected different combinations of features based on clinical importance, lacked comparisons with traditional tools, or were not conducted in an ICU setting. Therefore, further investigation is needed to clarify this point [18–21].

Our goal is to use machine learning algorithms to analyze the vast amount of ICU data to predict mortality risk after TBI, which is more tailored to patients in our country. Additionally, it is essential to compare these ML models with the existing APACHE II and SOFA scores. We also use the SHAP technique to explain which clinical features are important for predicting various diseases or patient outcomes.

2. Materials and Methods

2.1. Ethics

This research received ethical approval (revision: 11106-013) from the institutional review board at Chi Mei Medical Center in Tainan, Taiwan. The authors conducted the study in accordance with appropriate guidelines and regulations. Since the study was retrospective in nature, the Ethics Committee waived the requirement for informed consent.

2.2. Flow Chart and AI Device of Current Study

Our study followed the guidelines specified in the Transparent Reporting of a Multivariable Prediction Model for Individual Prognosis or Diagnosis (TRIPOD) standard. Figure 1 illustrates the flowchart detailing the ML training process and its integration into the hospital system. The ML model was trained using a total of 42 selected features identified based on their statistically significant differences (p-value < 0.05) between the mortality and non-mortality groups.

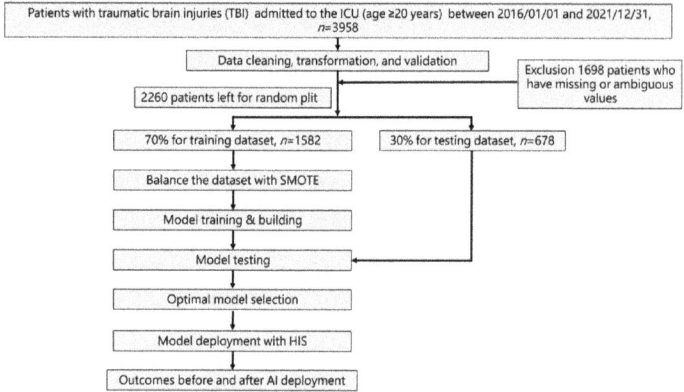

Figure 1. Workflow diagram for data collection and machine learning model training.

To assess model performance, a 70% training dataset was used, while the remaining 30% formed the test set via random splitting. As a result, four models were developed to predict mortality risk.

Statistical analysis involved t-tests for numerical variables and Chi-square tests for categorical variables. Additionally, Spearman correlation analysis was conducted to evaluate the strength of the correlation between each feature and the outcome. Recognizing the imbalanced outcome classes, particularly in mortality cases, we employed the synthetic minority oversampling technique (SMOTE) [22]. This oversampling technique was applied to balance the number of positive outcome cases (mortality) with the negative cases (survival) during the final model training with each machine learning algorithm.

Figure 2 illustrates the utilization of the hospital backend system to collect data from various assessment modules, including the ICU evaluation module, vital signs module, health status module, and medical history module. These modules provide input to the central computer for integrated processing, and the data are then fed into the ML training model for simulation.

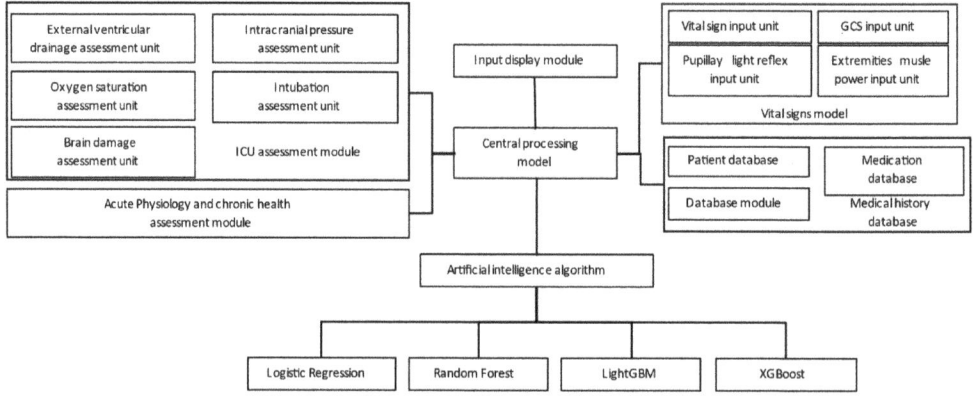

Figure 2. System training architecture.

2.3. Patient Selection

From January 2016 to December 2021, a retrospective collection of patients aged 20 years and older who were diagnosed with TBI and admitted to the ICU was conducted using the electronic medical records of Chi Mei Medical Center. The inclusion criteria included neurosurgical patients who have been admitted to the ICU with the following diagnostic codes. ICD-9: 800*–804*, 850*–854*, 959.0, 959.01, and 959.8–959.9; ICD-10: S00*-T07*. Patients with missing or ambiguous values were excluded.

2.4. Feature Selection and Model Building

Under the consensus of several neurosurgeons and intensive care physicians, we identified parameters that met the following criteria: (1) representation of the clinical status of traumatic brain injury patients, (2) objective assessability, and (3) generalizability. Subsequently, we employed univariate filter methods for feature selection, considering both continuous and categorical variables. A significance level of 0.05 or lower was used for selection. Additionally, Spearman's correlation coefficient and expert opinions were considered during the finalization of the feature selection process. The study utilized 42 features, as listed in Table 1. We employed four machine learning algorithms, including Logistic Regression [23], Random Forest [24], LightGBM [25], and XGBoost [26], to construct predictive models for mortality in ICU. To reduce concerns of overfitting that might arise from a small dataset, we utilized the cross-validation technique to build the models.

Table 1. Characteristics and significance of traumatic brain injury patients.

Feature	Overall $n = 2260$	Non-Mortality $n = 2020$	Mortality $n = 240$	p-Value
Female, n (%)	813 (35.97)	735 (36.39)	78 (32.50)	0.265
male, n (%)	1447 (64.03)	1285 (63.61)	162 (67.50)	
Age, mean (SD)	63.89 (17.74)	63.26 (17.76)	69.22 (16.65)	<0.001
height, mean (SD)	162.74 (11.24)	162.75 (10.95)	162.60 (13.43)	0.862
weight, mean (SD)	63.00 (14.16)	63.24 (14.23)	61.00 (13.42)	0.016
Systolic blood pressure (SBP), mean (SD)	142.36 (29.41)	143.33 (28.40)	134.22 (35.86)	<0.001
Diastolic blood pressure (DBP), mean (SD)	78.02 (17.02)	78.72 (16.36)	72.13 (20.90)	<0.001
Mean Arterial Pressure (MAP), mean (SD)	100.04 (20.67)	100.99 (19.86)	92.06 (25.24)	<0.001
Body temperature (BT), mean (SD)	36.55 (0.63)	36.57 (0.56)	36.39 (1.01)	0.005
pulse, mean (SD)	86.48 (16.95)	85.93 (15.90)	91.10 (23.57)	0.001
Respiratory rate (RR), mean (SD)	17.67 (4.06)	17.73 (3.95)	17.10 (4.83)	0.054
Glasgow Coma Scale_eye opening (GCS_E), mean (SD)	3.13 (1.26)	3.31 (1.15)	1.69 (1.18)	<0.001
Glasgow Coma Scale_verbal response (GCS_V), mean (SD)	3.52 (1.75)	3.75 (1.66)	1.65 (1.30)	<0.001
Glasgow Coma Scale_motor response (GCS_M), mean (SD)	4.99 (1.77)	5.21 (1.60)	3.08 (1.97)	<0.001
Glasgow Coma Scale (GCS), mean (SD)	11.64 (4.48)	12.27 (4.11)	6.41 (4.03)	<0.001
Left Pupil				
Pupil reflex (−), n (%)	230 (10.18)	104 (5.15)	126 (52.50)	<0.001
Pupil reflex (+), n (%)	2030 (89.82)	1916 (94.85)	114 (47.50)	
Pupil size (L), mean (SD)	3.23 (0.99)	3.10 (0.77)	4.29 (1.70)	<0.001
Right Pupil				
Pupil reflex (−), n (%)	231 (10.22)	103 (5.10)	128 (53.33)	<0.001
Pupil reflex (+), n (%)	2029 (89.78)	1917 (94.90)	112 (46.67)	
Pupil size (R), mean (SD)	3.22 (0.99)	3.09 (0.76)	4.34 (1.74)	<0.001
Muscle power_left upper extremity (Muscle_LUE), mean (SD)	3.03 (1.66)	3.24 (1.54)	1.30 (1.59)	<0.001
Muscle power_left lower extremity (Muscle_LLEE), mean (SD)	2.93 (1.67)	3.13 (1.58)	1.24 (1.48)	<0.001
Muscle power_right upper extremity (Muscle_RUE), mean (SD)	3.04 (1.66)	3.25 (1.54)	1.30 (1.57)	<0.001
Muscle power_right lower extremity (Muscle_RLE), mean (SD)	2.94 (1.67)	3.14 (1.58)	1.22 (1.46)	<0.001
Inspired fraction of oxygen (FiO2), mean (SD)	27.80 (11.52)	26.49 (9.08)	38.84 (20.50)	<0.001
APACHE II, mean (SD)	12.92 (7.44)	11.71 (6.44)	23.10 (7.49)	<0.001
Sequential Organ Failure Assessment (SOFA score), mean (SD)	3.10 (2.72)	2.64 (2.26)	6.94 (3.17)	<0.001
Endotracheal tube (Endo)				
No, n (%)	1283 (56.77)	1229 (60.84)	54 (22.50)	<0.001
Yes, n (%)	977 (43.23)	791 (39.16)	186 (77.50)	
External ventricular drain (EVD)				
No, n (%)	2045 (90.49)	1823 (90.25)	222 (92.50)	0.313
Yes, n (%)	215 (9.51)	197 (9.75)	18 (7.50)	

Table 1. Cont.

Feature	Overall n = 2260	Non-Mortality n = 2020	Mortality n = 240	p-Value
Intracranial pressure (ICP), n (%)				
No, n (%)	2025 (89.60)	1835 (90.84)	190 (79.17)	<0.001
Yes, n (%)	235 (10.40)	185 (9.16)	50 (20.83)	
Cerebral perfusion pressure (CPP), n (%)				
No, n (%)	2025 (89.60)	1835 (90.84)	190 (79.17)	<0.001
Yes, n (%)	235 (10.40)	185 (9.16)	50 (20.83)	
surgery, n (%)	310 (13.72)	247 (12.23)	63 (26.25)	<0.001
Drugs				
vasopressors, n (%)	293 (12.96)	157 (7.77)	136 (56.67)	<0.001
sedative_hypnotic, n (%)	950 (42.04)	787 (38.96)	163 (67.92)	<0.001
Perdipine, n (%)	354 (15.66)	295 (14.60)	59 (24.58)	<0.001
Underlying disease				
Hypertension, n (%)	954 (42.21)	829 (41.04)	125 (52.08)	0.001
Diabetes mellitus, n (%)	581 (25.71)	510 (25.25)	71 (29.58)	0.169
heart disease, n (%)	363 (16.06)	320 (15.84)	43 (17.92)	0.462
Cerebrovascular disease, n (%)	206 (9.12)	181 (8.96)	25 (10.42)	0.534
Gastrointestinal disease, n (%)	168 (7.43)	151 (7.48)	17 (7.08)	0.929
Liver Disease, n (%)	161 (7.12)	135 (6.68)	26 (10.83)	0.026
kidney disease, n (%)	133 (5.88)	100 (4.95)	33 (13.75)	<0.001
cancer, n (%)	110 (4.87)	97 (4.80)	13 (5.42)	0.795
Thyroid disease, n (%)	55 (2.43)	53 (2.62)	2 (0.83)	0.139
epilepsy, n (%)	45 (1.99)	40 (1.98)	5 (2.08)	0.809
asthma, n (%)	41 (1.81)	39 (1.93)	2 (0.83)	0.310
pneumonia, n (%)	38 (1.68)	32 (1.58)	6 (2.50)	0.286

Note. A t-test was used for numerical variables and the Chi-square test was used for categorical variables. Surgical procedures are as follows: decompressive craniectomy, acute epidural hematoma removal, acute subdural hematoma removal, acute intracerebral hematoma removal, and intracranial pressure monitor placement. A patient who undergoes one of the above five surgical procedures is said to have undergone surgery.

2.5. Model Performance Measurement

In this study, we evaluated the performance of the machine learning models using accuracy, sensitivity, specificity, and area under the curve (AUC) of the receiver operating characteristic curve (ROC).

Specificity is an important metric to assess the ability of a test or diagnostic method to correctly identify normal results (non-patients), while sensitivity evaluates the ability to correctly identify positive outcomes (patients). These metrics are mutually influencing and should be considered comprehensively in research [27].

Accuracy measures the correctness of predictions made by a classification model or testing method and represents the proportion of correct predictions among all predictions made. However, in certain imbalanced datasets, accuracy can be misleading and lead to poor prediction performance for minority classes [28].

The AUC, representing the area under the ROC curve, which represents the trade-off between sensitivity and specificity (false positive rate) at different thresholds, serves as an effective "summary" of the ROC curves' performance [29,30].

To assess the superiority of each machine learning model compared to traditional tools, we specifically used the DeLong test [31].

3. Results

3.1. Characteristics and Clinical Presentations of Individuals with Traumatic Brain Injury

A total of 2260 patients were retrospectively included from the electronic medical records system of Chi-Mei Hospital. Among them, there were 1447 males (64.03%) and 813 females (35.97%). The average age was approximately 63.89 ± 17.74 (mean $\pm$ SD) years old. The characteristics of the patients are listed in Table 1, comprising 42 features, including vital signs, coma scale, pupillary reflex, intubation status, external ventricular drainage, and comorbidities. Among these, 29 features showed a significant difference in relation to mortality (p-value < 0.05).

3.2. The Correlation between Factors and Mortality (Spearman Correlation Coefficient)

To accurately quantify the impact of each factor on prediction within the ML model, we conducted an analysis using the Spearman correlation coefficient. Among the factors, 22 had coefficients greater than 0.1 (italic) and showed a significant correlation with mortality, indicating their substantial influence on prediction. Moreover, among these features, 14 had coefficients greater than 0.2 (bold) and demonstrated a significant correlation with mortality (Table 2). The top five variables exhibiting high correlation coefficients include pupil_reflex + (R), pupil_reflex + (L), vasopressors, GCS_M, and GCS_E. Notably, while SOFA and APACHE II were employed to compare predictive performances with the AI model, they were not utilized as features in the AI model itself.

Table 2. The Spearman correlation coefficient for each factor.

Feature	Mortality	Feature	Mortality
Gender	0.025	FiO2	**0.294**
Age	*0.108*	**APACHE II**	**0.397**
Hight	0.008	**SOFA**	**0.398**
Weight	−0.045	**Endo**	**0.238**
SBP	−0.066	EVD	−0.024
DBP	*−0.108*	*ICP*	*0.118*
MAP	*−0.110*	*CPP*	*0.118*
BT	−0.088	*surgery*	*0.126*
pulse	0.079	**vasopressors**	**0.448**
RR	−0.066	*Sedative−hypnotic drugs*	*0.181*
GCS_E	**−0.371**	Perdipine	0.085
GCS_V	**−0.348**	Hypertension	0.069
GCS_M	**−0.398**	Diabetes mellitus	0.031
GCS	**−0.363**	Cerebrovascular disease	0.016
pupil_reflex + (L)	**−0.483**	heart disease	0.017
pupil_size(L)	**0.235**	asthma	−0.025
pupil_reflex + (R)	**−0.491**	pneumonia	0.022
pupil_size(R)	**0.241**	Gastrointestinal disease	−0.005
Muscle_LUE	**−0.325**	cancer	0.009
Muscle_LLEE	**−0.326**	Liver Disease	0.050
Muscle_RUE	**−0.328**	epilepsy	0.002
Muscle_RLE	**−0.331**	*kidney disease*	*0.115*
		Thyroid disease	−0.036

Note. *Italicized* text: absolute value greater than 0.1; **Bold** text: absolute value greater than 0.2.

3.3. Predictive Models with Different Features Combinations

Table 3 presents the predictive outcomes obtained from various feature combinations and artificial intelligence learning. Initially, there were 42 features, which were then categorized based on their significant difference with mortality and their Spearman correlation coefficient. This resulted in three groups: 29 features significantly correlated with mortality, 22 features with a Spearman correlation coefficient greater than 0.1, and 14 features with a Spearman correlation coefficient greater than 0.2. It should be noted that the original 15-feature model includes four features: GCS_E, GCS_V, GCS_M, and GCS. Since GCS is the sum of GCS_E, GCS_V, and GCS_M, we therefore excluded the GCS feature and built the 14-feature model. The results show that the impact on the model's quality is not significant.

Table 3. Model performance with different feature combinations.

Algorithm	Accuracy	Sensitivity	Specificity	AUC
42 features				
Logistic Regression	0.799	0.806	0.799	0.901
Random Forest	0.829	0.833	0.828	0.914
LightGBM	**0.832**	**0.833**	**0.832**	**0.916**
XGBoost	0.794	0.806	0.792	0.900
29 significant features				
Logistic Regression	0.771	0.833	0.764	0.895
Random Forest	**0.844**	**0.847**	**0.843**	**0.918**
LightGBM	0.835	0.833	0.835	0.913
XGBoost	0.783	0.792	0.782	0.901
22 significant features and Spearman correlation coefficient > 0.1				
Logistic Regression	0.833	0.819	0.835	0.919
Random Forest	**0.830**	**0.833**	**0.830**	**0.921**
LightGBM	0.851	0.819	0.855	0.909
XGBoost	0.785	0.806	0.782	0.896
14 significant features and Spearman correlation coefficient > 0.2				
Logistic Regression	0.814	0.819	0.814	0.877
Random Forest	0.832	0.833	0.832	0.902
LightGBM	**0.878**	**0.806**	**0.886**	**0.914**
XGBoost	0.794	0.806	0.794	0.897

Note. AUC = Area under receiver operating characteristic curve. Algorithms in bold indicate the model with the highest AUC.

Each feature combination was assessed across four different machine learning models, and the performance of each model was evaluated using the AUC of the ROC curve to determine the best predictive model. Regardless of the feature combination, the best-performing machine learning model achieved an AUC greater than 0.9.

Among the 42 features, the LightGBM model performed the best with an AUC of 0.916. In the combination of 29 features, the Random Forest model achieved the highest AUC of 0.918. For the 22-feature combination, the Random Forest model again outperformed others with an AUC of 0.921. Lastly, in the combination of 14 features, the LightGBM model had the highest AUC of 0.914 (Figure 3a–d).

3.4. Comparing the Best-Performing Model with Traditional ICU Assessment Tools in Different Feature Combinations

In the DeLong test, no significant differences (>0.05) were observed in any of the feature combinations when compared to the combination of 42 features and the LightGBM model. For the sake of clinical convenience, we believe that using a combination of 14 features is easier to execute. When compared to APACHE II and SOFA scores, the *p*-values obtained were 0.0180 and 0.0156, respectively, indicating significant differences (Table 4).

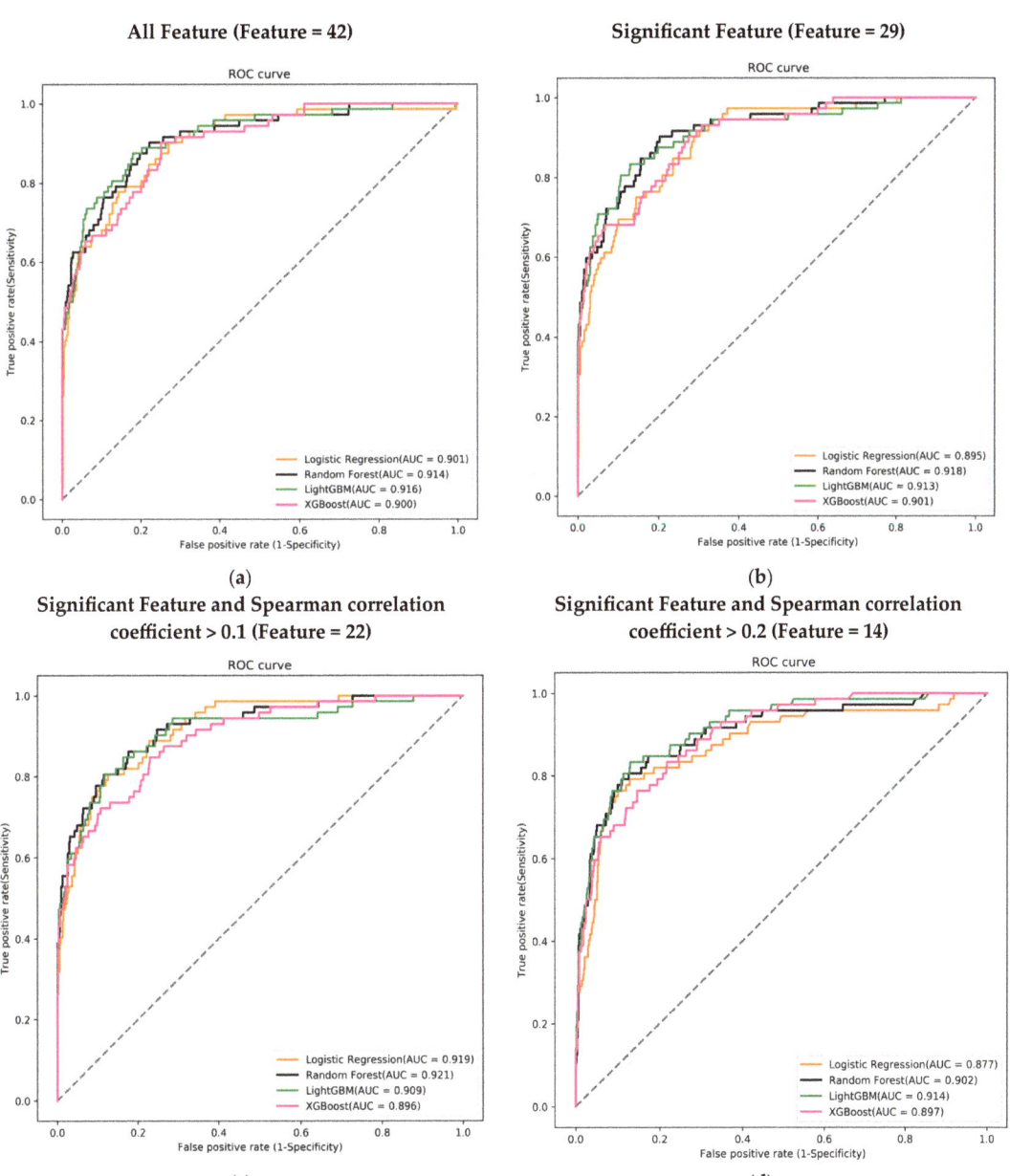

Figure 3. Receiver operating characteristic curves (ROC), area under the curve (AUC), for mortality prediction in the training course. (**a**) Using 42 features to train the ML model; (**b**) using 29 features that were significant in the mortality; (**c**) using 22 features that were significant and Spearman correlation coefficient >0.1; and (**d**) using 14 features that were significant and Spearman correlation coefficient >0.2. Logistic regression (LR) (orange), random forest (black), LightGBM (green), and XGBoost (pink) using the 14 feature variables.

Table 4. The DeLong test of ML models with different feature combinations and conventional tools (APACH II and SOFA scores).

Algorithm	Accuracy	Sensitivity	Specificity	AUC	Delong Test
Feature = 42 (LightGBM)	0.832	0.833	0.832	0.916	-
Feature = 29 (Random Forest)	0.844	0.847	0.843	0.918	0.8376
Feature = 22 (Random Forest)	0.830	0.833	0.830	0.921	0.5641
Feature = 14 (LightGBM)	0.878	0.806	0.886	0.914	0.8198
APACH II	0.768	0.847	0.759	0.872	0.0180
SOFA	0.801	0.778	0.804	0.853	0.0156

3.5. Feature Importance of AI Algorithm LightGBM Using 14 Feature Variables

Feature importance was used to rank the most important attributes that significantly contribute to the accuracy of the final prediction models [32]. To better interpret how each feature contributes to the associated outcome, we performed SHAP (SHapley Additive exPlanations) [33].

We ranked the significance of all variables in the LightGBM model to comprehend the role of each better (Figure 4). In Figure 4a, the color of the SHAP plot represents the size of the original feature values, with red indicating positive variable values and blue indicating negative ones. The SHAP value signifies the degree of a feature's impact on the outcome (a positive SHAP value indicates a positive effect). A wider Feature SHAP value suggests a more extensive influence on the outcome. As depicted, patients using vasopressors (represented by red dots) have an increased risk of death (SHAP value is positive), whereas the impact of GCS_M and GCS_V is the opposite. Figure 4b displays the ranking of features' influence on the outcome based on the absolute values of the SHAP values. The figure shows that the top five influential feature variables are vasopressors, GCS_M, GCS_V, pupil reflex + (R), and Muscle_RLE.

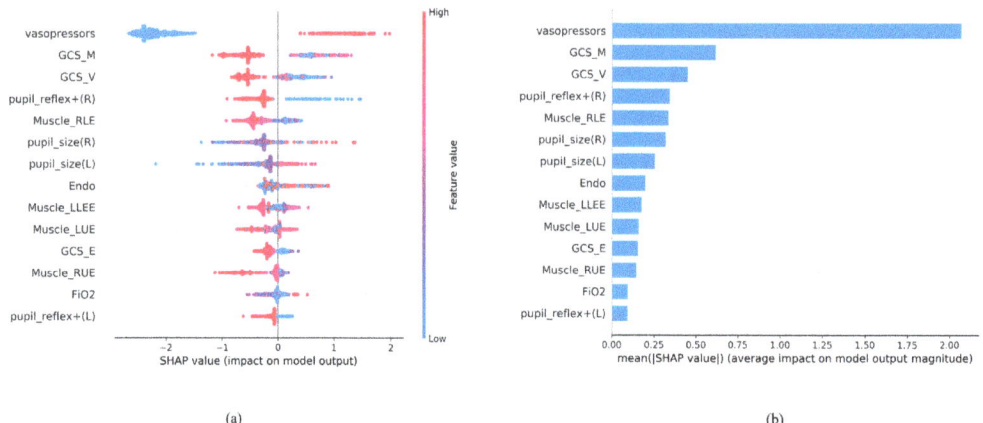

Figure 4. SHAP analysis results. (**a**) SHAP global explanation on the 14-feature model (LightGBM model); (**b**) SHAP absolute value of each feature on the 14-feature model (LightGBM model).

Based on the contribution of each predictor to the machine learning method, it can be presented in the form of feature importance (Figure 4).

3.6. Integration and Application of AI with Clinical Systems

After a series of analyses, we concluded that the LightGBM model with a combination of 14 features was more lightweight. Therefore, we integrated it into the hospital system to assist clinical doctors and nurses in treatment and facilitate communication with patients' families. The "Original" column represents data for current status. Currently, it displays data from the time of admission to the ICU. The "Adjust" column allows the observer to adjust the values of each feature to understand the effect of each feature on the risk of mortality as a reference for treatment. (Figure 5).

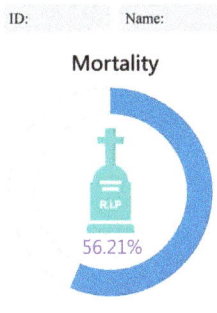

Figure 5. Interface presentation of AI in practical application within the Chi Mei Hospital healthcare system.

4. Discussion

This is the first study to demonstrate the mortality risk of TBI in ICU using a machine learning model and compare it to the present prediction model. The novelty of the current study is as follows. The simplified model using 14 features with the LightGBM algorithm for mortality prediction proved to be the most practical and excellent, achieving an AUC of 0.914. The study made significant achievements in several aspects: (a) specialized ICU parameters improved the credibility of prediction results; (b) different feature combinations were chosen based on clinical importance and correlation with mortality significance; (c) a comparison was made between ML techniques and commonly used ICU prognostic indicators and mortality assessment tools, such as APACHE II and SOFA scores (4). The observer can adjust the values of each feature to understand the effect of each feature on the risk of mortality as a reference for treatment.

This study employed artificial intelligence (AI) for data analysis, offering numerous advantages. ML can handle complex interactions in vast datasets, leading to more accurate outcome predictions. However, ML models require a larger number of input-output pairings for training, and interpretability may be sacrificed compared to standard statistics [18]. In this study, we utilized AI to identify suitable models and clinically examine the mortality of patients with brain injury admitted to the ICU.

The data from 2260 patients, including electronic medical records, clinical physiological values, and laboratory tests, were collected and analyzed. Initially, 42 features were included, but not all of them showed a correlation with mortality. Therefore, we performed a direct analysis of the features and mortality, comparing their significance, and found that 29 parameters exhibited a significant difference in relation to mortality as Table 1 shows. Further analysis involved considering Spearman's correlation coefficient values, which led us to identify 14 features from LightGBM that still possessed a high AUC, making it the most accurate prediction model. Utilizing the mortality risk provided by AI, clinicians can be assisted in making informed medical decisions.

At our hospital, we primarily use the APACHE II and SOFA assessment tools to assist with clinical decision-making and effectively communicate with patients and their families to explain their medical condition in the ICU. Despite the existence of more precise and updated versions such as APACHE III and IV, APACHE II continues to be the predominant severity grading system and mortality risk in use [34]. The SOFA score is also widely used by critical-care physicians due to its ability to provide rapid and accurate mortality predictions [35]. To compare the AI models with APACHE II and SOFA scores, we employed the DeLong test. The results revealed that the ML models generally outperformed the traditional tools. This finding suggests the potential clinical utility of AI in this study. For ease of clinical practice and completeness of data acquisition, we chose to use a 14-feature LightGBM predictive model for clinical use.

Figure 4 shows that the use of vasopressors predominated and significantly influenced the mortality risk in the LightGBM model. Maintaining the stability of mean arterial pressure and cerebral perfusion pressure (CPP) has always been crucial in brain injury care. The judicious use of vasopressors helps balance intracranial pressure and maintain a constant CPP [36]. For intubated patients, motor evaluation was relatively more important due to the inability to assess verbal function. The focus was primarily on the unaffected side's functionality to determine the patient's prognosis [37]. A GCS score below 8 indicates severe brain injury, often requiring intubation to protect the airway. According to the study by Hsu SD et al., not only GCS but also systolic blood pressure (SBP) is an important prognostic factor. In the emergency department, if a patient has a GCS < 6 or an SBP < 84 mmHg, immediate life-saving measures need to be taken [19,38]. Monitoring blood pressure and tracking changes in the GCS can be beneficial for predicting prognosis. However, in Hsu SD's study [19], they utilized features from the emergency department, whereas we utilized features from the ICU, where patients have already received treatment. Consequently, the mortality risk prediction based on ICU features tends to be more accurate at that stage.

Table 5 presents the literature comparison we conducted. In comparison to other literature, our study examines the impact of different feature combinations on mortality risk prediction and suggests that the predictive capability of the machine learning model outperforms traditional tools (APACH II, and SOFA scores). In addition, the model is currently being applied in ICU. We believe that this model can serve as an alternative choice for routine assessment in the ICU.

Table 5. A comparative analysis of the mortality rate among patients with brain injury over the past five years, as reviewed in our study.

Study	Current Study, 2023	Abujaber et al. [18], 2020	Hsu et al. [19], 2021	Wang et al. [20], 2022	Wu et al. [21], 2023
Setting	ICU	In-hospital	In-hospital	In-hospital	In-hospital
Patient number	2260	1620	3331	368	2804
Study models	Four ML models	Two ML models	Seven ML models	Two ML models	4 ML models
Features	Different features (42, 29, 22, 14) combination	20	8	21	26
Outcome	Mortality	Mortality	Mortality	Mortality	Mortality
Testing result (AUC)	0.915	0.96	0.82	0.955	0.87
Comparing with other prediction models	APACHE II score, SOFA score	Nil.	Nil.	Nil.	IMPACT, CRASH
The best prediction model	LightGBM (14 features)	SVM	J48	XGBoost	XGBoost

Generally, IMPACT and CRASH are commonly used prognostic tools for predicting outcomes and mortality in clinical TBI cases [39,40]. In Han J et al.'s report, these two traditional tools were found to have an AUC of 0.86 and 0.87, which is significantly lower compared to our ML approach [41]. Wu X et al. compared XGBoost, a machine learning algorithm, with traditional prediction tools such as IMPACT and CRASH. The results demonstrated that machine learning (ML), specifically XGBoost, outperformed IMPACT and CRASH the traditional tools in terms of predictive accuracy [21]. In Table 5, our AUC is greater than Wu's model, indicating that our model is more suitable for clinical use.

Moreover, the AI predictive tool we propose is intended as a clinical aid, not a replacement for a doctor's judgment. Before implementing policies based on AI predictions, it is essential to conduct comprehensive evaluations in terms of ethics, society, and policy. For example, protecting patients' data privacy and rights and ensuring they are not treated unfairly because of AI predictions.

Despite the robust ML algorithms demonstrating promising predictive performance, this study still has some limitations. First, it is a retrospective study, and prospective research is needed to validate the experimental results. Second, the diagnosis of brain injuries relies on Taiwan's National Health Insurance regulations, which may have a small number of miscoded diagnosis codes. However, the impact of these miscodings is relatively minor in terms of overall influence. Third, imaging parameters such as midline shift and presence/absence of brain ventricles have not been quantitatively incorporated into our ML model. Fourth, the potential confounding effects of the numerous features utilized require further exploration. Fifth, additional confounding variables such as smoking, alcohol intake, shifts in treatment guidelines, and emerging medical practices could not be comprehensively assessed due to the constraints of the retrospective database. Last, the current ML training is limited to various medical centers and laboratories, and due to differences in treatment guidelines, the generalization of ML from a single center to other regions is not yet possible. However, we provide the logical framework for ML, and the iterative process validates the effectiveness and value of such predictive models. Based on this foundation, further research can be conducted to improve upon these findings.

5. Conclusions

Our research primarily focuses on training AI using ICU data and utilizing various feature combinations to identify suitable ML models. In the end, we obtained 14 feature combinations (with a significant correlation to mortality and Spearman > 0.2), among which LightGBM performed exceptionally well. Not only does it demonstrate mortality prediction capabilities on par with models using more features but it also outperforms traditional models. These research findings can be applied in critical clinical settings to assist physicians in assessing patients' conditions and providing more data-driven explanations during communication with family members. In the future, we advocate for more studies that focus on incorporating additional variables to enhance model performance. The application of AI predictions in other healthcare settings, such as emergency care and long-term care, warrants deeper exploration.

Author Contributions: K.-C.T., C.-L.K. and E.n.t.T. conceived and designed the experiments.; C.-L.K. and C.-F.L. performed the experiments; C.-L.K. and C.-F.L. analyzed the data; C.-C.W., N.-C.C., M.-C.C. and T.-C.Y. contributed reagents/materials/analysis tools; K.-C.T., C.-L.K. and E.n.t.T. wrote the paper. All authors have read and agreed to the published version of the manuscript.

Funding: This research was supported by ChiMei Medical CMFHR 11034.

Institutional Review Board Statement: This study obtained ethics approval (11106-013) from the institutional review board of Chi Mei Medical Center, Tainan, Taiwan.

Informed Consent Statement: Patient consent was waived due to the retrospective nature of the study.

Data Availability Statement: Based on the privacy of patients within the Chi Mei Medical Center's Health Information Network, the primary data underlying this article cannot be shared publicly. However, de-identified data will be shared upon reasonable request to the corresponding author.

Acknowledgments: The authors would like to thank all of the researchers, especially Yu-Ting Shen, who extended her unwavering support in this study.

Conflicts of Interest: The authors declare no conflict of interest.

References

1. GBD 2016 Traumatic Brain Injury and Spinal Cord Injury Collaborators. Global, regional, and national burden of traumatic brain injury and spinal cord injury, 1990–2016: A systematic analysis for the Global Burden of Disease Study 2016. *Lancet Neurol.* **2019**, *18*, 56–87, Erratum in *Lancet Neurol.* **2021**, *20*, e7.
2. Majdan, M.; Plancikova, D.; Brazinova, A.; Rusnak, M.; Nieboer, D.; Feigin, V.L.; Maas, A. Epidemiology of traumatic brain injuries in Europe: A cross-sectional analysis. *Lancet Public Health* **2016**, *1*, e76–e83. [CrossRef] [PubMed]
3. Taylor, C.A.; Bell, J.M.; Breiding, M.J.; Xu, L. Traumatic Brain Injury-Related Emergency Department Visits, Hospitalizations, and Deaths—United States, 2007 and 2013. *MMWR Surveill. Summ.* **2017**, *66*, 1–16. [CrossRef] [PubMed]
4. Prasanthi, P.; Adnan, A.H. The burden of traumatic brain injury in asia: A call for research. *Pak. J. Neurol. Sci.* **2009**, *4*, 27–32.
5. Hukkelhoven, C.W.; Steyerberg, E.W.; Rampen, A.J.; Farace, E.; Habbema, J.D.F.; Marshall, L.F.; Murray, G.D.; Maas, A.I.R. Patient age and outcome following severe traumatic brain injury: An analysis of 5600 patients. *J. Neurosurg.* **2003**, *99*, 666–673. [CrossRef]
6. Ozyurt, E.; Goksu, E.; Cengiz, M.; Yilmaz, M.; Ramazanoglu, A. Retrospective Analysis of Prognostic Factors of Severe Traumatic Brain Injury in a University Hospital in Turkey. *Turk. Neurosurg.* **2015**, *25*, 877–882.
7. Okidi, R.; Ogwang, D.M.; Okello, T.R.; Ezati, D.; Kyegombe, W.; Nyeko, D.; Scolding, N.J. Factors affecting mortality after traumatic brain injury in a resource-poor setting. *BJS Open* **2020**, *4*, 320–325. [CrossRef]
8. Maas, A.I.; Steyerberg, E.W.; Butcher, I.; Dammers, R.; Lu, J.; Marmarou, A.; Mushkudiani, N.A.; McHugh, G.S.; Murray, G.D. Prognostic value of computerized tomography scan characteristics in traumatic brain injury: Results from the IMPACT study. *J. Neurotrauma* **2007**, *24*, 303–314. [CrossRef]
9. Perel, P.; Edwards, P.; Wentz, R.; Roberts, I. Systematic review of prognostic models in traumatic brain injury. *BMC Med. Inform. Decis. Mak.* **2006**, *6*, 38. [CrossRef]
10. Carter, E.L.; Hutchinson, P.J.; Kolias, A.G.; Menon, D.K. Predicting the outcome for individual patients with traumatic brain injury: A case-based review. *Br. J. Neurosurg.* **2016**, *30*, 227–232. [CrossRef]
11. Vincent, J.L.; Moreno, R.; Takala, J.; Willatts, S.; De Mendonça, A.; Bruining, H.; Reinhart, C.K.; Suter, P.M.; Thijs, L.G. The SOFA (Sepsis-related Organ Failure Assessment) score to describe organ dysfunction/failure. On behalf of the Working Group on Sepsis-Related Problems of the European Society of Intensive Care Medicine. *Intensive Care Med.* **1996**, *22*, 707–710. [CrossRef] [PubMed]
12. Singer, M.; Deutschman, C.S.; Seymour, C.W.; Shankar-Hari, M.; Annane, D.; Bauer, M.; Bellomo, R.; Bernard, G.R.; Chiche, J.-D.; Coopersmith, C.M.; et al. The Third International Consensus Definitions for Sepsis and Septic Shock (Sepsis-3). *JAMA* **2016**, *315*, 801–810. [CrossRef] [PubMed]
13. Knaus, W.A.; Draper, E.A.; Wagner, D.P.; Zimmerman, J.E. APACHE II: A severity of disease classification system. *Crit. Care Med.* **1985**, *13*, 818–829. [CrossRef] [PubMed]
14. Raj, R.; Skrifvars, M.; Bendel, S.; Selander, T.; Kivisaari, R.; Siironen, J.; Reinikainen, M. Predicting six-month mortality of patients with traumatic brain injury: Usefulness of common intensive care severity scores. *Crit. Care* **2014**, *18*, R60. [CrossRef]
15. Ley, C.; Martin, R.K.; Pareek, A.; Groll, A.; Seil, R.; Tischer, T. Machine learning and conventional statistics: Making sense of the differences. *Knee Surg. Sports Traumatol. Arthrosc.* **2022**, *30*, 753–757. [CrossRef]
16. Loh, H.W.; Ooi, C.P.; Seoni, S.; Barua, P.D.; Molinari, F.; Acharya, U.R. Application of Explainable Artificial Intelligence for Healthcare: A Systematic Review of the Last Decade (2011–2022). *Comput. Methods Programs Biomed.* **2022**, *226*, 107161. [CrossRef]
17. Courville, E.; Kazim, S.F.; Vellek, J.; Tarawneh, O.; Stack, J.; Roster, K.; Roy, J.; Schmidt, M.; Bowers, C. Machine learning algorithms for predicting outcomes of traumatic brain injury: A systematic review and meta-analysis. *Surg. Neurol. Int.* **2023**, *14*, 262. [CrossRef]
18. Abujaber, A.; Fadlalla, A.; Gammoh, D.; Abdelrahman, H.; Mollazehi, M.; El-Menyar, A. Prediction of in-hospital mortality in patients with post traumatic brain injury using National Trauma Registry and Machine Learning Approach. *Scand. J. Trauma Resusc. Emerg. Med.* **2020**, *28*, 44. [CrossRef]
19. Hsu, S.D.; Chao, E.; Chen, S.J.; Hueng, D.Y.; Lan, H.Y.; Chiang, H.H. Machine Learning Algorithms to Predict In-Hospital Mortality in Patients with Traumatic Brain Injury. *J. Pers. Med.* **2021**, *11*, 1144. [CrossRef]
20. Wang, R.; Wang, L.; Zhang, J.; He, M.; Xu, J. XGBoost Machine Learning Algorism Performed Better Than Regression Models in Predicting Mortality of Moderate-to-Severe Traumatic Brain Injury. *World Neurosurg.* **2022**, *163*, e617–e622. [CrossRef]
21. Wu, X.; Sun, Y.; Xu, X.; Steyerberg, E.W.; Helmrich, I.R.A.R.; Lecky, F.; Guo, J.; Li, X.; Feng, J.; Mao, Q.; et al. Mortality Prediction in Severe Traumatic Brain Injury Using Traditional and Machine Learning Algorithms. *J. Neurotrauma* **2023**, *40*, 1366–1375. [CrossRef] [PubMed]
22. Chawla, N.V.; Bowyer, K.W.; Hall, L.O.; Kegelmeyer, W.P. SMOTE: Synthetic minority over-sampling technique. *J. Artif. Intell.* **2002**, *16*, 321–357. [CrossRef]
23. Hosmer, D.W.; Lemeshow, S., Jr.; Sturdivant, R.X. *Applied Logistic Regression*; John Wiley & Sons, Inc.: Hoboken, NJ, USA, 2013.
24. Breiman, L. Random forests. *Mach. Learn.* **2001**, *45*, 5–32. [CrossRef]
25. Ke, G.; Meng, Q.; Finley, T.; Wang, T.F.; Chen, W.; Ma, W.D.; Ye, Q.; Liu, T.Y. LightGBM: A highly efficient gradient boosting decision tree. In Proceedings of the 31st Conference on Neural Information Processing Systems, Long Beach, CA, USA, 4–9 December 2017.
26. Chen, T.; Guestrin, C. Xgboost: A scalable tree boosting system. In Proceedings of the 22nd ACM SIGKDD International Conference on Knowledge Discovery and Data Mining, Long Beach, CA, USA, 6–10 August 2016; pp. 785–794.

27. Parikh, R.; Mathai, A.; Parikh, S.; Sekhar, G.C.; Thomas, R. Understanding and using sensitivity, specificity and predictive values. *Indian J. Ophthalmol.* **2008**, *56*, 45–50. [CrossRef] [PubMed]
28. Patorno, E.; Najafzadeh, M.; Pawar, A.; Franklin, J.M.; Déruaz-Luyet, A.; Brodovicz, K.G.; Ortiz, A.J.S.; Bessette, L.G.; Kulldorff, M.; Schneeweiss, S. The EMPagliflozin compaRative effectIveness and SafEty (EMPRISE) study programme: Design and exposure accrual for an evaluation of empagliflozin in routine clinical care. *Endocrinol. Diabetes Metab.* **2019**, *3*, e00103. [CrossRef] [PubMed]
29. Swets, J.A. Measuring the accuracy of diagnostic systems. *Science* **1988**, *240*, 1285–1293. [CrossRef]
30. Jin, H.; Ling, C.X. Using AUC and accuracy in evaluating learning algorithms. *Knowl. Data Eng.* **2005**, *17*, 299–310.
31. Hasraddin, G.; Eldayag, M. Predicting the changes in the WTI crude oil price dynamics using machine learning models. *Resour. Policy* **2022**, *77*, 102664.
32. Inui, A.; Nishimoto, H.; Mifune, Y.; Yoshikawa, T.; Shinohara, I.; Furukawa, T.; Kato, T.; Tanaka, S.; Kusunose, M.; Kuroda, R. Screening for Osteoporosis from Blood Test Data in Elderly Women Using a Machine Learning Approach. *Bioengineering* **2023**, *10*, 277. [CrossRef]
33. Lundberg, S.M.; Lee, S.I. A Unified Approach to Interpreting Model Predictions. In Proceedings of the 31st International Conference on Neural Information Processing Systems, Red Hook, NY, USA, 4–9 December 2017.
34. Breslow, M.J.; Badawi, O. Severity scoring in the critically ill: Part 1—Interpretation and accuracy of outcome prediction scoring systems. *Chest* **2012**, *141*, 245–252. [CrossRef]
35. Lambden, S.; Laterre, P.F.; Levy, M.M.; Francois, B. The SOFA Score—Development, Utility and Challenges of Accurate Assessment in Clinical Trials. *Crit. Care* **2019**, *23*, 374. [CrossRef] [PubMed]
36. Pinto, V.L.; Tadi, P.; Adeyinka, A. *Increased Intracranial Pressure*; [Updated 2022 Aug 1]; StatPearls Publishing: St. Petersburg, FL, USA, 2023.
37. Saika, A.; Bansal, S.; Philip, M.; Devi, B.I.; Shukla, D.P. Prognostic value of FOUR and GCS scores in determining mortality in patients with traumatic brain injury. *Acta Neurochir.* **2015**, *157*, 1323–1328. [CrossRef] [PubMed]
38. Huang, J.F.; Tsai, Y.C.; Rau, C.S.; Hsu, S.Y.; Chien, P.C.; Hsieh, H.Y.; Hsieh, C.H. Systolic blood pressure lower than the heart rate indicates a poor outcome in patients with severe isolated traumatic brain injury: A cross-sectional study. *Int. J. Surg.* **2019**, *61*, 48–52. [CrossRef] [PubMed]
39. Steyerberg, E.W.; Mushkudiani, N.; Perel, P.; Butcher, I.; Lu, J.; McHugh, G.S.; Murray, G.D.; Marmarou, A.; Roberts, I.; Habbema, J.D.F.; et al. Predicting outcome after traumatic brain injury: Development and international validation of prognostic scores based on admission characteristics. *PLoS Med.* **2008**, *5*, 1251–1261. [CrossRef] [PubMed]
40. MRC CRASH Trial Collaborators; Perel, P.; Arango, M.; Clayton, T.; Edwards, P.; Komolafe, E.; Poccock, S.; Roberts, I.; Shakur, H.; Steyerberg, E.; et al. Predicting outcome after traumatic brain injury: Practical prognostic models based on large cohort of international patients. *BMJ* **2008**, *336*, 425–429.
41. Han, J.; King, N.; Neilson, S.; Gandhi, M.; Ng, I. External validation of the CRASH and IMPACT prognostic models in severe traumatic brain injury. *J. Neurotrauma* **2014**, *31*, 1146–1152. [CrossRef]

Disclaimer/Publisher's Note: The statements, opinions and data contained in all publications are solely those of the individual author(s) and contributor(s) and not of MDPI and/or the editor(s). MDPI and/or the editor(s) disclaim responsibility for any injury to people or property resulting from any ideas, methods, instructions or products referred to in the content.

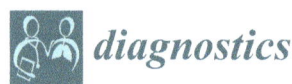

Article

Implementing AI Models for Prognostic Predictions in High-Risk Burn Patients

Chin-Choon Yeh [1], Yu-San Lin [1], Chun-Chia Chen [1] and Chung-Feng Liu [2,*]

[1] Department of Plastic Surgery, Chi Mei Medical Center, Tainan 711, Taiwan; frankyeh1977@gmail.com (C.-C.Y.); plastylin@mail.chimei.org.tw (Y.-S.L.); chenjica@msa.hinet.net (C.-C.C.)
[2] Department of Medical Research, Chi Mei Medical Center, Tainan 711, Taiwan
* Correspondence: chungfengliu@gmail.com; Tel.: +886-6-2812811 (ext. 52590)

Abstract: Background and Objectives: Burn injuries range from minor medical issues to severe, life-threatening conditions. The severity and location of the burn dictate its treatment; while minor burns might be treatable at home, severe burns necessitate medical intervention, sometimes in specialized burn centers with extended follow-up care. This study aims to leverage artificial intelligence (AI)/machine learning (ML) to forecast potential adverse effects in burn patients. Methods: This retrospective analysis considered burn patients admitted to Chi Mei Medical Center from 2010 to 2019. The study employed 14 features, comprising supplementary information like prior comorbidities and laboratory results, for building models for predicting graft surgery, a prolonged hospital stay, and overall adverse effects. Overall, 70% of the data set trained the AI models, with the remaining 30% reserved for testing. Three ML algorithms of random forest, LightGBM, and logistic regression were employed with evaluation metrics of accuracy, sensitivity, specificity, and the area under the receiver operating characteristic curve (AUC). Results: In this research, out of 224 patients assessed, the random forest model yielded the highest AUC for predictions related to prolonged hospital stays (>14 days) at 81.1%, followed by the XGBoost (79.9%) and LightGBM (79.5%) models. Besides, the random forest model of the need for a skin graft showed the highest AUC (78.8%), while the random forest model and XGBoost model of the occurrence of adverse complications both demonstrated the highest AUC (87.2%) as well. Based on the best models with the highest AUC values, an AI prediction system is designed and integrated into hospital information systems to assist physicians in the decision-making process. Conclusions: AI techniques showcased exceptional capabilities for predicting a prolonged hospital stay, the need for a skin graft, and the occurrence of overall adverse complications for burn patients. The insights from our study fuel optimism for the inception of a novel predictive model that can seamlessly meld with hospital information systems, enhancing clinical decisions and bolstering physician–patient dialogues.

Keywords: burn patient; prognosis; prolonged hospital stay; skin graft needed; adverse complications; artificial intelligence; machine learning; hospital information systems

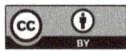

1. Introduction

A burn injury refers to the damage to the skin or underlying tissues caused by exposure to heat, fire, chemicals, electricity, or radiation. Burn injuries can vary in severity, ranging from mild superficial burns to severe deep burns that can be life-threatening [1,2].

Burns are typically classified into different degrees based on their depth and severity:

First-degree burns: These are superficial burns that only affect the outer layer of the skin (epidermis). They usually result in redness, pain, and minor swelling, but do not typically cause blistering.

Second-degree burns: These burns affect both the outer layer of the skin (epidermis) and the underlying layer (dermis). They are characterized by blistering, severe pain, redness, and swelling.

Third-degree burns: These burns extend through all layers of the skin, damaging nerve endings and underlying tissues. They may appear white, charred, leathery, or blackened. Third-degree burns often result in numbness due to nerve damage and may require surgical intervention for treatment [3–5].

The severity of a burn injury can also be assessed using the "Rule of Nines", which divides the body into different regions, each accounting for a specific percentage of the total body surface area (TBSA). This helps in estimating the extent of the burn and determining the need for specialized care [6].

Immediate first aid for burns typically involves removing the source of heat, cooling the burn with running cool (not cold) water, and covering it with a clean cloth or dressing. However, for more severe burns or burns involving critical areas such as the face, hands, feet, or genitals, immediate medical attention is essential.

Treatment for burn injuries often includes wound cleaning, the application of topical medications, pain management, and, in some cases, surgical procedures like skin grafting to promote healing [4]. Additionally, rehabilitation and long-term care may be necessary for individuals with extensive burns to regain functionality and manage potential complications such as scarring, contractures, and emotional trauma [7,8]. Furthermore, burns occurring in specific delicate regions, such as the eyelids or penis, pose significant challenges for healthcare practitioners in terms of both treatment and care [9].

However, the hospital faces limitations in its resources to effectively treat burns and scalds. This becomes particularly challenging when dealing with a diverse range of burn patients, including those who have been affected by indoor fires and outdoor dust storms, such as the colored power fire. Therefore, it is crucial to determine the severity of each individual's condition and allocate appropriate medical resources accordingly. To address this urgency, the Baux score, also referred to as the "Baux index", was developed by Dr. Jean Baux in 1960 [10].

The Baux score takes into account the patient's age and the percentage of total body surface area (TBSA) affected by burns. It is calculated using the following formula:

$$\text{Baux score} = \text{age (years)} + \text{burned area (\%)}$$

$$\text{rBaux score} = \text{age (years)} + \text{burned area (\%)} + (17 \times I)$$

In which: I = 1 if the patient suffered inhalation injury; and I = 0 if patients did not suffer inhalation injury.

For example, for a 35-year-old burn patient who suffered burns covering 20% of their total body surface area (TBSA), his/her Baux score and rBaux are:

$$\text{Baux score} = \text{age} + \text{burned area} = 35 + 20 = 55$$

$$\text{rBaux score} = \text{age} + \text{burned area} + (17 \times I) = 35 + 20 + (17 \times 1) = 35 + 20 + 17 = 72$$

The rBaux score ranges from 0 to 216. A higher Baux score indicates a greater risk of mortality. The score is used as a prognostic tool to assess the severity of burn injuries and help guide treatment decisions. Scoring systems like the Baux score and its variations provide a standardized method for assessing burn severity and predicting outcomes [11].

The rBaux scoring system has been widely and extensively utilized in clinical settings, garnering widespread acceptance for its effectiveness in predicting the likelihood of mortality in patients suffering from burns and scalds. According to Lam et al. [12], the revised Baux score has been found to be more accurate than the Baux score. However, they recommend its application solely for prognosis purposes in adult and elderly burn patients within developing countries [13,14]. Nevertheless, there have been studies indicating that the predictive power of the Baux score is limited, suggesting its inadequacy in accurately predicting burn outcomes. One such study conducted by Roberts et al. [15] (2012) found that the Baux score had a low sensitivity and specificity in predicting mortality in a cohort of burn patients in the US. Similarly, a study by Kirimi et al. [16] (2013) demonstrated that the Baux score exhibited poor discrimination in predicting complications such as infections and organ dysfunction.

Furthermore, alternative scoring systems, such as the Anesthesiologists Physical Status (ASA PS) Score [17] and body mass index (BMI) [18], are employed to forecast mortality in cases of burn injuries.

However, the aforementioned scoring methods can only provide limited clinical predictive information and may not effectively handle the variability of changing medical conditions and the diverse consultation requests from patients and their families, leading to a communication and information gap between healthcare providers and patients.

Moreover, the condition of severely burned patients typically exhibits rapid fluctuations, sometimes even on the scale of hours or minutes. Therefore, acquiring real-time clinical data, such as the information provided by Volumeview [19], and effectively integrating and interpreting these data, pose significant challenges and are of paramount importance. Consequently, we seek to harness the power of AI/ML to fully leverage this invaluable information, thereby making a valuable contribution to the enhancement of clinical care quality.

In view of this, it is urgent and necessary to develop more real-time and high-quality burn prediction tools to meet the requirements of modern precision medicine. Therefore, our study aims to develop a prediction model for high-risk burn patients and identify the factors that potentially increase the risk for mortalities and complications using AI/ML approaches based on a large database of burn patients in a Taiwanese center. We made a comparison of the prediction quality with the Baux score, and a prediction system based on our best model was implemented into practice as well.

2. Materials and Methods

2.1. Study Design, Setting, and Samples

All inpatients with burn of any degree (ICD-9: 948.XX or ICD-10: T31.XX) in the first 6 diagnosis codes from 1 January 2010 to 31 December 2019 were included, but those aged ≤6 years old (5 cases) were excluded. Overall, 348 raw cases were used in the study. Figure 1 shows our research flow.

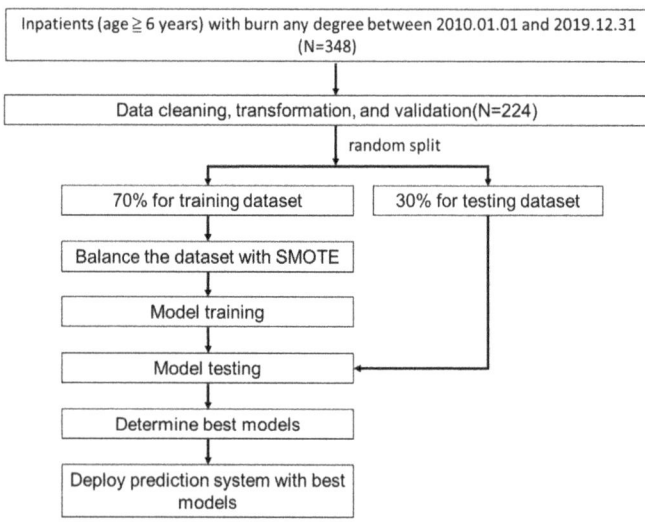

SMOTE, synthetic minority oversampling technique

Figure 1. Research flow.

The study was approved by the Institutional Review Board of the Chi Mei Medical Center (IRB Serial No.: 11206-014). All methods were carried out following relevant guidelines and regulations. Informed consent from patients was waived due to the retrospective nature of the study.

2.2. Feature and Outcome Variables

We chose three outcome variables for the prediction models: (1) graft surgery (operation code 62015), (2) prolonged hospital stay (hospitalization days >14 days), and (3) overall adverse effects (sepsis, use of respirator, pneumonia, chronic kidney disease (CKD), mortality, and prolonged hospital stay).

Furthermore, we chose 12 feature variables, based on literature review and clinical experience, for building these prediction models:

(1) Basic information: gender, age, body mass index (BMI), smoking history, and escharotomy;
(2) Burn data: burn area, burn site—perineum, and burn site—extremities;
(3) Lab information: white blood cell (WBC), hemoglobin, creatinine, and glutamate pyruvate transaminase (GPT).

2.3. Model Building and Performance Evaluation

We used all the variables to build the prediction models to maximize model performance without performing any feature selection preprocessing. The data were randomly stratified into a training dataset (70%) and a testing dataset (30%). The SMOTE method (synthetic minority oversampling technique) [20] was used to deal with the data imbalance due to the fewer related positive classes (outcomes to be predicted, such as mortality) in the training dataset. The model of each outcome was built with 4 machine-learning algorithms, including (1) logistic regression, (2) random forest, (3) LightGBM, and (4) XGBoost.

We used a grid search with 5-fold cross-validation to build the best models based on the training dataset. We, then, used the testing dataset to evaluate the performance of the built models with indicators of accuracy, sensitivity, specificity, and AUC (area under the receiver operating characteristic curve).

2.4. Implementation and Deployment of the Best Models

The models with the highest AUCs were judged as the best and were used to implement a web-based prediction application and deployed into practice for physicians' decision making. The web-based predictive application was developed with the Microsoft Visual Studio® tool (v 17.7).

3. Results

3.1. Demographics

From 1 January 2010 to 31 December 2019, a total of 384 burn inpatients who are above 6 years old were enrolled in the study. After data cleaning and missing-value deletion, 224 cases underwent analysis. Overall, 70% of the data were randomly split for model training, and 30% for model evaluating.

Tables 1–3 show the demographics and characteristics of the patients with graft surgery, prolonged hospital stay (>14 days), and overall adverse effects, respectively. In total, the mean age was 45.8, and most patients were males (66.1%); about 50.4% of them were categorized as the least mild condition of burned area rank 1, while 18.8% of them were categorized as the most severe condition of burned area rank 4. The mean Baux score was 69.2.

Table 1. Demographics—patients with graft surgery.

Feature	Overall	Graft Surgery No	Graft Surgery Yes	p-Value
	N = 224	N = 124	N = 100	
Age, mean (SD)	45.8 (20.3)	46.1 (20.8)	45.4 (19.9)	0.813
Gender_Female, n (%)	76 (33.9)	42 (33.9)	34 (34.0)	1
Gender_male, n (%)	148 (66.1)	82 (66.1)	66 (66.0)	
Burned area rank 1 (area <10%), n (%)	113 (50.4)	90 (72.6)	23 (23.0)	<0.001
Burned area rank 2 (area 10–19%), n (%)	24 (10.7)	4 (3.2)	20 (20.0)	
Burned area rank 3 (area 20–29%), n (%)	45 (20.1)	19 (15.3)	26 (26.0)	
Burned area rank 4 (area >30%), n (%)	42 (18.8)	11 (8.9)	31 (31.0)	
BMI (body mass index), mean (SD)	24.5 (4.8)	24.3 (4.4)	24.7 (5.3)	0.546
GPT (glutamate pyruvate transaminase), mean (SD)	38.7 (95.2)	43.0 (124.6)	33.2 (32.5)	0.4
WBC (white blood cell), mean (SD)	11.5 (6.3)	10.3 (5.0)	12.9 (7.5)	0.003
Hemoglobin, mean (SD)	14.4 (1.8)	14.2 (1.7)	14.6 (1.9)	0.081
Creatinine, mean (SD)	1.1 (1.1)	1.1 (1.2)	1.1 (0.9)	0.988
Smoking, n (%)	32 (14.3)	16 (12.9)	16 (16.0)	0.641
Burned perineum, n (%)	37 (16.5)	22 (17.7)	15 (15.0)	0.713
Burned limb, n (%)	62 (27.7)	42 (33.9)	20 (20.0)	0.031
Underwent escharotomy, n (%)	27 (12.1)	7 (5.6)	20 (20.0)	0.002
Baux score, mean (SD)	69.2 (27.7)	64.2 (28.5)	75.4 (25.4)	0.002

Note. Significance testing approaches (p value): Chi-square test for categorical variables; t-test for continuous variables.

Table 2. Demographics—patients with prolonged hospital stay.

Feature	Overall	Prolonged Hospital Stay No	Prolonged Hospital Stay Yes	p-Value
	N = 224	N = 95	N = 129	
Age, mean (SD)	45.8 (20.3)	45.8 (20.5)	45.8 (20.3)	0.994
Gender_Female, n (%)	76 (33.9)	36 (37.9)	40 (31.0)	0.351
Gender_male, n (%)	148 (66.1)	59 (62.1)	89 (69.0)	
Burned area rank 1 (area <10%), n (%)	113 (50.4)	77 (81.1)	36 (27.9)	<0.001
Burned area rank 2 (area 10–19%), n (%)	24 (10.7)	3 (3.2)	21 (16.3)	
Burned area rank 3 (area 20–29%), n (%)	45 (20.1)	7 (7.4)	38 (29.5)	
Burned area rank 4 (area >30%), n (%)	42 (18.8)	8 (8.4)	34 (26.4)	
BMI (body mass index), mean (SD)	24.5 (4.8)	23.8 (4.0)	25.0 (5.3)	0.044
GPT (glutamate pyruvate transaminase), mean (SD)	38.7 (95.2)	42.1 (139.7)	36.1 (37.7)	0.687
WBC (white blood cell), mean (SD)	11.5 (6.3)	10.1 (5.1)	12.5 (6.9)	0.002
Hemoglobin, mean (SD)	14.4 (1.8)	14.2 (1.6)	14.5 (1.9)	0.219
Creatinine, mean (SD)	1.1 (1.1)	1.0 (0.2)	1.2 (1.4)	0.033
Smoking, n (%)	32 (14.3)	12 (12.6)	20 (15.5)	0.679
Burned perineum, n (%)	37 (16.5)	16 (16.8)	21 (16.3)	1
Burned limb, n (%)	62 (27.7)	33 (34.7)	29 (22.5)	0.061
Underwent escharotomy, n (%)	27 (12.1)	5 (5.3)	22 (17.1)	0.013
Baux score, mean (SD)	69.2 (27.7)	62.6 (30.1)	74.1 (24.9)	0.003

Note. Significance testing approaches (p value): Chi-square test for categorical variables; t-test for continuous variables.

Table 3. Demographics—patients with overall adverse effects.

Feature	Overall	Overall Adverse No	Overall Adverse Yes	p-Value
	N = 224	N = 86	N = 138	
Age, mean (SD)	45.8 (20.3)	44.4 (20.4)	46.6 (20.3)	0.439
Gender_Female, n (%)	76 (33.9)	33 (38.4)	43 (31.2)	0.335
Gender_male, n (%)	148 (66.1)	53 (61.6)	95 (68.8)	
Burned area rank 1 (area <10%), n (%)	113 (50.4)	76 (88.4)	37 (26.8)	<0.001
Burned area rank 2 (area 10–19%), n (%)	24 (10.7)	3 (3.5)	21 (15.2)	
Burned area rank 3 (area 20–29%), n (%)	45 (20.1)	6 (7.0)	39 (28.3)	
Burned area rank 4 (area >30%), n (%)	42 (18.8)	1 (1.2)	41 (29.7)	
BMI, mean (SD)	24.5 (4.8)	23.6 (4.0)	25.0 (5.2)	0.027
GPT, mean (SD)	38.7 (95.2)	28.4 (17.9)	45.1 (120.1)	0.111
WBC, mean (SD)	11.5 (6.3)	9.3 (4.0)	12.8 (7.1)	<0.001
Hemoglobin, mean (SD)	14.4 (1.8)	14.1 (1.5)	14.5 (1.9)	0.091
Creatinine, mean (SD)	1.1 (1.1)	0.9 (0.2)	1.2 (1.3)	0.014
Smoking, n (%)	32 (14.3)	11 (12.8)	21 (15.2)	0.758
Burned perineum, n (%)	37 (16.5)	14 (16.3)	23 (16.7)	1
Burned limb, n (%)	62 (27.7)	33 (38.4)	29 (21.0)	0.008
Underwent escharotomy, n (%)	27 (12.1)	1 (1.2)	26 (18.8)	<0.001
Baux score, mean (SD)	69.2 (27.7)	56.2 (22.8)	77.3 (27.5)	<0.001

Note. Significance testing approaches (p value): Chi-square test for categorical variables; t-test for continuous variables.

3.2. Machine-Learning Modeling Results

The model performance of each predicted outcome was summarized in Table 4. In model of graft surgery, the highest AUC was found in the random forest model with a value of 0.757, followed by the logistic regression model, LightGBM model, and XGBoost model with values of 0.755, 0.745, and 0.738, respectively. In the model of prolonged hospital stay, the highest AUC was found in the XGBoost model with a value of 0.815, followed by the random forest model, LightGBM model, and logistic regression model with values of 0.801, 0.797, and 0.720, respectively (see Table 4). Finally, in the model of overall adverse effects, the highest AUC was found in the LightGBM model with a value of 0.845, followed by the logistic regression model, random forest model, and XGBoost model with values of 0.832, 0.822, and 0.816, respectively.

Table 4. Model performance.

Model	Algorithm	Accuracy	Sensitivity	Specificity	AUC	AUC 95%CI
Graft surgery	Random forest	0.765	0.833	0.711	0.756	0.639–0.874
	Logistic regression	0.706	0.7	0.711	0.755	0.638–0.873
	LightGBM	0.706	0.733	0.684	0.745	0.625–0.864
	XGBoost	0.721	0.733	0.711	0.738	0.616–0.859
Model	Algorithm	Accuracy	Sensitivity	Specificity	AUC	AUC 95%CI
Prolonged hospital stay	XGBoost	0.779	0.795	0.759	0.815	0.710–0.920
	Random forest	0.794	0.795	0.793	0.801	0.690–0.912
	LightGBM	0.706	0.769	0.621	0.797	0.688–0.905
	Logistic regression	0.676	0.718	0.621	0.720	0.595–0.844
Model	Algorithm	Accuracy	Sensitivity	Specificity	AUC	AUC 95%CI
Overall adverse effects	LightGBM	0.779	0.786	0.769	0.845	0.751–0.939
	Logistic regression	0.765	0.714	0.846	0.832	0.734–0.929
	XGBoost	0.765	0.786	0.731	0.822	0.724–0.921
	Random forest	0.765	0.738	0.808	0.816	0.716–0.916

3.3. Interpreting the Feature Importance

Furthermore, for a better interpretation of how each feature contributes to the associated outcome, we performed a SHAP (SHapley Additive exPlanations) [21] analysis for each best AI model. In the SHAP global explanation plot, dots in red and blue indicate higher and lower feature values, respectively. A dot distribution to the left of the horizontal axis point 0 represents a negative correlation to the outcome, while a distribution to the right represents a positive correlation. The y-axis indicates the feature name, in order of importance from the top to the bottom of the plot. The wider the dots of the feature distributed, the greater the influence of the feature on the outcome. Figures 2 and 3 depict global explanations of the best models and mean absolute SHAP values, respectively. As shown in Figure 2A, the x-axis represents the SHAP values of each of the features by which the model predicts the graft surgery. The interpretation of the summary plot shows that a higher burn area rank (higher values visible in red on the horizontal bar) implies an increase in the predicted outcome; conversely, a smaller burn area rank (visible in blue) is associated with a decrease in the predicted outcome. The feature of burn area rank was similarly explained in predicting a prolonged hospital stay and adverse effects. The same interpretation can be applied to the rest of the features.

Figure 3 shows the absolute SHAP value of each feature, presenting its importance on the associated outcome. It can be interpreted that the top three critical features on graft surgery are burned area rank, WBC, and GPT; the top three critical features on a prolonged hospital stay are burned area rank, BMI, and creatinine; and the top three critical features on overall adverse effects are burned area rank, WBC, and age.

3.4. Performance Comparison of AI Model and Baux Score

We compared the best AI-based model with the Baux score by the performance indicators. For this, we first calculated the indicators of accuracy, sensitivity, specificity, and AUC for AI models and Baux score models. We, then, performed the DeLong test for figuring out the significance of the model difference. As shown in Table 5, AI models have higher values for all indicators than Baux score models. AI models of prolonged hospital stay and overall adverse effects outperformed Baux score models in a statistically significant manner ($p < 0.05$).

Table 5. Comparisons of AI models and Baux score models.

Outcome	Model	Accuracy	Sensitivity	Specificity	AUC	AUC95%CI	DeLong Test (p)
Graft surgery	AI model (random forest)	0.765	0.833	0.711	0.756	0.639–0.874	0.206
	Baux score	0.574	0.433	0.684	0.641	0.509–0.774	
Prolonged hospital stay	AI model (XGBoost)	0.779	0.795	0.759	0.815	0.710–0.920	0.023
	Baux score	0.588	0.487	0.724	0.657	0.515–0.800	
Overall adverse effects	AI model (LightGBM)	0.779	0.786	0.769	0.845	0.751–0.939	0.008
	Baux score	0.559	0.524	0.615	0.619	0.484–0.754	

3.5. Clinical Prediction Application Development and Deployment and User Preliminary Evaluation

For clarifying the feasibility and acceptance of our AI models, we developed an AI risk prediction system based on the three best models and deployed it in a burn critical care center for assisting with the physician's decisions. Figure 4 showed a snapshot of the AI system (a probability $\geq 50\%$ indicates a high probability of causing the adverse outcome). Models were built in the Python programming language and the Web-based interface was built in MS Visual Studio® with VB (v 17.7).

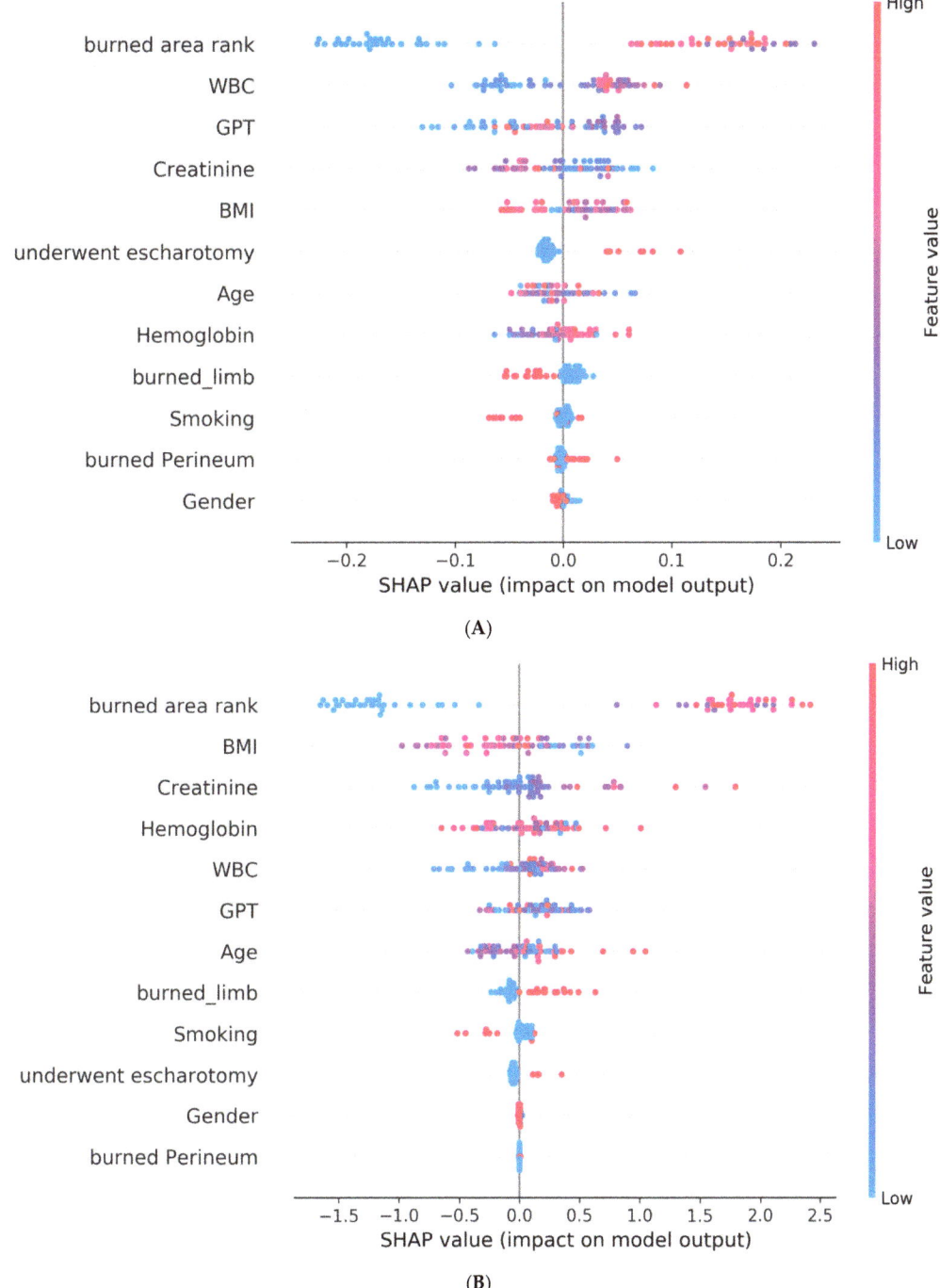

Figure 2. *Cont.*

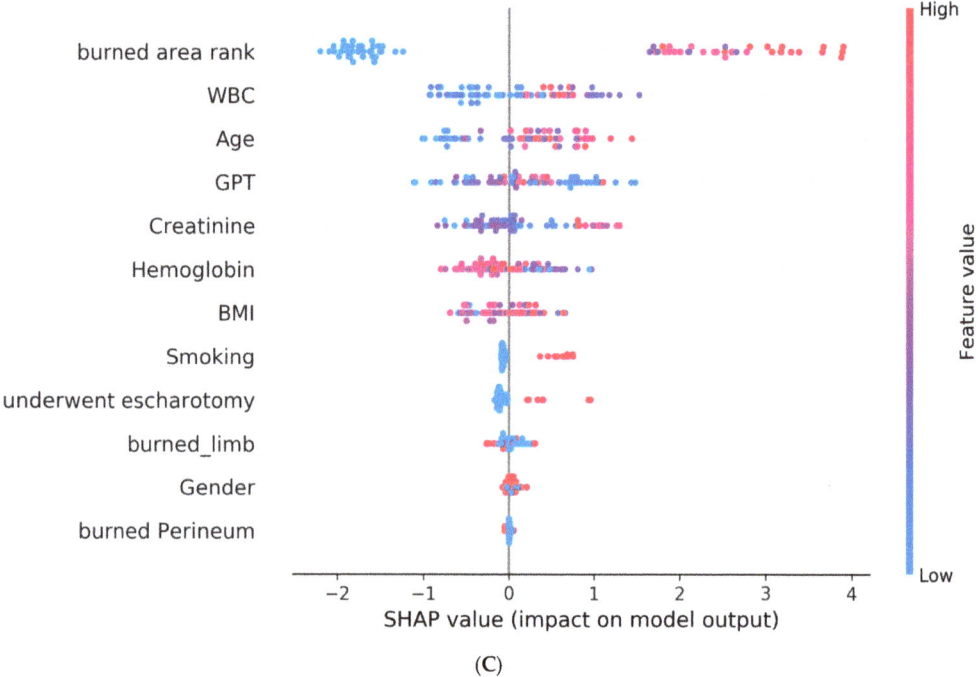

(C)

Figure 2. SHAP global explanation on the best model: (**A**) SHAP plot for model of graft surgery (random forest); (**B**) SHAP plot for model of prolonged hospital stay (XGBoost); (**C**) SHAP plot for model of overall adverse effects (LightGBM).

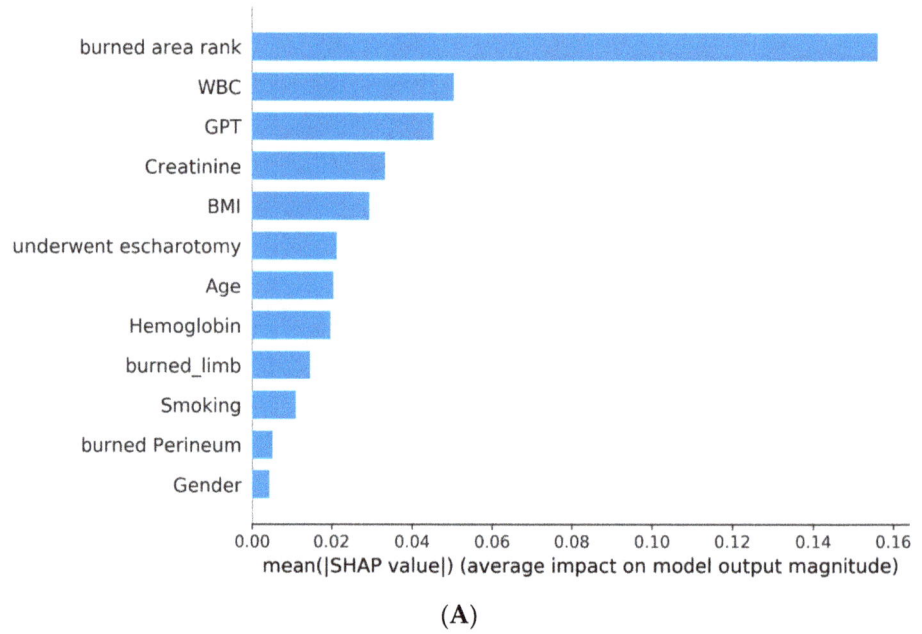

(A)

Figure 3. *Cont.*

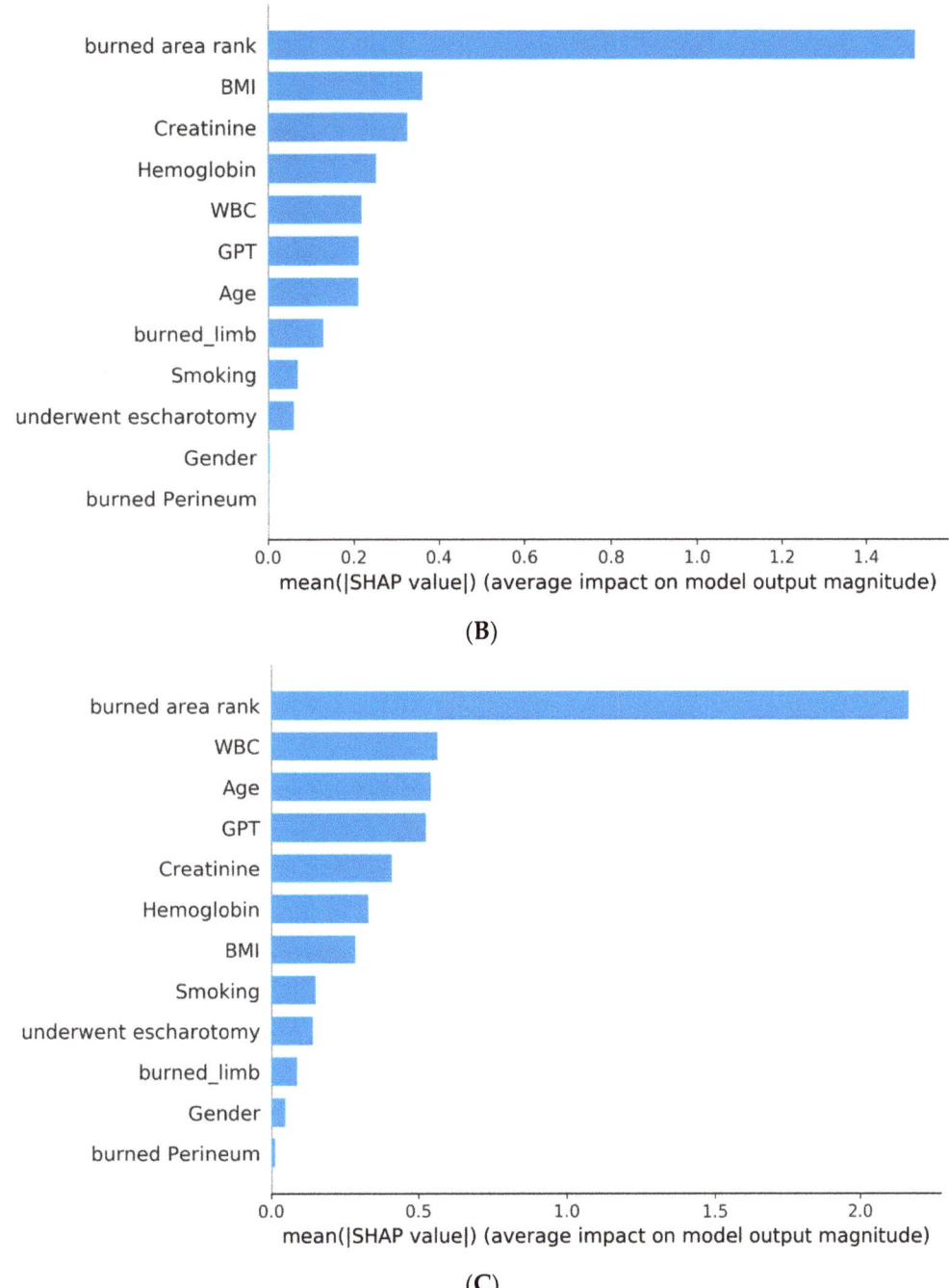

Figure 3. Absolute SHAP value of each feature on the best model: (**A**) SHAP plot for model of graft surgery (random forest); (**B**) SHAP plot for model of prolonged hospital stay (XGBoost); (**C**) SHAP plot for model of overall adverse effects (LightGBM).

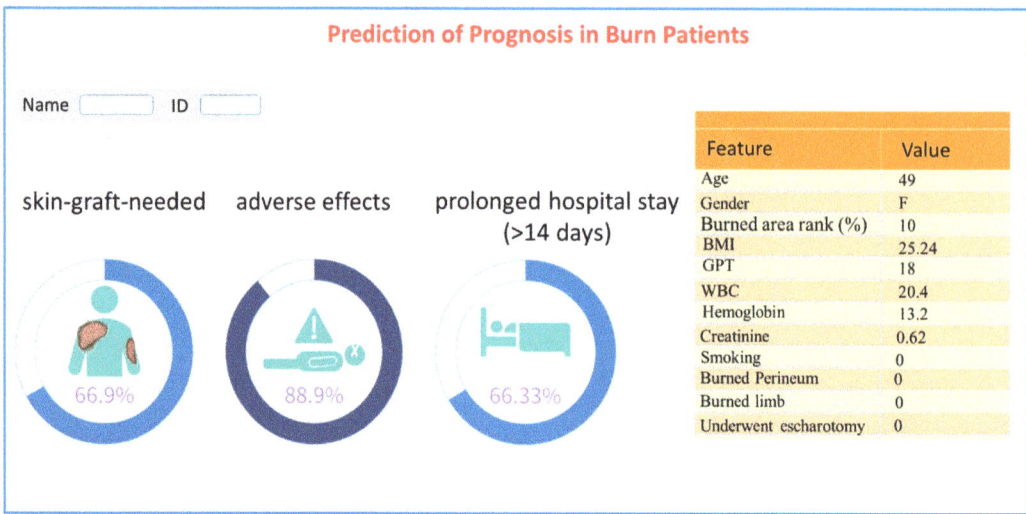

Figure 4. A snapshot of the prediction system.

We, then, demonstrated the AI system to the pilot burn care staff (three nurses and two physicians) and received positive feedback. They see this as a useful tool for the timely identification of high-risk burn patients. According to the risk probability, care staff can consider appropriate treatment plans to optimize the utilization of medical resources. It can greatly improve the quality and efficiency of burn patient care.

4. Discussion

In this study, we collected and analyzed a comprehensive set of laboratory data and clinical information to gain valuable insights. Our research encompassed crucial factors such as body mass index, gender, age, blood pressure, body temperature (BT), total body surface area (TBSA), hemoglobin levels, alanine transaminase levels, glucose levels, platelet count, blood urea nitrogen levels, creatinine levels, and more.

By including these significant parameters in our analysis, we aimed to capture a holistic view of the subjects and their health profiles. The diverse range of data points allowed us to explore the relationships between various variables and draw meaningful conclusions.

In summary, our study employed a robust dataset consisting of crucial laboratory measurements and clinical information. By considering these factors, we aimed to enhance the depth and accuracy of our findings, providing a comprehensive understanding of the subject population.

Moreover, we took into consideration several prevalent and significant comorbidities, including diabetes, hypertension, and cardiovascular disease. These conditions play a crucial role in determining patient outcomes.

We utilized all the aforementioned features to develop predictive models for various outcomes, such as in-hospital mortality, acute respiratory failure during hospitalization, ventilator dependence, renal failure, a prolonged hospital stay, and the need for skin grafting. To obtain the necessary data, we primarily relied on the routine emergency department (ED) charts and regular medical records. This approach eliminated the need for additional examinations while ensuring we had an ample amount of relevant data at our disposal.

By leveraging these readily available sources, we were able to capture a comprehensive range of information essential for our analysis. This streamlined approach allowed us to focus on utilizing the existing data to develop robust predictive models, saving time and resources without compromising the quality of our study.

This study stands out as one of the rare tools that aim to predict the severity of burn injuries in patients by leveraging diverse clinical characteristic data. By employing various statistical models and machine-learning approaches (i.e., logistic regression, random forest, SVM, KNN, LightGBM, ML, and Xgboost), we successfully achieved positive predictive outcomes. These results were anticipated, and we firmly believe that they hold significant value in terms of predicting and managing patients' conditions effectively.

In the context of predicting the necessity of skin graft surgery using a machine-learning model (random forest), Figures 2A and 3A indicate that the total body surface area (TBSA) has the most significant impact on the requirement for skin graft surgery, followed by the white blood cell count (WBC) and GPT (a liver enzyme), whereas gender has minimal influence. Higher values in the burn area rank correlate with an increased risk of undergoing skin graft surgery, indicating a greater likelihood of needing the procedure. Similarly, WBC levels also influence the risk of requiring skin graft surgery. Therefore, early and adequate fluid resuscitation is crucial in reducing the necessity of surgery.

Figures 2B and 3B reveal that the total body surface area (TBSA) has the most significant impact on prolonged hospitalization, followed by the body mass index (BMI) and creatinine levels. The location of the burn or scald and gender have minimal influence. Higher TBSA values indicate a higher risk of prolonged hospitalization (exceeding 14 days). This suggests that obesity and impaired renal function are both risk factors associated with prolonged hospital stays.

Figures 2C and 3C highlight the factors influencing different complications during hospitalization, as indicated by the LightGBM model. Notably, the total body surface area (TBSA) exhibits the most significant impact on overall adverse outcomes, followed by white blood cell count (WBC) and age. On the other hand, the location of the burn or scald and gender have minimal influence. Higher values in TBSA, WBC, and age are associated with an increased risk of overall adverse outcomes. These findings emphasize the importance of implementing specific preventive measures for elderly patients with extensive burn areas and a heightened risk of dehydration.

In Table 5, we compared the predictive results of the ML models we utilized (random forest, XGBoost, and LightGBM) with the Baux scoring in predicting the necessity of surgery, prolonged hospitalization, and the occurrence of complications. The ML models demonstrate superior performance over the Baux score in terms of accuracy, sensitivity, specificity, and AUC. Notably, the results for prolonged hospitalization and occurrence of complications exhibit significant differences based on the DeLong test.

The Baux score has traditionally been commonly employed to primarily predict the mortality probability of burn patients, while also implying the severity of the burn injury, with the result that it is of significant reference value and sees widespread use. However, our model, when compared to the Baux score, demonstrates superior performance in predicting prolonged hospital stays and complications. Consequently, it is expected to complement the shortcomings of the Baux score in clinical settings, thus offering a synergistic effect.

Next, we conducted a thorough review of several relevant and comparable studies. In Stylianou et al. [22]'s study, an established logistic mortality model was compared to machine-learning methods (artificial neural network, support vector machine, random forests, and naive Bayes) using a population-based (England and Wales) case-cohort registry. They presented the following findings: Random forests were marginally better for a high positive predictive value and reasonable sensitivity. Neural networks yielded slightly better prediction overall. Logistic regression gives an optimal mix of performance and interpretability.

Liu and colleagues [23] reviewed several databases such as MEDLINE, the Cochrane Database of Systematic Reviews, and ScienceDirect, and performed a citation review of relevant primary and review articles—the databases were searched for studies involving burn care/research and machine learning in the year 2015. The review conducted by Liu and colleagues highlighted the potential of machine-learning techniques in burn care and research. The studies reviewed in 2015 demonstrated the effectiveness of machine-learning algorithms in various aspects of burn care, including diagnosis, treatment planning, prognostic prediction, and wound assessment. The findings underscore the importance of continued research and development in this area, as the integration of machine learning holds great promise for enhancing patient outcomes and improving the overall quality of burn care.

A few years later, Huang et al. [24] conducted a systemic review in which thirty articles were included. Nine studies used machine learning and automation to estimate the percent total body surface area (%TBSA) burned, four calculated fluid estimations, nineteen estimated the burn depth, five estimated the need for surgery, and two evaluated scarring. In their conclusion, the utilization of machine learning as an adjunct for evaluating burn wound severity has demonstrated promising results in improving diagnostic accuracy. These techniques provide an objective approach by leveraging diverse data points to enhance the assessment process. However, it is crucial to conduct further research to validate and refine existing models, ensuring their clinical feasibility and applicability. The integration of machine learning into burn wound evaluation has the potential to advance the field, empowering clinicians with valuable insights and, ultimately, enhancing patient care.

We summarized the comparison of these works in Table 6.

Table 6. A comparison with related studies.

Study	This Study	[22]	[23]	[24]
Sample size	224	66,611	6059	3264
Types of samples	High-risk patient admitted to our burn center	Population-based (England and Wales) case-cohort registry	Image in majority Patient data in minority	Image Animal models Simulated patient data
Outcome	Prolonged hospital stay (>14 days) Skin graft needed Adverse complications including mortality	Mortality	(%TBSA) Fluid estimations Burn depth Need for surgery Scarring	(%TBSA) Fluid requirements Burn depth Surgical candidacy
Study method	Seven machine-leaning methods	Four machine-leaning methods	Systemic review	Systemic review
Real-world implementation	Yes A predictive application with AI models was implemented and integrated into the existing HIS	N/A	N/A	N/A
Input data	Fourteen patient demographic features, TBSA, burned part, vital signs, laboratory results, comorbidities	Age, TBSA, type of burn, comorbidities	Vital signs Burn photos TBSA Inhalation TBSA	Simulated patient data 2D image Animal models
Testing results (AUC)	Prolonged hospital stay (>14 days) (0.795–0.811) Skin graft needed (0.788) Occurrence of adverse complications (0.872)	Mortality (0.945)	Burn depth (0.83)	Burn depth (0.662–0.925) Surgery determination (0.793–1.000)
Year	2023	2015	2015	2021

In recent years, global scholars have extensively utilized machine learning to aid in judgment and decision making by utilizing various sources of information, such as burn wound photos [25–27], patient demographics, vital signs, underlying diseases, total burn areas, and more [28,29]. Furthermore, the utilization of animal models for comparative prediction is extensively practiced across numerous prominent research institutions [30,31]. These advancements have significantly contributed to both basic research and clinical applications.

Moreover, we conducted a comprehensive comparison of our study with other similar research endeavors, which we have succinctly summarized in Table 7.

Table 7. A comparison with similar studies.

Study	This Study	[28]	[32]
Patient number	224	1585	1080
Types of patient origin	High-risk patient admitted to our burn center	Burn center inpatient in a medical center in the US	A regional burn center inpatient
Outcome	Prolonged hospital stay (>14 days) Skin graft needed Adverse complications including mortality	LOS (length of hospital stay) Survival	LOS (length of hospital stay)
Study method	Seven machine-leaning methods	An artificial neural network	Two machine-leaning methods
Real-world implementation	Yes A predictive application with AI models was implemented and integrated into the existing HIS	N/A	N/A
Input data	Fourteen patient demographic features, TBSA, burned part, vital signs, laboratory results, comorbidities	TBSA, burned part, type of transportation, burn mechanism	Sixteen patient demographic features, TBSA, burned part, vital signs, laboratory results, comorbidities, operation, burn depth
Testing results (AUC)	Prolonged hospital stay (>14 days) (0.795–0.811) Occurrence of adverse complications including mortality (0.872) Skin graft needed (0.788)	LOS (length of hospital stay) (0.72) Survival (0.98)	LOS (length of hospital stay) (0.487–0.718)
Year	2023	1996	2010

Based on the above comparison, it can be observed that our predictive model performs better in estimating the extended length of hospital stays. However, when it comes to predicting mortality/survival and complications, both our predictive method and Frye et al.'s method [28] have their own merits. This difference in estimation is likely due to slight variations in the extraction of clinical information and analysis methods.

In accordance with the achievements of previous studies, we have envisioned extracting a wider range of patient data and have employed seven machine-learning methods to generate more detailed predictions for various outcomes. By integrating this approach with the hospital information system (HIS) [32], our research not only assists clinical healthcare professionals in their decision-making processes but also provides objective references for explaining medical conditions to and predicting outcomes for patients and their families.

The clinical advantages of integrating our system with the hospital information system (HIS) lie in the enhanced convenience and efficiency of medical record and nursing record management. This integration enables the direct retrieval of computational results and medical staff–patient communication logs, effectively reducing the time spent on documentation tasks. Consequently, it leads to improved operational efficiency.

We acknowledge that our study is subject to certain limitations that warrant careful consideration. Firstly, the data for our analysis were exclusively sourced from a singular burn care unit located in Tainan, Taiwan. To enhance the robustness and generalizability of our findings, it is imperative that subsequent investigations incorporate data from a broader range of medical facilities. Secondly, it is plausible that certain granular data points may not have been collected in their entirety, underscoring the potential for additional insights. Thus, it becomes evident that further endeavors are essential to refine this model and elevate its overall performance.

5. Conclusions

This study aimed to develop a versatile machine-learning model to aid physicians in diagnosing disease progression and predicting the risk of death for burn patients. The model utilized a combination of patients' basic health indicators, comorbidity indicators, and specific laboratory data as features. Additionally, we have successfully implemented and seamlessly integrated a web-based predictive application into the existing hospital information system (HIS) without requiring complex computational operations. This integration was well-received by physicians during the initial usage phase, indicating a high level of acceptance. We firmly believe that utilizing machine-learning algorithms to predict adverse outcomes in burn patients is a promising research approach that can assist physicians in promptly assessing disease severity following hospital admission. This early assessment enables them to select the most suitable and personalized treatment strategies, thereby improving patient prognosis.

Furthermore, in addressing the dynamic fluctuations in injury conditions, we can harness objective data acquisition to facilitate AI assistance in comprehensively interpreting information and subsequently delivering it to clinical caregivers and patients. This approach enables us to respond more promptly to changes in the patient's medical condition.

For future studies, researchers can consider incorporating additional potential variables and conducting a feature selection process to enhance the quality of the models. With the continual emergence of novel physiological monitoring tools and laboratory diagnostic instruments, we anticipate the ability to gather a greater volume of valuable data for utilization. Simultaneously, the accumulation of clinical cases through real-world usage will further enhance the system's performance in future operations.

Author Contributions: Conceptualization, C.-C.Y. and C.-F.L.; methodology, Y.-S.L. and C.-F.L.; formal analysis, C.-F.L.; writing—original draft preparation, C.-C.Y. and C.-F.L.; writing—review and editing, C.-C.Y., Y.-S.L., C.-C.C. and C.-F.L. All authors have read and agreed to the published version of the manuscript.

Funding: This research received no external funding.

Institutional Review Board Statement: This study was conducted according to the guidelines of the Declaration of Helsinki and approved by the Institutional Review Board of Chi Mei Medical Center (IRB No. 11206-014; 5 July 2023).

Informed Consent Statement: Informed consent from patients was waived due to the retrospective nature of the study.

Data Availability Statement: The dataset used for this study is available upon request from the corresponding author.

Conflicts of Interest: The authors declare no conflict of interest.

References

1. Artz, C.P. The burn injury—A summary. *J. Trauma* **1966**, *6*, 420–421. [CrossRef] [PubMed]
2. Wang, Y.; Beekman, J.; Hew, J.; Jackson, S.; Issler-Fisher, A.C.; Parungao, R.; Lajevardi, S.S.; Li, Z.; Maitz, P.K.M. Burn injury: Challenges and advances in burn wound healing, infection, pain and scarring. *Adv. Drug Deliv. Rev.* **2018**, *123*, 3–17. [CrossRef] [PubMed]
3. Brodie, N. Plastic reconstruction following third degree burn of forearm. *Am. J. Surg.* **1947**, *74*, 834–837. [CrossRef]
4. Davis, S.C.; Mertz, P.M.; Bilevich, E.D.; Cazzaniga, A.L.; Eaglstein, W.H. Early debridement of second-degree burn wounds enhances the rate of epithelization--an animal model to evaluate burn wound therapies. *J. Burn Care Rehabil.* **1996**, *17*, 558–561. [CrossRef] [PubMed]
5. Pencle, F.J.; Mowery, M.L.; Zulfiqar, H. *First Degree Burn*; StatPearls: Treasure Island, FL, USA, 2023.

6. Hahn, B.; Roh, S.A.; Price, C.; Fu, W.; Dibello, J.; Berwald, N.; Greenstein, J.; Chacko, J. Estimates of Total Burned Surface Area by Emergency Department Clinicians and Burn Specialists. *Cureus* **2020**, *12*, e9362. [CrossRef]
7. Miri, S.; Mobayen, M.; Aboutaleb, E.; Ezzati, K.; Feizkhah, A.; Karkhah, S. Exercise as a rehabilitation intervention for severe burn survivors: Benefits & barriers. *Burns* **2022**, *48*, 1269–1270. [CrossRef] [PubMed]
8. Zal, M.; Deldar, K.; Froutan, R.; Ahmadabadi, A.; Mazlom, S.R. Rehabilitation of Burn Victims: Improving Quality of Life in Victims With Face and Neck Burn Through an Augmented Reality Coupled Pamphlet. *J. Burn Care Res.* **2023**, *44*, 311–319. [CrossRef] [PubMed]
9. Yeh, C.C.; Lin, Y.S.; Huang, K.F. Resurfacing of total penile full-thickness burn managed with the Versajet hydrosurgery system. *J. Burn Care Res.* **2010**, *31*, 361–364. [CrossRef] [PubMed]
10. Christofides, C.; Moore, R.; Nel, M. Baux Score as a Predictor of Mortality at the CHBAH Adult Burns Unit. *J. Surg. Res.* **2020**, *251*, 53–62. [CrossRef] [PubMed]
11. Heng, J.S.; Clancy, O.; Atkins, J.; Leon-Villapalos, J.; Williams, A.J.; Keays, R.; Hayes, M.; Takata, M.; Jones, I.; Vizcaychipi, M.P. Revised Baux Score and updated Charlson comorbidity index are independently associated with mortality in burns intensive care patients. *Burns* **2015**, *41*, 1420–1427. [CrossRef] [PubMed]
12. Lam, N.N.; Hung, N.T.; Duc, N.M. Prognosis value of revised Baux score among burn patients in developing country. *Int. J. Burn. Trauma* **2021**, *11*, 197–201.
13. Osler, T.; Glance, L.G.; Hosmer, D.W. Simplified estimates of the probability of death after burn injuries: Extending and updating the baux score. *J. Trauma* **2010**, *68*, 690–697. [CrossRef] [PubMed]
14. Dokter, J.; Meijs, J.; Oen, I.M.; van Baar, M.E.; van der Vlies, C.H.; Boxma, H. External validation of the revised Baux score for the prediction of mortality in patients with acute burn injury. *J. Trauma Acute Care Surg.* **2014**, *76*, 840–845. [CrossRef]
15. Roberts, G.; Lloyd, M.; Parker, M.; Martin, R.; Philp, B.; Shelley, O.; Dziewulski, P. The Baux score is dead. Long live the Baux score: A 27-year retrospective cohort study of mortality at a regional burns service. *J. Trauma Acute Care Surg.* **2012**, *72*, 251–256. [CrossRef] [PubMed]
16. Karimi, H.; Motevalian, S.A.; Rabbani, A.; Motabar, A.R.; Vasigh, M.; Sabzeparvar, M.; Mobayen, M. Prediction of mortality in pediatric burn injuries: R-baux score to be applied in children (pediatrics-baux score). *Iran. J. Pediatr.* **2013**, *23*, 165–170. [PubMed]
17. Choi, K.J.; Pham, C.H.; Collier, Z.J.; Mert, M.; Ota, R.K.; Li, R.; Yenikomshian, H.A.; Singh, M.; Gillenwater, T.J.; Kuza, C.M. The Predictive Capacity of American Society of Anesthesiologists Physical Status (ASA PS) Score in Burn Patients. *J. Burn Care Res.* **2020**, *41*, 803–808. [CrossRef] [PubMed]
18. Saadat, G.H.; Toor, R.; Mazhar, F.; Bajani, F.; Tatebe, L.; Schlanser, V.; Kaminsky, M.; Messer, T.; Starr, F.; Dennis, A.; et al. Severe burn injury: Body Mass Index and the Baux score. *Burns* **2021**, *47*, 72–77. [CrossRef] [PubMed]
19. Bendjelid, K.; Giraud, R.; Siegenthaler, N.; Michard, F. Validation of a new transpulmonary thermodilution system to assess global end-diastolic volume and extravascular lung water. *Crit. Care* **2010**, *14*, R209. [CrossRef] [PubMed]
20. Chawla, N.V.B.; Bowyer, K.W.; Hall, L.O.; Kegelmeyer, W.P. SMOTE: Synthetic minority over-sampling technique. *J. Artif. Intell. Res.* **2002**, *16*, 321–357. [CrossRef]
21. Lundberg, S.M.; Lee, S.I. A Unified Approach to Interpreting Model Predictions. In Proceedings of the 31st International Conference on Neural Information Processing Systems, Red Hook, NY, USA, 4 December 2017; pp. 4768–4777.
22. Stylianou, N.; Akbarov, A.; Kontopantelis, E.; Buchan, I.; Dunn, K.W. Mortality risk prediction in burn injury: Comparison of logistic regression with machine learning approaches. *Burns* **2015**, *41*, 925–934. [CrossRef] [PubMed]
23. Liu, N.T.; Salinas, J. Machine learning in burn care and research: A systematic review of the literature. *Burns* **2015**, *41*, 1636–1641. [CrossRef] [PubMed]
24. Huang, S.; Dang, J.; Sheckter, C.C.; Yenikomshian, H.A.; Gillenwater, J. A systematic review of machine learning and automation in burn wound evaluation: A promising but developing frontier. *Burns* **2021**, *47*, 1691–1704. [CrossRef] [PubMed]
25. Serrano, C.; Acha, B.; Gomez-Cia, T.; Acha, J.I.; Roa, L.M. A computer assisted diagnosis tool for the classification of burns by depth of injury. *Burns* **2005**, *31*, 275–281. [CrossRef]
26. Acha, B.; Serrano, C.; Acha, J.I.; Roa, L.M. Segmentation and classification of burn images by color and texture information. *J. Biomed. Opt.* **2005**, *10*, 034014. [CrossRef] [PubMed]
27. Ganapathy, P.; Tamminedi, T.; Qin, Y.; Nanney, L.; Cardwell, N.; Pollins, A.; Sexton, K.; Yadegar, J. Dual-imaging system for burn depth diagnosis. *Burns* **2014**, *40*, 67–81. [CrossRef] [PubMed]
28. Frye, K.E.; Izenberg, S.D.; Williams, M.D.; Luterman, A. Simulated biologic intelligence used to predict length of stay and survival of burns. *J. Burn Care Rehabil.* **1996**, *17*, 540–546. [CrossRef] [PubMed]
29. Estahbanati, H.K.; Bouduhi, N. Role of artificial neural networks in prediction of survival of burn patients-a new approach. *Burns* **2002**, *28*, 579–586. [CrossRef] [PubMed]
30. Iyoho, A.; Ng, L.; Chan, P. The Development of a Probabilistic Dose-Response for a Burn Injury Model. *Mil. Med.* **2017**, *182*, 202–209. [CrossRef] [PubMed]

31. Rowland, R.; Ponticorvo, A.; Baldado, M.; Kennedy, G.T.; Burmeister, D.M.; Christy, R.J.; Bernal, N.P.; Durkin, A.J. Burn wound classification model using spatial frequency-domain imaging and machine learning. *J. Biomed. Opt.* **2019**, *24*, 056007. [CrossRef]
32. Yang, C.S.; Wei, C.P.; Yuan, C.C.; Schoung, J.Y. Predicting the length of hospital stay of burn patients: Comparisons of prediction accuracy among different clinical stages. *Decis. Support. Syst.* **2010**, *50*, 325–335. [CrossRef]

Disclaimer/Publisher's Note: The statements, opinions and data contained in all publications are solely those of the individual author(s) and contributor(s) and not of MDPI and/or the editor(s). MDPI and/or the editor(s) disclaim responsibility for any injury to people or property resulting from any ideas, methods, instructions or products referred to in the content.

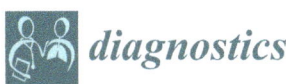

Article

Clinical Decision Support System to Detect the Occurrence of Ventilator-Associated Pneumonia in Pediatric Intensive Care

Jerome Rambaud [1,2,*], Masoumeh Sajedi [3], Sally Al Omar [3], Maryline Chomtom [4], Michael Sauthier [1], Simon De Montigny [3,5] and Philippe Jouvet [1]

1. Pediatric Intensive Care Unit, Sainte-Justine Hospital, Montreal, QC H3T 1C5, Canada; michael.sauthier.med@ssss.gouv.qc.ca (M.S.); philippe.jouvet.med@ssss.gouv.qc.ca (P.J.)
2. Pediatric and Neonatal Intensive Care Unit, Armand-Trousseau Hospital, Sorbonne University, 75012 Paris, France
3. Research Center, Sainte-Justine Hospital, Montreal, QC H3T 1C5, Canada; masoumeh.sajedi.hsj@ssss.gouv.qc.ca (M.S.); sally.alomar@hotmail.com (S.A.O.); simon.de.montigny@umontreal.ca (S.D.M.)
4. Pediatric Intensive Care Unit, Caen University Hospital, 14000 Caen, France; chomtom-m@chu-caen.fr
5. School of Public Health, Montréal University, Montreal, QC H2X 3E4, Canada
* Correspondence: jerome.rambaud@aphp.fr; Tel.: +33-1-71-73-85-27

Abstract: Objectives: Ventilator-associated pneumonia (VAP) is a severe care-related disease. The Centers for Disease Control defined the diagnosis criteria; however, the pediatric criteria are mainly subjective and retrospective. Clinical decision support systems have recently been developed in healthcare to help the physician to be more accurate for the early detection of severe pathology. We aimed at developing a predictive model to provide early diagnosis of VAP at the bedside in a pediatric intensive care unit (PICU). Methods: We performed a retrospective single-center study at a tertiary-care pediatric teaching hospital. All patients treated by invasive mechanical ventilation between September 2013 and October 2019 were included. Data were collected in the PICU electronic medical record and high-resolution research database. Development of the clinical decision support was then performed using open-access R software (Version 3.6.1®). Measurements and main results: In total, 2077 children were mechanically ventilated. We identified 827 episodes with almost 48 h of mechanical invasive ventilation and 77 patients who suffered from at least one VAP event. We split our database at the patient level in a training set of 461 patients free of VAP and 45 patients with VAP and in a testing set of 199 patients free of VAP and 20 patients with VAP. The Imbalanced Random Forest model was considered as the best fit with an area under the ROC curve from fitting the Imbalanced Random Forest model on the testing set being 0.82 (95% CI: (0.71, 0.93)). An optimal threshold of 0.41 gave a sensitivity of 79.7% and a specificity of 72.7%, with a positive predictive value (PPV) of 9% and a negative predictive value of 99%, and with an accuracy of 79.5% (95% CI: (0.77, 0.82)). Conclusions: Using machine learning, we developed a clinical predictive algorithm based on clinical data stored prospectively in a database. The next step will be to implement the algorithm in PICUs to provide early, automatic detection of ventilator-associated pneumonia.

Keywords: pneumonia; ventilator associated; clinical decision system; PICU

1. Introduction

Ventilator-associated pneumonia (VAP) is a common and severe complication in intensive care units. VAP, as a care-related complication leads to a worsening prognosis for the affected patients and its early diagnosis remain an ongoing challenge in intensive care. In an attempt to enhance VAP detection, the Centers for Disease Control (CDC) issued diagnosis criteria allowing the identification of VAP after 48h of clinical alteration (defined by worsening gas exchange, fever >38 °C or hypothermia, leukocytosis >15,000/mm^3 or leukopenia <4000/mm^3, new onset of purulent sputum, apnea or tachypnea, wheezing/rales/rhonchi,

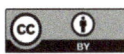

cough and bradycardia <100/min or tachycardia >170/min) [1]. However, delays in VAP diagnosis and, to some extent, in initiating anti-infectious therapy are observed and associated with worse outcomes [2–4]. Furthermore, subjective criteria included in the CDC pediatric definition for VAP results in a variability of VAP diagnosis and incidence (changes in the appearance and amount of sputum, worsening of an existing cough) [5–7]. To help physicians to prospectively diagnose VAP, the CDC developed the concept of Ventilator-Associated Events (VAE) in adults, but children have long been excluded from this definition [1]. It is usual that for adult recommendations, children are excluded mainly because of physiological differences between populations (normal respiratory parameters for an adult are very different from those of a child). Cirulis et al. [8] proposed a pediatric modified VAE definition. Chomton et al. [9] evaluated the pediatric modified VAE definition to detect VAP, but the sensitivity (66%) to identify this ICU-related complication remained disappointing.

In recent years, the number of publications dealing with the development of computerized clinical decision support systems (CDSS) to improve disease diagnosis increased and was shown to be useful for several disease in ICUs [10–14]. The emergence of high-resolution databases supports these developments [15] which allow for a precise and continuous analysis of clinical and biological parameters. Leisman et al. [16] recently reported several recommendations for the development and reporting of predictive models. They identified two categories of predictive models: (1) clinical prediction models for bedside use, and (2) other prediction models intended for deployment across populations for research, benchmarking, and administrative purposes. The usefulness of CDSS had already been highlighted by Mack et al. [17] but no reports on VAP are available currently. To that effect, our project has been developed with the main objective of developing a predictive model to provide early diagnosis of VAP at the bedside in a pediatric intensive care unit (PICU).

2. Materials and Methods

This single-center retrospective study was performed using the data collected in the PICU electronic medical record (Intelligence Critical Care and Anesthesia (ICCA®); Philips Medical, version F0.1) of a tertiary-care pediatric teaching hospital (Sainte-Justine Hospital, Montréal, QC, Canada). To improve data quality, ICCA® was configured with drop-down menus and critical values alerts. Furthermore, all data entered in ICCA® benefited from a medically-endorsed validation.

The hospital database was queried using SQL Server Management Studio 18® (Microsoft, Redmond, WA, USA) to select patients who were aged from 1 day to 18 years at PICU admission and were mechanically ventilated for more than 48 h, between September 2013 and October 2019. We analyzed the first 30 days of invasive mechanical ventilation.

During the first step of the study, all medical files were reviewed by two senior pediatric intensive care experts (JR and PJ) to classify patients into two groups: VAP patients and free-of-VAP patients. VAP was defined according to the 2021 CDC criteria [1]: The 1st context criteria: invasive mechanical ventilation for more than 48 h, 2nd radiological criteria: new or progressive and persistent infiltrate/consolidation/cavitation, 3rd clinical criteria: worsening gas exchange, fever >38 °C or hypothermia, leukocytosis >15,000/mm^3 or leukopenia <4000/mm^3, new onset of purulent sputum, apnea or tachypnea, wheezing/rales/rhonchi, cough and bradycardia <100/min or tachycardia >170/min.

The second step of the study consisted in the extraction of data coming from the electronic medical record (ICCA®, Philips, Toronto, ON, Canada) and high-resolution database (database collecting and storing data from medical devices in real time) [15]. The queried data were date, time, weight (kg), white blood cell count (/mm^3), neutrophil count (/mm^3), partial pressure of carbon dioxide (PaCO$_2$ in mmHg), partial pressure of oxygen (PaO$_2$ in mmHg), inspired fraction of oxygen (FiO$_2$ in %), positive end-expiratory pressure (PEEP in cmH$_2$O), peak inspiratory pressure (PIP in cmH$_2$O), mean airway pressure (MAwP in cmH$_2$O), respiratory rate (/rpm), tidal volume (mL), subjective amount of respiratory tract secretion (0, +, ++, +++), oxygenation (OI) and oxygen saturation index (OSI) [18], calculated pulmonary dynamic compliance (in barometric ventilation mode: tidal volume/(PIP–PEEP); and in volumetric ventilation mode: tidal volume/(peak pressure–PEEP)). We also gathered PIM 2 [19] and PELOD-2 scores [20,21].

Data formatting. The data was formatted using R (version 3.6.1) as a preparation step to train the prediction models based on different algorithms.

All times were expressed as a relative duration since ICU admission.

Data cleaning and Missing data. Incoherent data were identified and corrected according to the scheme described in Supplementary Data S1 "Data Cleaning". Variables consisting of data streams of continuous values were imputed following the last observation carried forward method. For missing data at the beginning of the stream, the first valid observation was carried backward.

Segmenting Variables in Time Blocks. The variables data streams were first segmented into time blocks of 6 h and then for each variable the median (mode for the discrete variable) was calculated over each 6 h time block to avoid aberrant or missing data. Then, the 6 h blocks were aggregated into 48 h time blocks. We chose to aggregate into 48 h time blocks to be as close as possible to the actual VAP timing definition. For each variable, two columns were generated. One consisted of the first non-missing value among the 6 h time blocks and the other one the last non-missing value among the 6 h time blocks, if there was any, in each 48 h time block (if there was no observation, the data was considered missing). For the development of the algorithms, for each variable, the first non-missing values and the actual difference or relative change of the values of the two columns were considered (more details are available in Supplementary Data S2 "Segmenting variables in time blocks").

Stratified train-test split at a patient level. VAP patients and non-VAP patients were split into the training set (70% of each class) and the testing set (remaining 30% of each class). Since some patients had more than one stay in the PICU, all stays of a patient in the training set were kept in the training set (and the same for patients in the testing set). All details for the train-test split are available in Supplementary Data S3 "train-test split".

Imputation. Preliminary inspection of the dataset showed that around 50% of data was missing for the variables "pulmonary dynamic compliance" and "minute ventilation". Missing values imputation in the training dataset was performed by 'randomForest' (v4.6-14) with the function 'rfImpute' [22]. The imputed values were the weighted average of the non-missing observations, where the weights were the proximities from randomForest. For data in the testing set, the missing values in each variable were replaced by the mean of the imputed values for the variables with missing values in the training set (more details are available in Supplementary Data S4 "Imputation").

Predictive models. We applied six different learning algorithms to generate predictive models. The algorithms were: Random Forest with the function 'rfsrc' and error rate as the measure of performance, Imbalanced Random Forest with the function 'imbalanced' and G-means as the measure of performance, Stepwise Regression and Random Forest using 5-fold cross validation (5-CV) with the 'train' function; 'glmStepAIC' and 'rf' methods and accuracy were used to select the optimal model using the largest value [23]. Finally, we implemented Elastic Net Regression (5-CV) and Weighted Elastic Net Regression (5-CV) with the 'glmnet' method and ROC was used to select the optimal model using the largest value. The hyperparameters for the Random Forest, Imbalanced Random Forest and stepwise regression (5-CV) algorithms were 'ntree' (number of trees used at the tuning step) and 'mtry' (number of variables randomly selected as candidates for the division of a node) [24]. The parameters in Elastic Net regression were alpha, which controls the relative balance between the lasso and ridge regularization, and lambda, which controls the amount of the penalty. All these models used readily available implementations in R [25,26]. Here, cross-validation was performed inside the training set only (more details are available in Supplementary Data S5 "Predictive models").

Performance measure and model choice. Models resulting from the different algorithms were evaluated, at the level of 48 h time blocks, on the train and the test set by calculating their AUC score and by determining classification thresholds reaching predetermined levels of sensitivity (80%, 85%, 90%, 95%). The final model was chosen based on the capacity to [1] maximize specificity under these sensitivity levels, and [2] generalize the sensitivity and specificity from the test set. The area under the ROC curve (AUC) was considered as the primary measure of performance to choose the best model.

Per patient validation. The final model was evaluated on its capacity to correctly assess the infection status of patients over time. The predictions' results obtained after setting different classification thresholds were taken. The number of patients with accurate predictions (i.e., predicted class = observed VAP status) and inaccurate predictions (i.e., predicted class ≠ observed VAP status) were computed over time. The number of patients for whom the predictions contained at least one error were identified. We looked at the accuracy of predictions by stratifying patients into two groups. We identified the patients for whom the predictions contained at least one error for each subgroup. The global error rates were calculated for each subgroup.

Statistics

Development of the clinical decision support was performed using open-access R software, Version 3.6.1® (R Foundation for Statistical Computing, Vienna, Austria). Statistical analysis of patients' characteristics was performed using Prism X® software (version 7.05) (GraphPad Inc. San Diego, CA, USA). Kolmogorov analysis was performed to test the normal distribution of continuous variables. Population description used categorical variables expressed as frequency with corresponding proportion and quantitative variables presented as mean and standard deviation. Performance evaluation was conducted using ROC curves, AUC and their confidence intervals, and derived measures of sensitivity and specificity. The ethical committee of Sainte-Justine University hospital approved the study and waived the need for informed consent given the retrospective design.

The Saint-Justine ethical committee approved the study as a retrospective study and waived the need for written consent (n°2020–2454).

3. Results

3.1. General Description of the Population

A total of 5153 children had been hospitalized in Saint-Justine PICU during the study period of which 40% (2077) were mechanically ventilated and 1235 episodes with more than 48 h of mechanical invasive ventilation were identified (Figure 1). Seventy-seven patients had at least one VAP event. Seventy-eight VAP events (6%) were diagnosed by two experts. The patients' general characteristics are described in Table 1.

Table 1. Population characteristics.

Population Characteristics	Global Population (N: 827)	VAP Patients (N: 77)	No VAP Patients (N: 750)	p:
Weight (kg)	15.8 ± 1.6	20.99 ± 2.7	15.25 ± 0.7	0.01
Age (days)	1308 ± 1904	1806 ± 250	1256 ± 69	0.02
Gender male (%)	475 (57%)	41 (53%)	434 (58%)	0.4
Pelod 2 score	10.1 ± 4.8	10.4 ± 0.6	9.9 ± 0.2	0.47
Pelod 2 mortality risk (%)	0.3 ± 0.3	0.3 ± 0.1	0.2 ± 0.01	0.15
Bronchoscopie (%)	70 (8%)	14 (18%)	56 (8%)	0.04
Neuromuscular blocker (%)	279 (34%)	43 (55%)	236 (31%)	<0.0001
Mechanical Ventilation duration (days)	12.5 ± 30.9	29.3 ± 5.1	10.9 ± 1.5	<0.0001
PICU length of stay (days)	26.1 ± 52.5	48.3 ± 7.1	23.4 ± 1.8	<0.0001
Survival rate (%)	740 (90%)	65 (84%)	675 (90%)	0.16

PICU: Pediatric intensive care unit; VAP: Ventilator-associated pneumonia.

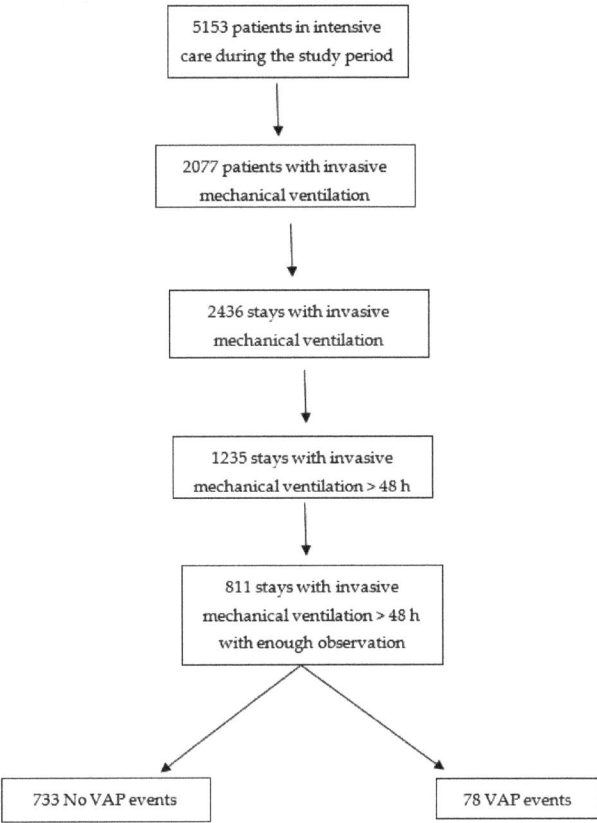

Figure 1. Flow chart. VAP: Ventilator-associated event.

Patients with less than 4 days of mechanical ventilation were removed (see Supplementary Data S2 "Segmenting variables") to achieve 811 episodes of invasive mechanical ventilation. The training set (70% of each class) and testing set (remaining 30% of each class), resulted in a training set of 461 patients free of VAP and 45 patients with VAP and in a testing set of 199 patients free of VAP and 20 patients with VAP. Since some patients had more than one stay in the ICU, there could be different events for the same patient. The training set thus had 513 stays with no VAP event and 45 stays with a VAP event, and the testing set had 231 stays with no VAP event and 22 stays with a VAP event. The segmenting of variables in 48 h non-overlapping time blocks generated, from these datasets, 1852 time blocks free of VAP and 45 time blocks with VAP in the training set, and 788 time blocks free of VAP and 22 time blocks with VAP in the testing set.

We observed similar characteristics in the train and test groups (Table 2).

Table 2. Train and test groups' characteristics.

Train and Test Groups Characteristics	Test Group (n: 261)	Train Group (n: 572)	p:
Weight (kg)	16.9 ± 1.3	15.6 ± 0.8	0.40
Age (days)	1387 ± 129	1268 ± 84	0.43
Gender male, (n, %)	146 (60)	284 (58)	0.69
Pelod 2 score	10.4 ± 0.2	9.7 ± 0.5	0.16

Table 2. *Cont.*

Train and Test Groups Characteristics	Test Group (*n*: 261)	Train Group (*n*: 572)	*p*:
Pelod 2 mortality risk (%)	0.3 ± 0.1	0.2 ± 0.1	0.13
Proportion of VAP patients (*n*, %)	25 (10)	50 (10)	0.99
Length of mechanical ventilation before VAP (days)	9.9 ± 2.7	9.6 ± 1.9	0.66
Length of mechanical ventilation duration (days)	12.1 ± 1.6	11.2 ± 1.1	0.64
PICU length of stay (days)	21.3 ± 2.4	22.3 ± 2.0	0.81

Pelod: Pediatric logistic organ dysfunction, PICU: Pediatric intensive care unit; VAP: Ventilator-associated pneumonia.

3.2. Missing Data

We observed two missing values for "sf ratio" and "oxygen saturation index (OSI)" in the test set (0.1% of total observations). For the variable "pulmonary dynamic compliance" the proportion of missing values in the train and test sets were 0.49 and 0.54, respectively. For the variable "minute ventilation", the proportion of missing values in the train and test sets were 0.49 and 0.54, respectively.

3.3. Results of Training Algorithm

The Imbalanced Random Forest model was considered as the best fit with an area under the ROC curve of 0.86 from the train set.

Thresholds and specificities corresponding to the predetermined levels of sensitivity are presented in Table 3. Variable importance obtained from the Imbalanced Random Forest model are presented in Figure 2.

Table 3. Imbalanced Random Forest model. Threshold and specificity from predetermined sensitivity for the train set.

Threshold	Specificity	Sensitivity
0.41	0.79	0.80
0.29	0.64	0.87
0.25	0.58	0.91
0.22	0.52	0.96

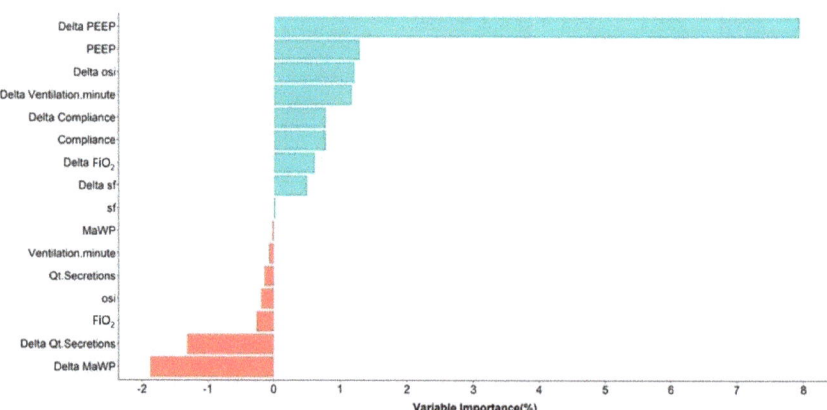

Figure 2. Variable importance used in the clinical decision system.

3.4. Performance on Test Dataset

The area under the ROC curve from fitting the Imbalanced Random Forest model on the test set was 0.82 (95% CI: (0.71, 0.93)) (Figure 3).

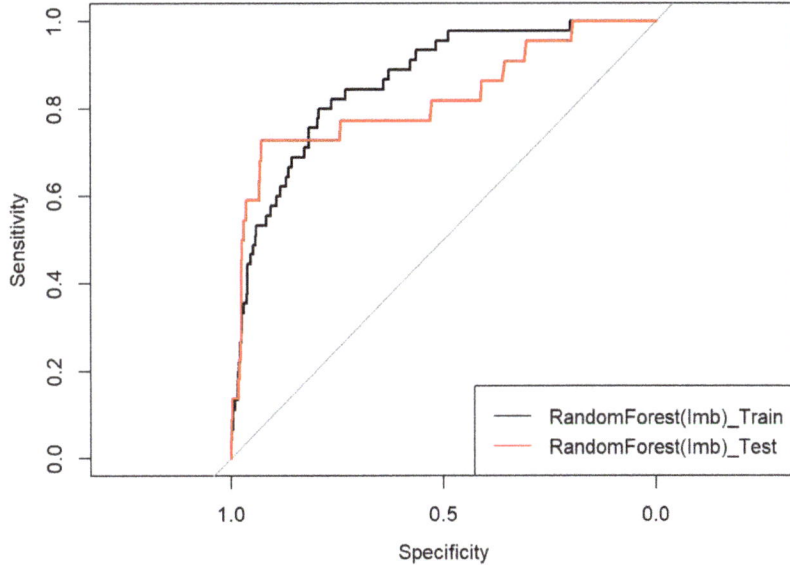

Figure 3. ROC Curve. Black curve represent the efficiency of the training of the algorithm on 2/3 of the dataset. Red curve represents the efficiency of the test of the algorithm on the rest of the data set.

The specificity and sensitivity obtained after setting different classification thresholds are presented in Table 4. An optimal threshold of 0.41 gave a sensitivity of 79.7% and a specificity of 72.7%, with a positive predictive value (PPV) of 9% and a negative predictive value of 99%, with an accuracy of 79.5% (95% CI: (0.77, 0.82)).

Table 4. Imbalanced Random Forest model. Sensitivity and specificity for the test set corresponding to different thresholds.

Threshold	Specificity	Sensitivity
0.41	0.797	0.73
0.28	0.66	0.77
0.25	0.59	0.77
0.22	0.53	0.82

3.5. Per Patient Validation

Performance of the final model was evaluated over different time periods. Time periods were defined starting from the first time block and going up to a given time block in the future. The confusion matrices for all the time periods were constructed. False positive rates (FPR), true positive rates (TPR), and area under the curve (AUC) were calculated. The results are presented in Figure 4. The procedure is explained in detail in Supplementary Data S6 "Per patient validation".

The global error rate is presented in Table 5. We observed a lower error rate for patients with at most three time blocks of observations, compared to the ones with at least four time blocks of observations.

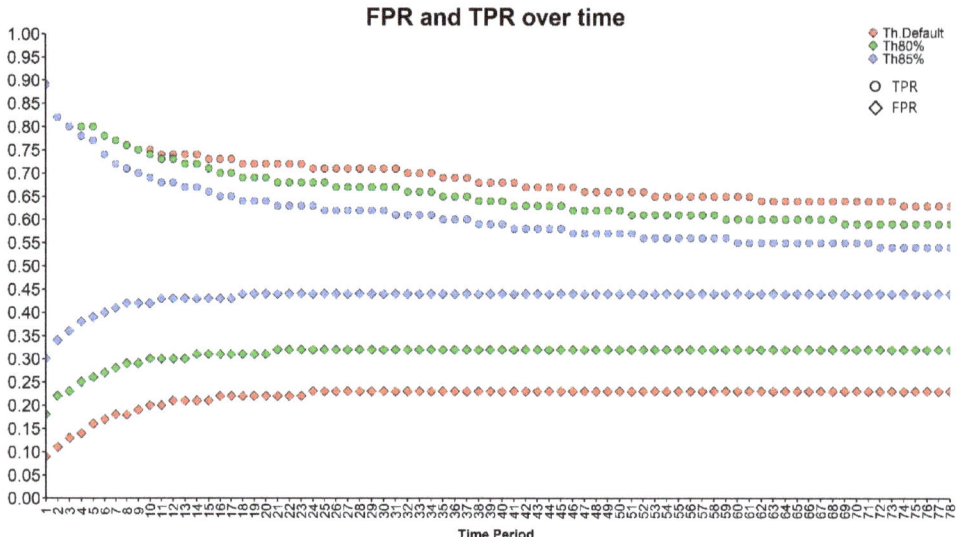

Figure 4. False positive rate and true positive rate over different time periods for different thresholds. Th.Default: default threshold of the model; Th80%: threshold correspond to the 80% sensitivity; Th85%: threshold correspond to the 85% sensitivity.

Table 5. Error rates (%) for predicted classes.

	G1			G2		
	ER.Pred	ER.Pred.th80	ER.Pred.th85	ER.Pred	ER.Pred.th80	ER.Pred.th85
All	11.56	19.60	31.66	79.59	83.67	95.92
VAP	23.08	23.08	23.08	66.67	66.67	88.89
NoVAP	10.75	19.35	32.26	82.50	87.50	97.50

G1: Patients with at most 3 time blocks of observations; G2: Patients with at least 4 time-blocks of observations. E.Pred: Error rate for prediction; E.Pred.the80%: Error rate for prediction with threshold correspond to the 80% sensitivity; E.Pred.th85%: Error rate for prediction with threshold correspond to the 85% sensitivity.

4. Discussion

Using an electronic medical record, an algorithm supporting clinicians in the early diagnosis of ventilator-associated pneumonia in PICU had a sensitivity of 80% and specificity of 73%, with the threshold of 0.41. To date, it is the most accurate sensitivity achieved by a CDSS system to provide early detection of VAP.

Ventilator-associated pneumonias is a severe health care disease [2,27,28]. To improve the delay and accuracy of this challenging diagnosis, Cirulis et al. [8] evaluated the accuracy of adults' ventilator-associated events (VAE) to early diagnose pediatric VAP and developed modified pediatric criteria for VAE (increase in FiO_2 by 20% or PEEP by 2 cm H_2O sustained for more than one day). VAE and modified pediatric VAE both had a disappointing sensitivity of 23% and 56% for Cirulis et al. [8] and 56% and 66% for Chomton et al. [9], respectively. Our algorithm was based on machine learning methods and improved the sensitivity in this study and could be implemented to screen in real-time patient's data to provide early detection of VAP in children. The prediction of the test set using the Imbalanced Random Forest model is stored in a file and is available on Github [29].

Implementation of a clinical decision system to help physicians is a promising technology aimed at helping the physician to take medical decision [10,30], to analyze chest X-rays [31], or to increases diagnosis sensitivity [32]. The development methodology starts with a retrospective classification of analyzed patients to define whether they develop the studied conditions (e.g., VAP). This step is crucial to develop an accurate algorithm and rely on the quality of the classification method. In a large review of published CDSS, Ostropolets et al. [33] highlight that only one manuscript addressed confounding and bias due to misclassification. Our classification methodology included all the relevant data from the electronic medical record clinically collected and is the best accuracy that can be obtained currently.

In addition to the classification methodology, the main strength of this study includes the use of continuous vital signs and the ventilatory parameters monitoring database, limiting the number of missing data and allowing the use of the algorithm in real time in the future [15]. The variables extracted from this monitoring included the OSI ratio, the variation of pulmonary compliance, minute ventilation, and ventilatory median pressures. However, the algorithm identified the variation of PEEP during the last 48 h preceding the VAP as the most important criteria as suggested by the CDC definition. Nevertheless, the variation of the ventilatory mean airway pressure was the second most important variable. This result seems crucial because the ventilatory mean airway pressure that not only includes PEEP but also the PIP, I/E ratio and instantaneous gas flow is not included in the CDC diagnosis criteria for VAP.

Nonetheless, we noticed that our algorithm has a better efficacy to diagnose early VAP (before day 6 of the PICU stay) versus late VAP (after day 6 of the PICU stay), with the error rate in prediction of 23.08% vs. 66.67%, respectively. We can hypothesize that the more time the patient stays in the PICU, the more discrete are the variations to be detected due to the potential alteration of the patient's condition.

This study has several strengths. First, this is the first study with a CDSS system reaching over 80% sensitivity. Second, despite this being a single-center study, we report one of the largest number of patients included in a study in children. Finally, we report the highest sensitivity and specificity to diagnose VAP.

Despite these promising results, this work suffers from several limitations. First, the invasive procedures were not considered in our algorithm (bronchoscopy, transportations) due to the lack of data concerning the timing between these procedures and the VAP. Second, data on the reason for invasive mechanical ventilation were not reported in all medical files, although it is well known that brain injury and neurological disorder with impaired swallowing predispose more to pneumonia. Third, the treatment of missing data was conducted using data-focused approaches (last observation carried forward for missing data mid-stream, first observation carried backward for data missing at the beginning of a stream) which did not model the missing data process; the classifications between the VAP and non-VAP patients were retrospectively performed which may have resulted in some misinterpretation of the clinical data. Fourth, for generalizability, a prospective validation of the algorithm in several PICU needs to be conducted.

5. Conclusions

We developed the first clinical predictive system dedicated to VAP diagnosis in PICUs using a high-fidelity database. The implementation of such an algorithm in PICUs could allow physicians to be alerted early in cases of respiratory function impairment and to decide whether to perform respiratory tract analysis and start anti-infective treatment. Although this algorithm achieves a promising sensitivity and specificity level, it is still lacking power and cannot be implanted in PICUs. Additionally, it still needs to be prospectively validated in other PICUs to confirm its reproductivity and external power.

Supplementary Materials: The following supporting information can be downloaded at: https://www.mdpi.com/article/10.3390/diagnostics13182983/s1, Supplementary Data S1 "Data Cleaning"; Supplementary Data S2 "Segmenting variables in time blocks"; Supplementary Data S3 "train-test split"; Supplementary Data S4 "Imputation"; Supplementary Data S5 "Predictive models"; Supplementary Data S6 "Per patient validation".

Author Contributions: Conceptualization, M.C., P.J. and J.R.; Methodology, J.R., S.A.O. and M.S. (Michael Sauthier); Software, S.A.O., M.S. (Michael Sauthier) and S.D.M.; Formal analysis, M.S. (Michael Sauthier) and S.D.M.; Investigation, J.R.; Data curation, M.S. (Masoumeh Sajedi) and S.D.M.; Writing—original draft, J.R.; Writing—review & editing, J.R. and M.C.; Supervision, P.J.; Project administration, P.J.; Funding acquisition, P.J. All authors have read and agreed to the published version of the manuscript.

Funding: J.R. received a studentship from the scholarship supplement program from the Quebec Respiratory Health Research Network. This work was supported in part by the Quebec Respiratory Health Research Network. J.P.'s scientific research funds from the Canadian Foundation for Innovation, Fonds de Recherche Québec, Quebec Ministry of Health and Sainte-Justine Hospital.

Institutional Review Board Statement: The Saint-Justine ethical committee approved the study as a retrospective study and waived the need for written consent (n°2020–2454).

Informed Consent Statement: Not applicable.

Data Availability Statement: Data are available on demand.

Acknowledgments: The authors want to thank the research center of Sainte-Justine University hospital and for their support.

Conflicts of Interest: The authors declare no conflict of interest.

Abbreviations

AUC	area under the curve
CDC	centers for disease control
CDSS	clinical decision support systems
FiO_2	inspired fraction of oxygen
FPR	false positive rates
ICCA	Intelligence Critical Care and Anesthesia®
MAwP	mean airway pressure
OI	oxygenation index
OSI	oxygenation and saturation index
$PaCO_2$	partial pressure of carbon dioxide
PaO_2	partial pressure of oxygen
PELOD-2	pediatric logistic organ dysfunction score
PEEP	positive end-expiratory pressure
PICU	pediatric intensive care unit
PIM 2	pediatric index of mortality
PIP	peak inspiratory pressure
ROC	receiving operator curve
TPR	true positive rates
VAE	ventilator-associated event
VAP	ventilator-associated pneumonia

References

1. Center for Disease Control. 2018. Available online: https://www.cdc.gov/nhsn/PDFs/pscManual/6pscVAPcurrent.pdf (accessed on 14 September 2023).
2. Chastre, J.; Fagon, J.-Y. Ventilator-associated pneumonia. *Am. J. Respir. Crit. Care Med.* **2002**, *165*, 867–903. [CrossRef] [PubMed]
3. Gutiérrez, J.M.M.; Borromeo, A.R.; Dueño, A.L.; Paragas, E.D.; Ellasus, R.O.; Abalos-Fabia, R.S.; Abriam, J.A.; Sonido, A.E.; Hernandez, M.A.; Generale, A.J.A.; et al. Clinical epidemiology and outcomes of ventilator-associated pneumonia in critically ill adult patients: Protocol for a large-scale systematic review and planned meta-analysis. *Syst. Rev.* **2019**, *8*, 180. [CrossRef] [PubMed]
4. Papazian, L.; Klompas, M.; Luyt, C.-E. Ventilator-associated pneumonia in adults: A narrative review. *Intensive Care Med.* **2020**, *46*, 888–906. [CrossRef]
5. Tullu, M.S.; Balasubramanian, P. Ventilator-Associated Pneumonia in Pediatric Intensive Care Unit: Correspondence. *Indian J. Pediatr.* **2015**, *82*, 662–663. [CrossRef]
6. Shaath, G.A.; Jijeh, A.; Faruqui, F.; Bullard, L.; Mehmood, A.; Kabbani, M.S. Ventilator-associated pneumonia in children after cardiac surgery. *Pediatr. Cardiol.* **2014**, *35*, 627–631. [CrossRef]

7. Ericson, J.E.; McGuire, J.; Michaels, M.G.; Schwarz, A.; Frenck, R.; Deville, J.G.; Agarwal, S.; Bressler, A.M.; Gao, J.; Spears, T.; et al. Hospital-acquired Pneumonia and Ventilator-associated Pneumonia in Children: A Prospective Natural History and Case-Control Study. *Pediatr. Infect. Dis. J.* **2020**, *39*, 658–664. [CrossRef] [PubMed]
8. Cirulis, M.M.; Hamele, M.T.; Stockmann, C.R.; Bennett, T.D.; Bratton, S.L. Comparison of the New Adult Ventilator-Associated Event Criteria to the Centers for Disease Control and Prevention Pediatric Ventilator-Associated Pneumonia Definition (PNU2) in a Population of Pediatric Traumatic Brain Injury Patients. *Pediatr. Crit. Care Med.* **2016**, *17*, 157–164. [CrossRef]
9. Chomton, M.; Brossier, D.; Sauthier, M.; Vallières, E.; Dubois, J.; Emeriaud, G.; Jouvet, P. Ventilator-Associated Pneumonia and Events in Pediatric Intensive Care: A Single Center Study. *Pediatr. Crit. Care Med.* **2018**, *19*, 1106–1113. [CrossRef] [PubMed]
10. Giannini, H.M.; Ginestra, J.C.; Chivers, C.; Draugelis, M.; Hanish, A.; Schweickert, W.D.; Fuchs, B.D.; Meadows, L.; Lynch, M.; Donnelly, P.J.; et al. A Machine Learning Algorithm to Predict Severe Sepsis and Septic Shock: Development, Implementation, and Impact on Clinical Practice. *Crit. Care Med.* **2019**, *47*, 1485–1492. [CrossRef]
11. Chen, C.-H.; Lee, Y.-W.; Huang, Y.-S.; Lan, W.-R.; Chang, R.-F.; Tu, C.-Y.; Chen, C.-Y.; Liao, W.-C. Computer-aided diagnosis of endobronchial ultrasound images using convolutional neural network. *Comput. Methods Programs Biomed.* **2019**, *177*, 175–182. [CrossRef] [PubMed]
12. Roggeveen, L.F.; Guo, T.; Driessen, R.H.; Fleuren, L.M.; Thoral, P.; van der Voort, P.H.J.; Girbes, A.R.J.; Bosman, R.J.; Elbers, P. Right Dose, Right Now: Development of AutoKinetics for Real Time Model Informed Precision Antibiotic Dosing Decision Support at the Bedside of Critically Ill Patients. *Front. Pharmacol.* **2020**, *11*, 646. [CrossRef] [PubMed]
13. Lauritsen, S.M.; Kalør, M.E.; Kongsgaard, E.L.; Lauritsen, K.M.; Jørgensen, M.J.; Lange, J.; Thiesson, B. Early detection of sepsis utilizing deep learning on electronic health record event sequences. *Artif. Intell. Med.* **2020**, *104*, 101820. [CrossRef]
14. Wulff, A.; Haarbrandt, B.; Tute, E.; Marschollek, M.; Beerbaum, P.; Jack, T. An interoperable clinical decision-support system for early detection of SIRS in pediatric intensive care using openEHR. *Artif. Intell. Med.* **2018**, *89*, 10–23. [CrossRef]
15. Brossier, D.; El Taani, R.; Sauthier, M.; Roumeliotis, N.; Emeriaud, G.; Jouvet, P. Creating a High-Frequency Electronic Database in the PICU: The Perpetual Patient. *Pediatr. Crit. Care Med.* **2018**, *19*, e189–e198. [CrossRef] [PubMed]
16. Leisman, D.E.; Harhay, M.O.; Lederer, D.J.; Abramson, M.; Adjei, A.A.; Bakker, J.; Ballas, Z.K.; Barreiro, E.; Bell, S.C.; Bellomo, R.; et al. Development and Reporting of Prediction Models: Guidance for Authors From Editors of Respiratory, Sleep, and Critical Care Journals. *Crit. Care Med.* **2020**, *48*, 623–633. [CrossRef]
17. Mack, E.H.; Wheeler, D.S.; Embi, P.J. Clinical decision support systems in the pediatric intensive care unit. *Pediatr. Crit. Care Med.* **2009**, *10*, 23–28. [CrossRef]
18. DesPrez, K.; McNeil, J.B.; Wang, C.; Bastarache, J.A.; Shaver, C.M.; Ware, L.B. Oxygenation Saturation Index Predicts Clinical Outcomes in ARDS. *Chest* **2017**, *152*, 1151–1158. [CrossRef]
19. Slater, A.; Shann, F.; Pearson, G.; Paediatric Index of Mortality (PIM) Study Group. PIM2: A revised version of the Paediatric Index of Mortality. *Intensive Care Med.* **2003**, *29*, 278–285. [CrossRef] [PubMed]
20. Leteurtre, S.; Duhamel, A.; Salleron, J.; Grandbastien, B.; Lacroix, J.; Leclerc, F.; Groupe Francophone de Réanimation et d'Urgences Pédiatriques (GFRUP). PELOD-2: An update of the PEdiatric logistic organ dysfunction score. *Crit. Care Med.* **2013**, *41*, 1761–1773. [CrossRef]
21. Sauthier, M.; Landry-Hould, F.; Leteurtre, S.; Kawaguchi, A.; Emeriaud, G.; Jouvet, P. Comparison of the Automated Pediatric Logistic Organ Dysfunction-2 Versus Manual Pediatric Logistic Organ Dysfunction-2 Score for Critically Ill Children. *Pediatr. Crit. Care Med.* **2020**, *21*, e160–e169. [CrossRef]
22. Breiman, L. Breiman and Cutler's Random Forests for Classification and Regression, R package version 4.6-14 [Internet]. 2018. Available online: https://cran.r-project.org/web/packages/randomForest/randomForest.pdf (accessed on 14 September 2023).
23. Available online: https://cran.r-project.org/web/packages/randomForestSRC/randomForestSRC.pdf (accessed on 14 September 2023).
24. Chen, C.; Liaw, A.; Breiman, L. *Using Random Forest to Learn Imbalanced Data*; University of California: Los Angeles, CA, USA, 2004.
25. Ishwaran, H. Fast Unified Random Forests for Survival, Regression, and Classification (RF-SRC). R Package Version 2.9.3. [Internet]. 2020. Available online: https://cran.rproject.org/web/packages/randomForestSRC/randomForestSRC.pdf (accessed on 14 September 2023).
26. Kuhn, M. Training on Classification and Regression, R Package Version 6.0.86. Available online: https://cran.r-project.org/web/packages/caret/caret.pdf (accessed on 14 September 2023).
27. Cernada, M.; Aguar, M.; Brugada, M.; Gutiérrez, A.; López, J.L.; Castell, M.; Vento, M. Ventilator-associated pneumonia in newborn infants diagnosed with an invasive bronchoalveolar lavage technique: A prospective observational study. *Pediatr. Crit. Care Med.* **2013**, *14*, 55–61. [CrossRef] [PubMed]
28. Elward, A.M.; Warren, D.K.; Fraser, V.J. Ventilator-associated pneumonia in pediatric intensive care unit patients: Risk factors and outcomes. *Pediatrics* **2002**, *109*, 758–764. [CrossRef] [PubMed]
29. Sajedi, M. VAP-Predictive-Model, GitHub repository [Internet]. 2021. Available online: https://github.com/SajediM/VAP-Predictive-Model (accessed on 30 September 2020).
30. Jouvet, P.A.; Payen, V.; Gauvin, F.; Emeriaud, G.; Lacroix, J. Weaning children from mechanical ventilation with a computer-driven protocol: A pilot trial. *Intensive Care Med.* **2013**, *39*, 919–925. [CrossRef]
31. Zaglam, N.; Jouvet, P.; Flechelles, O.; Emeriaud, G.; Cheriet, F. Computer-aided diagnosis system for the Acute Respiratory Distress Syndrome from chest radiographs. *Comput. Biol. Med.* **2014**, *52*, 41–48. [CrossRef] [PubMed]

32. Mazo, C.; Kearns, C.; Mooney, C.; Gallagher, W.M. Clinical Decision Support Systems in Breast Cancer: A Systematic Review. *Cancers* **2020**, *12*, 369. [CrossRef] [PubMed]
33. Ostropolets, A.; Zhang, L.; Hripcsak, G. A scoping review of clinical decision support tools that generate new knowledge to support decision making in real time. *J. Am. Med. Inform. Assoc.* **2020**, *27*, 1968–1976. [CrossRef]

Disclaimer/Publisher's Note: The statements, opinions and data contained in all publications are solely those of the individual author(s) and contributor(s) and not of MDPI and/or the editor(s). MDPI and/or the editor(s) disclaim responsibility for any injury to people or property resulting from any ideas, methods, instructions or products referred to in the content.

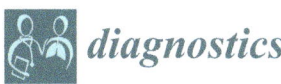

Article

Video-Based versus On-Site Neonatal Pain Assessment in Neonatal Intensive Care Units: The Impact of Video-Based Neonatal Pain Assessment in Real-World Scenario on Pain Diagnosis and Its Artificial Intelligence Application

Xiaofei Chen [1,†], Huaiyu Zhu [2,†], Linli Mei [3], Qi Shu [3], Xiaoying Cheng [4], Feixiang Luo [5], Yisheng Zhao [2], Shuohui Chen [3,*] and Yun Pan [2,*]

[1] Gastroenterology Department, The Children's Hospital, Zhejiang University School of Medicine, National Clinical Research Center for Child Health, Hangzhou 310052, China; hzxiao0914@163.com
[2] College of Information Science and Electronic Engineering, Zhejiang University, Hangzhou 310027, China; zhuhuaiyu@zju.edu.cn (H.Z.); zhaoys@zju.edu.cn (Y.Z.)
[3] Administration Department of Nosocomial Infection, The Children's Hospital, Zhejiang University School of Medicine, National Clinical Research Center for Child Health, Hangzhou 310052, China; 22018565@zju.edu.cn (L.M.); 22118788@zju.edu.cn (Q.S.)
[4] Quality Improvement Office, The Children's Hospital, Zhejiang University School of Medicine, National Clinical Research Center for Child Health, Hangzhou 310052, China; cxynicu@163.com
[5] Neonatal Intensive Care Unit, The Children's Hospital, Zhejiang University School of Medicine, National Clinical Research Center for Child Health, Hangzhou 310052, China; luofeixiang@zju.edu.cn
* Correspondence: chcsh2@zju.edu.cn (S.C.); panyun@zju.edu.cn (Y.P.)
† These authors contributed equally to this work.

Abstract: Background: Neonatal pain assessment (NPA) represents a huge global problem of essential importance, as a timely and accurate assessment of neonatal pain is indispensable for implementing pain management. Purpose: To investigate the consistency of pain scores derived through video-based NPA (VB-NPA) and on-site NPA (OS-NPA), providing the scientific foundation and feasibility of adopting VB-NPA results in a real-world scenario as the gold standard for neonatal pain in clinical studies and labels for artificial intelligence (AI)-based NPA (AI-NPA) applications. Setting: A total of 598 neonates were recruited from a pediatric hospital in China. Methods: This observational study recorded 598 neonates who underwent one of 10 painful procedures, including arterial blood sampling, heel blood sampling, fingertip blood sampling, intravenous injection, subcutaneous injection, peripheral intravenous cannulation, nasopharyngeal suctioning, retention enema, adhesive removal, and wound dressing. Two experienced nurses performed OS-NPA and VB-NPA at a 10-day interval through double-blind scoring using the Neonatal Infant Pain Scale to evaluate the pain level of the neonates. Intra-rater and inter-rater reliability were calculated and analyzed, and a paired samples t-test was used to explore the bias and consistency of the assessors' pain scores derived through OS-NPA and VB-NPA. The impact of different label sources was evaluated using three state-of-the-art AI methods trained with labels given by OS-NPA and VB-NPA, respectively. Results: The intra-rater reliability of the same assessor was 0.976–0.983 across different times, as measured by the intraclass correlation coefficient. The inter-rater reliability was 0.983 for single measures and 0.992 for average measures. No significant differences were observed between the OS-NPA scores and the assessment of an independent VB-NPA assessor. The different label sources only caused a limited accuracy loss of 0.022–0.044 for the three AI methods. Conclusion: VB-NPA in a real-world scenario is an effective way to assess neonatal pain due to its high intra-rater and inter-rater reliability compared to OS-NPA and could be used for the labeling of large-scale NPA video databases for clinical studies and AI training.

Keywords: neonatal pain assessment; inter-rater variability; neonatal intensive care units; neonatal nursing; pain management

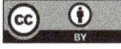

1. Introduction

Procedural pain in newborns represents a growing concern due to the increasing number of invasive procedures these patients undergo while receiving healthcare. Advances in neonatal care have promoted the survival of premature and sick infants; however, this has come at the cost of repeated episodes of acute and/or prolonged pain [1–3]. In neonatal intensive care units (NICUs), newborns are often subjected to injections and blood draws without the use of analgesia medication [4], which results in higher sensitivity to pain compared to older infants, children, and adults [5]. Pain can cause clinical instability, such as changes in cardiac and respiratory frequencies, and can even lead to complications, such as interventricular hemorrhages [6,7]. In order to ensure proper pain management, timely and accurate neonatal pain assessment (NPA) is of essential importance [8]. However, a cross-sectional study found that only 32.5% of pain records adopted pharmacological or non-pharmacological intervention for pain relief [9].

As newborns cannot self-report, caregivers must assess their pain by observing specific behavioral and physiological signs. This is usually conducted by using pediatric scales. Currently, there are more than 40 scales designed for this purpose; however, such an assessment approach is highly biased and is affected by several idiosyncratic factors, such as the observer's cognitive bias, identity, background, and culture, as well as gender, resulting in inconsistent assessment and treatment of pain [10]. In addition, current pain management of newborns in the NICU is manually performed, being subjective and discontinuous, with NICU nurses treating neonates with pain management plans based on intermittent, subjective ratings with poor inter-rater agreement [11]. Furthermore, the current practice for assessing infants' pain is time-consuming and requires many trained and professional laborers.

Pain is recognized as the fifth vital sign that should be monitored in NICUs [12]. Despite the growing body of literature on pain assessment and clinical practice guidelines that emphasize the importance of pediatric pain management, many pediatric patients still receive inadequate pain treatment. This is mainly due to the time and effort needed to evaluate pain, a lack of pain experts, and inadequate education on pain management among pediatric trainees. Additionally, cultural or personal beliefs such as negative attitudes towards pain treatment, the belief that pain builds character, and fear of adverse effects of pain medications can lead to improper pain management [13]. Despite numerous guidelines and standards requiring the use of standardized pain assessment tools in clinical practice, there is still poor compliance, posing a serious global issue [11,13].

To solve the above problems, both clinical NPA studies and new NPA technologies, such as artificial intelligence (AI)-based NPA (AI-NPA), should be developed to improve the quality and efficiency of current NPA for effective neonatal pain management. Those studies generally require large-scale neonatal pain data, e.g., neonatal images, videos, and physiological signals collected in pain, with precise pain diagnosis results for clinical statistical analysis or AI training, where neonatal pain videos with pain scores given by a consultation group of nursing experts using a pain scale is a common and feasible data form [11]. However, considering the real-world NICU scenario, it is difficult to carry out such labeling work with multiple experienced nurses on-site for large-scale data.

As the video-based NPA (VB-NPA) protocol could facilitate remote or after-the-event pain diagnosis by experts, it is widely used in clinical NPA and AI-NPA research as an equivalent alternative to the gold standard on-site NPA (OS-NPA) and has been proven feasible for ideal neonatal pain video data captured in controlled conditions; that is, intentional controls during the data collection phase or manual data selections at the pre-processing stage to ensure complete neonatal pain responses are captured with a correct perspective in neonatal pain videos. Yet neonatal pain videos captured in a real-world scenario could contain various disturbances, such as facial occlusion, pose variation, body occlusion, and movement interference from others. These real-world noises would cause information loss in videos, which might be crucial to NPA and further make VB-NPA lose its advantages, even its equivalence with OS-NPA.

In this paper, we investigated whether VB-NPA with neonatal pain videos captured in a real-world NICU scenario is with the consistency of OS-NPA and could be used for AI-NPA applications. A total of 598 neonates hospitalized in the NICU for more than 3 days and scheduled for a procedural pain procedure were randomly selected and included in the study. Both the OS-NPA and VB-NPA after 10 days were performed by two nurses in the form of a pain score and pain grade with reference to the Neonatal Infant Pain Scale (NIPS) [14]. Using the NIPS pain score of the OS-NPA as the golden standard, the result showed a high intraclass correlation coefficient (ICC) and inter-rater reliability for both single and average measures between the VB-NPA, with neonatal pain videos captured in a real-world NICU scenario, and OS-NPA, with a highly significant correlation ($p < 0.001$).

Compared with the on-site evaluation, the accuracy of the NIPS pain grade given by the VB-NPA was 96.98%, and the agreement between the two groups was compared, with a kappa value of 0.926 ($p < 0.001$), thus indicating that VB-NPA with neonatal pain videos captured in a real-world NICU scenario could cause inaccuracies in partial scoring due to the information loss in the videos, yet it was still not inferior to OS-NPA. Meanwhile, the test results of three state-of-the-art AI-NPA methods only showed an accuracy loss of 0.022–0.044, which was caused by the VB-NPA labels, indicating that there was just a limited impact of VB-NPA with neonatal pain videos captured in a real-world NICU scenario to AI-NPA. Therefore, VB-NPA in a real-world NICU scenario is an effective way to assess neonatal pain due to its high intra-rater and inter-rater reliability compared to OS-NPA and could be used for the labeling of large-scale NPA video databases for clinical studies and AI training.

2. Methods

2.1. Setting and Participants

This study was conducted at a tertiary class of a children's hospital in eastern China between 1 December 2021 and 30 May 2022. It was approved by the ethics committee of the Children's Hospital of Zhejiang University School of Medicine (2018-IRB-051) on 31 July 2018, and parental informed consent was obtained. The study flowchart is shown in Figure 1.

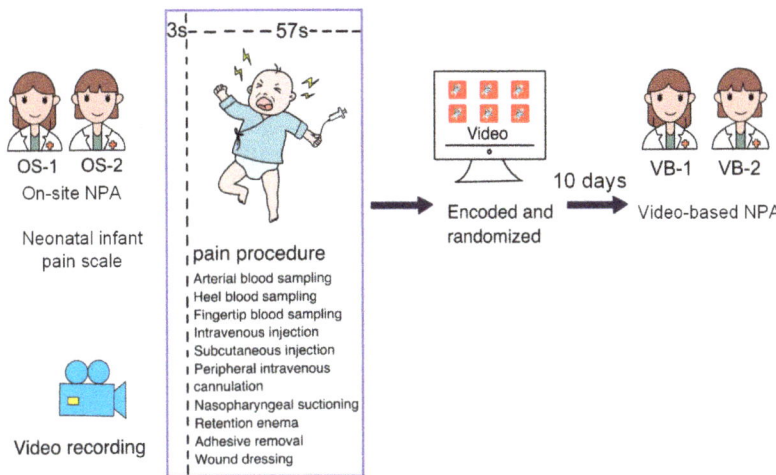

Figure 1. The study design of the neonatal pain assessment (NPA).

A total of 598 neonates hospitalized in the NICU for more than 3 days and already scheduled for a procedural pain procedure were randomly selected and included in the study. All hospitalized newborns underwent standard neonatal disposal after admission, including uniform clothing changing after admission. The procedures included arterial blood sampling, heel blood sampling, fingertip blood sampling, intravenous injection, subcutaneous injection, peripheral intravenous cannulation, nasopharyngeal suctioning, retention enema, adhesive removal, and wound dressing. These procedures were characterized as painful by doctors and nurses working in pediatrics and neonatology [3]. Exclusion criteria referred to serious illnesses such as birth injury, asphyxia, shock, metabolic encephalopathy, hypoxic-ischemic encephalopathy, severe cardiopulmonary disease, and conditions associated with facial image acquisition, such as severe congenital malformations.

Two experienced nurses were assigned to quantify the pain of 10 types of procedures for newborns using the NIPS on-site, with a third nurse recording the procedure simultaneously. The double-blind scoring results of OS-NPA performed by the two nurses were recorded as OS-1 and OS-2, respectively. All recorded videos were encoded and stored in the software, and the chronological sequence of the videos was randomized using a random number table to blind the assessors. After 10 days, the same two nurses performed VB-NPA on these randomized videos, and the double-blind scoring results were recorded as VB-1 and VB-2, of which the index numbers denoted the same nurse.

2.2. Video Recording in Real-World Scenario

The duration of painful procedures was limited to one minute. Meanwhile, a third nurse recorded the newborn's behavior in a 1-min video starting 3 s before the procedure. The video recordings were taken with a smartphone with automatic stabilization and a resolution of 1334 × 750 from 12 megapixels. There are no special restrictions during video shooting to guarantee recorded neonatal pain responses unaffected by occlusion, interference from other people's movements, or extreme postures of newborns. The sample key frames of these neonatal pain videos are shown in Figure 2.

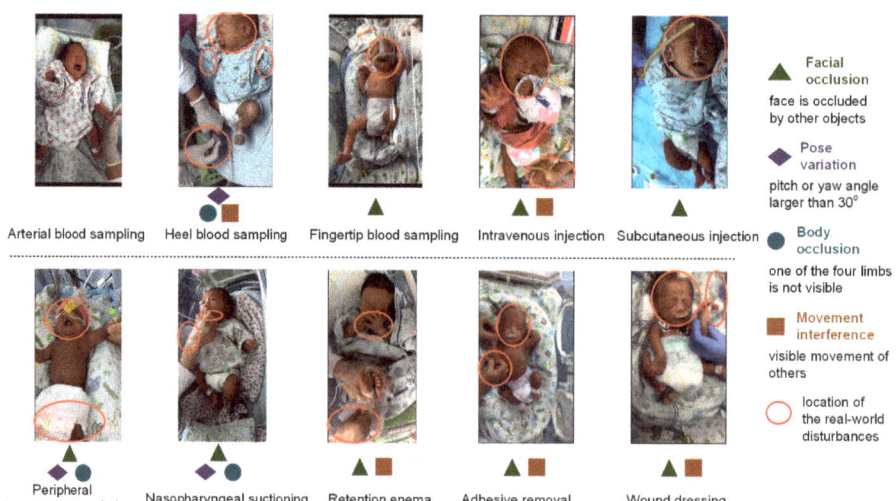

Figure 2. Visual representation of pain samples from neonatal pain videos captured in a real-world NICU scenario without control.

2.3. Pain Assessment

The NIPS was developed in the early 1990s at the Children's Hospital of Eastern Ontario to assess six behavioral reactions to painful procedures in preterm and full-term newborns [14]. Subsequently, the NIPS was successfully adapted and validated for use in other countries [15,16]. Its total score ranged from 0 to 7 points: facial expression (0–1 point), cry (0–2 points), breathing pattern (0–1 point), the position of arms (0–1 point), the position of legs (0–1 point), and state of arousal (0–1 point), with 0 being no pain and 7 being the most intense pain. The NIPS is easily understood and applied and is a useful tool for health professionals who work with neonates exposed to painful stimuli. Previous studies demonstrated that the scale has high inter-rater reliability and internal consistency [17]. It was also validated for construct and concurrent validity, making it a valid, reliable, and practical tool. Cronbach's alpha values of the Chinese version of the NIPS were found to be 0.97, 0.81, and 0.95 before, during, and after the heel lance, respectively [18].

2.4. OS-NPA and VB-NPA

In this study, we compared the consistency between the two NPA methods, i.e., OS-NPA, which involves medical staff observing the newborn's behavior on-site, and VB-NPA, which involves medical staff observing the newborn's behavior through a video recording. For the OS-NPA, two experienced nurses evaluated the pain scores of newborns undergoing painful procedures on-site using the NIPS. All videos captured in the real-world NICU scenario were randomized using a random number table to obfuscate the subject and timing information of the video. They were randomized and uploaded to in-hospital web-based video-rating software to ensure that the OS-NPA nurses were blinded during the VB-NPA. In order to minimize construct-irrelevant variance, VB-NPA training was conducted after the two nurses watched and assessed 5 videos, respectively, to increase the accuracy of the assessments, and after 10 days, the two OS-NPA nurses again evaluated neonatal pain using the NIPS through the recorded videos to derive their corresponding VB-NPA results.

2.5. Data Analysis

Intra-rater reliability was explored by comparing the NPA results under OS-NPA with the same assessor's results under VB-NPA (OS-1 vs. VB-1 and OS-2 vs. VB-2). Inter-rater reliability was explored by comparing assessments based on video recordings (VB-1 vs. VB-2). Reliability measures were calculated using the ICC for single and average measures. To investigate whether there was a Hawk–Dove effect between the two assessors, a paired samples *t*-test was conducted to compare NIPS pain scores given between OS-1 and OS-2; VB-1 and VB-2 statistical analysis was conducted using SPSS version 26.0 (IBM, Armonk, NY, USA).

The ICC was used to evaluate the repeatability or consistency of different measurement methods or assessors to the same certain measurement results. The randomized, double-blind method was applied, considering the influence of newborns and nurses in evaluating the reproducibility of diagnostic tests. The absolute agreement can be used to measure whether different investigators provide the same absolute value. The analysis unit of single measures is the results of each investigator, which can be used to estimate the situation of an individual investigator. Average measures are the mean of the research results of multiple investigators.

Furthermore, to investigate the impact of different label sources, i.e., OS-1, OS-2, VB-1, and VB-2, on artificial intelligence (AI) methods, we implemented three state-of-the-art AI-based NPA (AI-NPA) methods [19–21] to analyze the performance of these methods trained by the above four label sources. Zamzmi et al. [19] used an ensemble machine-learning framework to perform AI-NPA by fusing features of facial expressions, crying sounds, body movements, and vital signs; Min et al. [20] used a CNN-LSTM scheme to extract 2D features from neonatal videos and detect discomfort of neonates automatically; and Salekin et al. [21] proposed a multimodal spatio-temporal deep learning approach to analyze visual and vocal signals of neonatal videos to perform AI-NPA.

In this paper, we applied 5-fold cross-validation based on these three methods using the 598 video data we collected. The divided training and test video data were the same for the three methods in each fold. For each fold, we trained the methods using the training video data with the label given by OS-1, OS-2, VB-1, and VB-2, respectively, and evaluated the accuracy of each method using the test video data with the label given by OS-1 and OS-2, respectively, since the current common on-site scale rating is regarded as the gold standard for neonatal pain assessment.

3. Results

3.1. Study Population

A total of 598 neonates, with a mean birth weight of 2372.0 ± 1000.8 g, were recruited from a children's hospital in China. Among them, 252 were female, and 346 were male; 270 were born by spontaneous delivery, and 328 were delivered by cesarean section. Every newborn underwent one of the 10 kinds of the above-mentioned painful procedures. The detailed basic characteristics are listed in Table 1.

Table 1. Patients' characteristics in this study.

Variables	Total Amount (Proportion, %)
Gender	
Female	252 (42.14)
Male	346 (57.86)
Delivery mode	
Spontaneous delivery	270 (45.15)
Cesarean section	328 (54.85)
Pain procedure	
Arterial blood sampling	81 (13.55)
Heel blood sampling	61 (10.20)
Fingertip blood sampling	85 (14.21)
Intravenous injection	12 (2.01)
Subcutaneous injection	46 (7.69)
Peripheral intravenous cannulation	76 (12.7)
Nasopharyngeal suctioning	65 (10.87)
Retention enema	73 (12.21)
Adhesive removal	68 (11.37)
Wound dressing	31 (5.18)

3.2. Intra-rater Reliability and Inter-Rater Reliability

The goodness of fit for the linear regression model between VB-2 and OS-1 was 0.976, as shown in Figure 3. The NIPS pain scores are represented by the size and color of the circles, with the frequency of the ratings determining the size and darkness. The larger and darker the circles are, the more frequent the ratings, indicating a high level of consistency between the two. Additionally, when comparing the results from OS-1 with VB-1, we found an intra-rater reliability of 0.976, which was strongly significant ($p < 0.001$). When comparing the results from OS-1 with VB-2, the inter-rater reliability was 0.976 for single measures ($p < 0.001$) and 0.988 for average measures ($p < 0.001$). As shown in Table 2, there was no significant difference in the means between the two assessors' raters ($p > 0.05$). Both assessors had higher means in some types of scores, indicating a discriminative ability between the different procedures.

3.3. Comparison of the NIPS Pain Grades between OS-NPA and VB-NPA

According to the pain grade criteria of the NIPS, the OS-NPA showed no pain in 98 patients (16.38%), mild pain in 15 patients (2.50%), moderate pain in 36 patients (6.02%), and severe pain in 449 patients (75.08%). On the other hand, the VB-NPA showed no pain in 97 patients (16.22%), mild pain in 10 patients (1.67%), moderate pain in 42 patients (7.02%), and severe pain in 447 patients (74.74%). Compared with the on-site evaluation, the accuracy of the NIPS pain grade given by the VB-NPA was 96.98% (580/598), and the agreement between the two label sources was compared, with a kappa value of 0.926 ($p < 0.001$), as shown in Table 3.

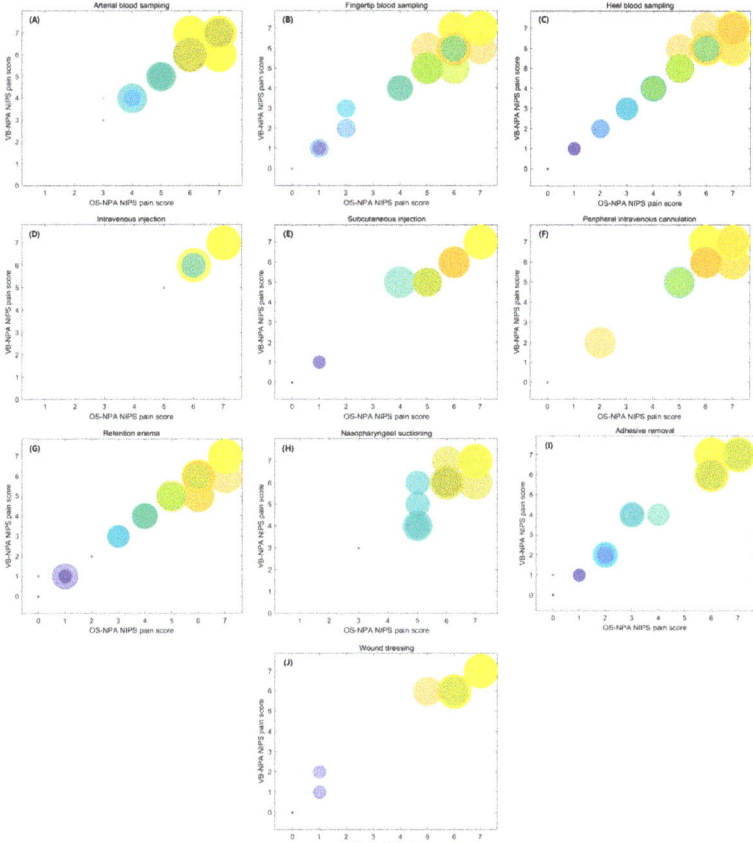

Figure 3. Scatter diagrams of NIPS pain scores of OS-NPA and VB-NPA: (**A**) arterial blood sampling, (**B**) fingertip blood sampling, (**C**) heel blood sampling, (**D**) intravenous injection, (**E**) subcutaneous injection, (**F**) peripheral intravenous cannulation, (**G**) retention enema, (**H**) nasopharyngeal suctioning, (**I**) adhesive removal, and (**J**) wound dressing. "NIPS" stands for the Neonatal Infant Pain Scale, "OS-NPA" refers to the on-site neonatal pain assessment, and "VB-NPA" refers to the video-based neonatal pain assessment.

Table 2. ICCs for scoring ratings given by OS-NPA and VB-NPA.

Label Source 1	Label Source 2	ICC	95% CI	p-Value
OS-1	VB-1	0.976 (single)	0.972–0.980	<0.001
		0.988 (averages)	0.986–0.990	<0.001
OS-2	VB-2	0.983 (single)	0.980–0.986	<0.001
		0.992 (averages)	0.990–0.993	<0.001
OS-1	VB-2	0.976 (single)	0.972–0.979	<0.001
		0.988 (averages)	0.986–0.990	<0.001
OS-1	OS-2	0.986 (single)	0.984–0.986	<0.001
		0.993 (averages)	0.992–0.994	<0.001
OS-2	VB-1	0.976 (single)	0.972–0.979	<0.001
		0.988 (averages)	0.986–0.990	<0.001
VB-1	VB-2	0.983 (single)	0.980–0.986	<0.001
		0.992 (averages)	0.990–0.993	<0.001

"ICC" stands for intraclass correlation coefficient, "CI" stands for the confidence interval, "OS-NPA" refers to the on-site neonatal pain assessment, and "VB-NPA" refers to the video-based neonatal pain assessment.

Table 3. Consistency analysis of NIPS pain grading by OS-NPA and VB-NPA.

		VB-NPA				Kappa Value	p-Value
		No Pain	Mild	Moderate	Severe		
OS-NPA	No pain	97	1	0	0		
	Mild	2	8	4	1	0.926	<0.001
	Moderate	0	1	32	3		
	Severe	0	0	6	443		

The background is highlighted for the diagonal of the confusion matrix.

3.4. Impact of Different Label Sources on AI Methods

The five-fold cross-validation accuracies for different AI-NPA methods trained and tested using different label sources, i.e., OS-1, OS-2, VB-1, and VB-2, for training with OS-1 and OS-2 for testing, are summarized in Table 4. For different AI algorithms, the highest average accuracies were all achieved when the training and testing labels were sourced from the same labeling conditions and labeling individuals (OS-1 training for the OS-1 test and OS-2 training for the OS-2 test), followed by the same labeling conditions and different labeling individuals (OS-1 training for the OS-2 test and OS-2 training for the OS-1 test), followed by different labeling conditions and the same labeling individuals (VB-1 training for the OS-1 test and VB-2 training for the OS-2 test), and the lowest accuracies were reached when the labeling conditions and labeling individuals were both different (VB-1 training for the OS-2 test and VB-2 training for the OS-1 test). However, considering the standard deviations of the accuracies for the five-fold cross-validation, the difference in the accuracies for the AI methods with different label sources was relatively small, with an accuracy loss of 0.022–0.044. Meanwhile, this phenomenon could be described as a domain migration problem in artificial intelligence and optimization based on mature domain migration methods. Therefore, we believed that the impact of different label sources on the AI methods was still limited in this study.

Table 4. Accuracies of different AI methods trained and tested using different label sources.

Label Source	Test	OS-1			OS-2		
Training	Method	[19]	[20]	[21]	[19]	[20]	[21]
OS-1	average	0.759	0.783	0.828	0.752	0.779	0.826
	std	0.044	0.040	0.036	0.034	0.031	0.028
OS-2	average	0.756	0.769	0.824	0.776	0.786	0.826
	std	0.036	0.039	0.035	0.028	0.024	0.035
VB-1	average	0.746	0.769	0.819	0.732	0.754	0.803
	std	0.038	0.038	0.028	0.022	0.023	0.027
VB-2	average	0.737	0.747	0.801	0.749	0.761	0.808
	std	0.037	0.042	0.023	0.019	0.031	0.021

'std' stands for standard deviation.

4. Discussion

4.1. High Evaluation Consistency of the VB-NPA

The above findings demonstrated that NPA could be accurately and reliably performed based on videos captured in a real-world NICU scenario, thus greatly advancing NICU pain management. This has important implications for the direct observation of neonatal care, as it could provide a more precise way to assess and manage pain in newborns. Pain assessment in newborns is often challenging due to their inability to communicate the discomfort, which can eventually result in inadequate pain management and serious consequences for the infant's health and well-being. Using the NIPS pain score of the OS-NPA as the golden standard, the ICC value of OS-1 and VB-2 was 0.976, with a highly significant correlation ($p < 0.001$). The inter-rater reliability was 0.983 for the single measures

($p < 0.001$) and 0.992 for the average measures ($p < 0.001$). The same result was seen between OS-2 and VB-1. The small difference between the two groups indicated that the NIPS is suitable for repeated measurements, consistent with previous studies [14,15]. The previous studies generally compared the differences between different assessors in the same clinical scenario. In this study, we still found a high consistency by comparing the OS-NPA score and the VB-NPA score, which indicated that the results obtained by the two NPA methods are equivalent, thus making it possible to use NIPS pain scores derived by VB-NPA with neonatal pain videos captured in a real-world NICU scenario in the future.

4.2. VB-NPA for NIPS Pain Grades

We included 598 children and 10 different procedures consistently evaluated as painful in the clinic. The results in Table 3 show that compared with the on-site evaluation, the accuracy of the NIPS pain grade given by the VB-NPA with neonatal pain videos captured in a real-world NICU scenario was 96.98%, and the agreement between the two groups was compared, with a kappa value of 0.926 ($p < 0.001$), thus indicating that, although the accuracy of VB-NPA was affected by real-world noises in the videos, it was not inferior to OS-NPA. Previous studies have shown that compared to OS-NPA, VB-NPA could significantly reduce the time spent on pain evaluation [22–25]. Meanwhile, with the advances in technology and operating equipment, it is easier to video-record painful procedures. The administrator staff can then use these recordings to review the pain level by observing the painful procedure video remotely for in-hospital nursing quality control purposes.

In addition, VB-NPA can reduce the stressful surroundings of a clinical setting, the contextual noise, and other elements that could shift the focus of the trainees from the rating. There has been an increasing interest in using machine-learning methods for understanding human behavioral responses to pain based on the analysis of facial expressions [26,27], crying sounds [28], and body movement. Several automated methods have been introduced to automatically assess infants' pain based on behavioral or physiological pain indicators analysis. By using AI-NPA, the nursing staff can also use these recordings to judge the pain level by observing the painful procedure video in the nurse station and taking timely intervention measures, which could greatly reduce the bedside observation time and improve work efficiency. We have already developed an artificial intelligence-based NPA (AI-NPA) tool in the early stage for 232 newborns during blood sampling in neonatal wards; the accuracies of the NIPS pain score and pain grade given by the automated NPA system were 88.79% and 95.25% [24].

4.3. VB-NPA for AI-NPA

In the clinical environment, one of the benefits of VB-NPA compared to OS-NPA is the possibility of using blinded assessments to reduce assessor bias. Various factors can affect the reliability and accuracy of the video rating of newborn pain assessment, such as video quality, shooting distance, shooting angle, shooting time, and the personal characteristics of the assessor [11]. While the personal factors associated with previous pain assessment experiences and the personality of the assessor cannot be removed with the blinding of VB-NPA, recording the procedure opens up the possibility of allowing multiple assessors to evaluate the same procedure to ensure the accuracy of the VB-NPA. Meanwhile, to reduce the risk of inaccurate scoring, we assigned two nurses to perform the OS-NPA in this study to avoid assessor bias, as one nurse may tend to score more strictly than others. After 10 days, the VB-NPA was conducted, allowing the nurses to forget the results of the OS-NPA and avoid any interference. These measures made the VB-NPA as accurate as possible, resulting in more reliable results. All video data were included in our pain identification database, providing the possibility of establishing a neonatal pain identification database for AI-NPA in the future.

However, considering the inaccuracy and uncertainty of data labels, which are inevitable when labels are conceptual entities and manually annotated [29] like in the NIPS, the results of this study indicate a high consistency between VB-NPA and OS-NPA, and we believe that in OS-NPA, experts can adjust their own observation perspectives appropriately and selectively evaluate whether the pain representations in the scale exist in individual newborns. While VB-NPA can be performed through multiple replays, the established shooting perspective cannot be changed after data collection, making it difficult for the experts to evaluate certain scale items. At the same time, we could see that the label sources of different labeling conditions and individuals would still introduce cross-domain problems in AI analysis, resulting in the loss of algorithm performance. Therefore, we believe that further studies for improving the accuracy of current VB-NPA to achieve a higher consistency with OS-NPA is still necessary.

4.4. Strengths and Limitations

The strength of this study is that it shows the real-world experience of a tertiary NICU, where the strain of everyday duties and work overload can sometimes lead to the omission of pain assessment. As a result, VB-NPA could provide a more reliable and accurate way to assess and manage pain in newborns, which could have important implications for the direct observation of neonatal care. Furthermore, it could reduce the burden on healthcare professionals, as it provides a more efficient way to assess and manage pain in newborns.

This study has some limitations. The recorded operation videos are limited by the environment, personnel, and shooting angle. Additionally, other pain operations in clinical practice were not recorded due to their low operating frequency. In the future, we hope to increase the sample size and expand the pain-causing operation database.

5. Conclusions

The accurate assessment of pain in the NICU is essential due to the high prevalence of painful experiences. Our results showed that the video-based assessment of neonatal pain could be reliably used, as confirmed by the high intra-rater and inter-rater reliability between direct observation and the video-based assessment, as well as the AI method-based performance evaluation, even with various disturbances in real-world NICUs. These results suggest that video-based assessment is viable for neonatal pain assessment in a clinical setting, and the extent of neonatal pain can be evaluated remotely in real-time, which can better identify and treat it and thus improve the neonatal pain condition.

Author Contributions: Conceptualization, X.C. (Xiaofei Chen), H.Z., S.C. and Y.P.; methodology, H.Z. and X.C. (Xiaofei Chen); software, H.Z. and Y.Z.; validation, F.L. and X.C. (Xiaoying Cheng); formal analysis, X.C. (Xiaofei Chen), H.Z., X.C. (Xiaoying Cheng) and F.L.; investigation, L.M. and Q.S.; resources, S.C. and Y.P.; data curation, L.M. and Q.S.; writing—original draft preparation, X.C. (Xiaofei Chen) and H.Z.; writing—review and editing, H.Z., Y.Z., Y.P. and S.C.; visualization, H.Z. and Y.Z.; supervision, S.C. and Y.P.; project administration, S.C. and Y.P.; funding acquisition, S.C., Y.P. and H.Z. All authors have read and agreed to the published version of the manuscript.

Funding: This research was funded in part by the Zhejiang Provincial Natural Science Foundation of China (Grant No. LGF20H040008 and LQ21F010016) and in part by the Zhejiang Provincial Key Research and Development Program of China (Grant No. 2021C03027).

Institutional Review Board Statement: This observational study was approved by the ethics committee of the Children's Hospital of Zhejiang University School of Medicine (2018-IRB-051) on 31 July 2018.

Informed Consent Statement: Informed Consents that include consent for research publication were obtained from all subjects (guardians) involved in the study.

Data Availability Statement: Data related to this study are stored at the Children's Hospital, the Zhejiang University School of Medicine. Requests for access to the data can be made to the corresponding authors, provided that the necessary ethical clearance has been obtained.

Conflicts of Interest: The authors declare no conflict of interest.

References

1. Carbajal, R.; Rousset, A.; Danan, C.; Coquery, S.; Nolent, P.; Ducrocq, S.; Saizou, C.; Lapillonne, A.; Granier, M.; Durand, P.; et al. Epidemiology and treatment of painful procedures in neonates in intensive care units. *JAMA* **2008**, *300*, 60–70. [CrossRef] [PubMed]
2. Courtois, E.; Droutman, S.; Magny, J.F.; Merchaoui, Z.; Durrmeyer, X.; Roussel, C.; Biran, V.; Eleni, S.; Vottier, G.; Renolleau, S.; et al. Epidemiology and neonatal pain management of heelsticks in intensive care units: EPIPPAIN 2, a prospective observational study. *Int. J. Nurs. Stud.* **2016**, *59*, 79–88. [CrossRef]
3. Cruz, M.D.; Fernandes, A.M.; Oliveira, C.R. Epidemiology of painful procedures performed in neonates: A systematic review of observational studies. *Eur. J. Pain* **2016**, *20*, 489–498. [CrossRef]
4. Meesters, N.J.; Simons, S.H.P.; van Rosmalen, J.; Holsti, L.; Reiss, I.K.M.; van Dijk, M. Acute pain assessment in prematurely born infants below 29 weeks: A long way to go. *Clin. J. Pain* **2019**, *35*, 975–982. [CrossRef]
5. Anand, K.J.S. Clinical importance of pain and stress in preterm neonates. *Neonatology* **1998**, *73*, 1–9. [CrossRef] [PubMed]
6. Slater, L.; Asmerom, Y.; Boskovic, D.S.; Bahjri, K.; Plank, M.S.; Angeles, K.R.; Phillips, R.; Deming, D.; Ashwal, S.; Hougland, K.; et al. Procedural pain and oxidative stress in premature neonates. *J. Pain* **2012**, *13*, 590–597. [CrossRef]
7. Walker, S.M. Long-term effects of neonatal pain. *Semin. Fetal Neonatal Med.* **2019**, *24*, 101005. [CrossRef]
8. Perry, M.; Tan, Z.; Chen, J.; Weidig, T.; Xu, W.; Cong, X.S. Neonatal pain: Perceptions and current practice. *Crit. Care Nurs. Clin.* **2018**, *30*, 549–561. [CrossRef]
9. Sposito, N.P.B.; Rossato, L.M.; Bueno, M.; Kimura, A.F.; Costa, T.; Guedes, D.M.B. Assessment and management of pain in newborns hospitalized in a neonatal intensive care unit: A cross-sectional study. *Rev. Lat.-Am. Enferm.* **2017**, *25*, e2931. [CrossRef]
10. Franck, L.S.; Bruce, E. Putting pain assessment into practice: Why is it so painful? *Pain Res. Manag.* **2009**, *14*, 13–20. [CrossRef]
11. Zamzmi, G.; Kasturi, R.; Goldgof, D.; Zhi, R.; Ashmeade, T.; Sun, Y. A review of automated pain assessment in infants: Features, classification tasks, and databases. *IEEE Rev. Biomed. Eng.* **2017**, *11*, 77–96. [CrossRef]
12. Merboth, M.K.; Barnason, S. Managing pain: The fifth vital sign. *Nurs. Clin. N. Am.* **2000**, *35*, 375–383. [CrossRef]
13. Grunauer, M.; Mikesell, C.; Bustamante, G.; Cobo, G.; Sánchez, S.; Román, A.M.; Icaza-Freire, A.P.; Gavilanes, A.W.D.; Wang, N.E.; PICU-MIC Research Group. Pain assessment and management in pediatric intensive care units around the world, an international, multicenter study. *Front. Pediatr.* **2021**, *9*, 746489. [CrossRef] [PubMed]
14. Lawrence, J.; Alcock, D.; McGrath, P.; Kay, J.; MacMurray, S.B.; Dulberg, C. The development of a tool to assess neonatal pain. *Neonatal Netw.* **1993**, *12*, 59–66. [CrossRef] [PubMed]
15. da Motta, G.d.C.P.; Schardosim, J.M.; da Cunha, M.L.C. Neonatal infant pain scale: Cross-cultural adaptation and validation in Brazil. *J. Pain Symptom Manag.* **2015**, *50*, 394–401. [CrossRef] [PubMed]
16. Napiórkowska-Orkisz, M.; Gutysz-Wojnicka, A.; Tanajewska, M.; Sadowska-Krawczenko, I. Evaluation of methods to minimize pain in newborns during capillary blood sampling for screening: A randomized clinical trial. *Int. J. Environ. Res. Public Health* **2022**, *19*, 870. [CrossRef]
17. Suraseranivongse, S.; Kaosaard, R.; Intakong, P.; Pornsiriprasert, S.; Karnchana, Y.; Kaopinpruck, J.; Sangjeen, K. A comparison of postoperative pain scales in neonates. *Br. J. Anaesth.* **2006**, *97*, 540–544. [CrossRef]
18. Yao, W.Y.; Petrini, M.; Deng, W.L.; Wu, H.L.; Tu, H.X. Effects of glucose administering approaches on reducing neonatal pain during heel lance procedures. *Chin. J. Nurs.* **2011**, *46*, 637–639. (In Chinese)
19. Zamzmi, G.; Pai, C.-Y.; Goldgof, D.; Kasturi, R.; Ashmeade, T.; Sun, Y. A comprehensive and context-sensitive neonatal pain assessment using computer vision. *IEEE Trans. Affect. Comput.* **2019**, *13*, 28–45. [CrossRef]
20. Min, L.; Sun, Y.; de With, P.H.N. Video-based infant monitoring using a CNN-LSTM scheme. *Proc. SPIE* **2021**, *11597*, 1159717.
21. Salekin, M.S.; Zamzmi, G.; Goldgof, D.; Kasturi, R.; Ho, T.; Sun, Y. Multimodal spatio-temporal deep learning approach for neonatal postoperative pain assessment. *Comput. Biol. Med.* **2021**, *129*, 104150. [CrossRef] [PubMed]
22. Dagnaes-Hansen, J.; Mahmood, O.; Bube, S.; Bjerrum, F.; Subhi, Y.; Rohrsted, M.; Konge, L. Direct observation vs. video-based assessment in flexible cystoscopy. *J. Surg. Educ.* **2018**, *75*, 671–677. [CrossRef] [PubMed]
23. Salekin, M.S.; Mouton, P.R.; Zamzmi, G.; Patel, R.; Goldgof, D.; Kneusel, M.; Elkins, S.L.; Murray, E.; Coughlin, M.E.; Maguire, D.; et al. Future roles of artificial intelligence in early pain management of newborns. *Paediatr. Neonatal Pain* **2021**, *3*, 134–145. [CrossRef] [PubMed]
24. Cheng, X.; Zhu, H.; Mei, L.; Luo, F.; Chen, X.; Zhao, Y.; Chen, S.; Pan, Y. Artificial intelligence based pain assessment technology in clinical application of real-world neonatal blood sampling. *Diagnostics* **2022**, *12*, 1831. [CrossRef]
25. Scaffidi, M.A.; Grover, S.C.; Carnahan, H.; Yu, J.J.; Yong, E.; Nguyen, G.C.; Ling, S.C.; Khanna, N.; Walsh, C.M. A prospective comparison of live and video-based assessments of colonoscopy performance. *Gastrointest. Endosc.* **2018**, *87*, 766–775. [CrossRef]
26. Sun, Y.; Kommers, D.; Wang, W.; Joshi, R.; Shan, C.; Tan, T.; Aarts, R.M.; van Pul, C.; Andriessen, P.; de With, P.H.N. Automatic and continuous discomfort detection for premature infants in a NICU using video-based motion analysis. In Proceedings of the 2019 41st Annual International Conference of the IEEE Engineering in Medicine and Biology Society (EMBC), Berlin, Germany, 23–27 July 2019; pp. 5995–5999.
27. Hoti, K.; Chivers, P.T.; Hughes, J.D. Assessing procedural pain in infants: A feasibility study evaluating a point-of-care mobile solution based on automated facial analysis. *Lancet Digit. Health* **2021**, *3*, e623–e634. [CrossRef]

28. Branco, A.; Fekete, S.M.W.; Rugolo, L.M.S.S.; Rehder, M.I. The newborn pain cry: Descriptive acoustic spectrographic analysis. *Int. J. Pediatr. Otorhinolaryngol.* **2007**, *71*, 539–546. [CrossRef]
29. Almeida, M.; Zhuang, Y.; Ding, W.; Crouter, S.E.; Chen, P. Mitigating class-boundary label uncertainty to reduce both model bias and variance. *ACM Trans. Knowl. Discov. Data* **2021**, *15*, 1–18. [CrossRef]

Disclaimer/Publisher's Note: The statements, opinions and data contained in all publications are solely those of the individual author(s) and contributor(s) and not of MDPI and/or the editor(s). MDPI and/or the editor(s) disclaim responsibility for any injury to people or property resulting from any ideas, methods, instructions or products referred to in the content.

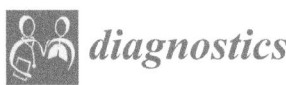

Article

Exploiting Machine Learning Technologies to Study the Compound Effects of Serum Creatinine and Electrolytes on the Risk of Acute Kidney Injury in Intensive Care Units

Hsin-Hung Liu [1], Yu-Tseng Wang [2], Meng-Han Yang [3], Wei-Shu Kevin Lin [1,4,*] and Yen-Jen Oyang [1,2,5,*]

1. Graduate Institute of Biomedical Electronics and Bioinformatics, National Taiwan University, Taipei City 10617, Taiwan; qi3800@yahoo.com.tw
2. Graduate Institute of Networking and Multimedia, National Taiwan University, Taipei City 10617, Taiwan; d05944001@ntu.edu.tw
3. Department of Computer Science and Information Engineering, National Kaohsiung University of Science and Technology, Kaohsiung City 807618, Taiwan; menghanyang@nkust.edu.tw
4. Department of Emergency Medicine, National Taiwan University Hospital, Taipei City 10002, Taiwan
5. Department of Computer Science and Information Engineering, National Taiwan University, Taipei City 10617, Taiwan
* Correspondence: booklin2@gmail.com (W.-S.K.L.); yjoyang@csie.ntu.edu.tw (Y.-J.O.)

Abstract: Assessing the risk of acute kidney injury (AKI) has been a challenging issue for clinicians in intensive care units (ICUs). In recent years, a number of studies have been conducted to investigate the associations between several serum electrolytes and AKI. Nevertheless, the compound effects of serum creatinine, blood urea nitrogen (BUN), and clinically relevant serum electrolytes have yet to be comprehensively investigated. Accordingly, we initiated this study aiming to develop machine learning models that illustrate how these factors interact with each other. In particular, we focused on ICU patients without a prior history of AKI or AKI-related comorbidities. With this practice, we were able to examine the associations between the levels of serum electrolytes and renal function in a more controlled manner. Our analyses revealed that the levels of serum creatinine, chloride, and magnesium were the three major factors to be monitored for this group of patients. In summary, our results can provide valuable insights for developing early intervention and effective management strategies as well as crucial clues for future investigations of the pathophysiological mechanisms that are involved. In future studies, subgroup analyses based on different causes of AKI should be conducted to further enhance our understanding of AKI.

Keywords: acute kidney injury; serum electrolyte; intensive care unit; machine learning

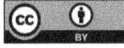

1. Introduction

Acute kidney injury (AKI) is a condition frequently encountered in medical care [1]. The underlying pathophysiological processes of AKI ultimately lead to a decline in renal function. As a result, the patients suffer from the accumulation of waste products, an imbalance of electrolytes, and a widespread inflammatory response that affects organs beyond the kidneys [2]. According to a recent study, 20% to 50% of the patients in an intensive care unit (ICU) suffered from AKI [3]. Therefore, how to assess the risk of AKI is a critical issue for clinicians in an ICU [4]. However, several early signs of AKI, including edema, hypertension, and oliguria, are non-specific. Therefore, the current practice only monitors the level of serum creatinine and the volume of urine output in order to assess the risk of AKI [5,6].

Due to the observation above, scientists have been investigating the physiological signs that may be associated with the development of AKI. Leaf et al. conducted a review of the pathophysiology of dysregulated mineral metabolism, specifically focusing on calcium, phosphate, parathyroid hormone, and vitamin D metabolites in the context of

AKI [7]. A review conducted by Yokota et al. found that the most common comorbidities associated with AKI in elderly patients included respiratory failure, cardiovascular disease, hypertension, diabetes, surgical complications, and liver disease [8].

As the kidneys play a crucial role in regulating the balance of calcium, phosphate, and magnesium, it is conceivable that an imbalance of serum electrolytes may be associated with the development of AKI. In this respect, a previous study reported that acute phosphate nephropathy was an early condition of AKI and might subsequently progress to chronic renal failure [9]. Furthermore, a number of studies were conducted to investigate how the levels of serum electrolytes, including chloride, phosphorus, magnesium, potassium, sodium, and calcium, were associated with the development of AKI [10–12]. Suetrong et al. observed a linear correlation between the concentration of serum chloride and the development of AKI among sepsis/septic shock patients [13]. Marttinen et al. reported a similar result and showed that the temporal chloride level was associated with an increased risk of AKI [14]. The work by Moon et al. revealed that a high level of serum phosphorus increased the risk of AKI [15]. Cheungpasitporn et al. showed that both hypomagnesemia and hypermagnesemia led to an increased risk of in-hospital AKI [16]. Thongprayoon et al. observed a U-shaped association between the level of serum ionized calcium and in-hospital AKI. Furthermore, both hypocalcemia and hypercalcemia were reported to be associated with an increased risk of hospital-acquired AKI [17,18], and Chen et al. discovered that abnormal levels of serum sodium or potassium before an AKI diagnosis were more likely to lead to AKI progression and a poor prognosis [19]. Nevertheless, Yessayan et al. reported that the concentration of hyperchloremia and the onset of AKI within 72 h of admission were not correlated [20]. Finally, Morooka et al. divided pediatric patients into three groups based on their serum magnesium values and investigated the association between magnesium levels and outcomes [21].

In addition to the studies addressed above, the latest trend is to exploit various machine learning algorithms, including artificial neural networks [22], support vector machines (SVMs) [23], Bayesian networks [24], random forests (RFs) [25], etc., to predict incidences of AKI, and Song et al. reviewed how the conventional logistic regression (LR) and various machine learning methods performed in this respect [26]. A representative study was conducted by Tomasev et al. [27]. In their study, the authors employed a recurrent neural network to build their prediction models based on a cohort of 703,782 cases collected from the medical facilities of the U.S. Department of Veterans Affairs.

Though the effects of several serum electrolytes on the development of AKI have been well reported, a comprehensive investigation into how these serum electrolytes interact in the context of the development of AKI has not been conducted [28–34]. It is conceivable that such studies can provide crucial clues for developing new clinical guidelines to assess the risk of AKI. Accordingly, we initiated this study aiming not only to illustrate how these factors interact with each other but also to provide new insights for developing new clinical practices. Our analyses focused on ICU patients who had no prior history of AKI and were free of AKI-related comorbidities such as diabetes and hypertension as well as common causes of AKI such as hypovolemia and heart failure. By focusing on this group of patients, we were able to eliminate the confounding influences of these conditions and examine the associations between the levels of serum electrolytes and renal function in a more controlled manner.

In this study, we exploited decision tree (DT) models [28–30] and RF models [31,32]. Compared to the other commonly exploited machine learning models, such as SVMs [23] and deep neural networks (DNNs) [22], DT and RF models are favorites in many applications due to the interpretable decision rules exhibited by these models. Figure 1 shows a DT structure that summarizes the main results of this study. A user can figure out the decision rules by traversing the tree structure from the root node, which is at the top of the structure and colored yellow. They can proceed by following the branch originating from the root node that matches the condition of the case. The path ends at one of the leaf nodes at the bottom level of the tree. The "n^+" and "n^-" symbols at each node denote the number of positive cases and the number of negative cases, respectively, in our study cohort that met the criteria specified along the path from the root node to this particular node. If a path ends at a red node, the prediction is positive. On the other hand, if a path ends at a green node, the prediction is negative. Based on these interpretable decision rules, physicians can have a comprehensive understanding of how these key factors interact with each other and develop new clinical guidelines accordingly. On the other hand, due to the non-linear transformations and the large number of coefficients involved in the prediction process, it is essentially impossible for a user to interpret the mathematics equations that an SVM or DNN model follows to make a prediction.

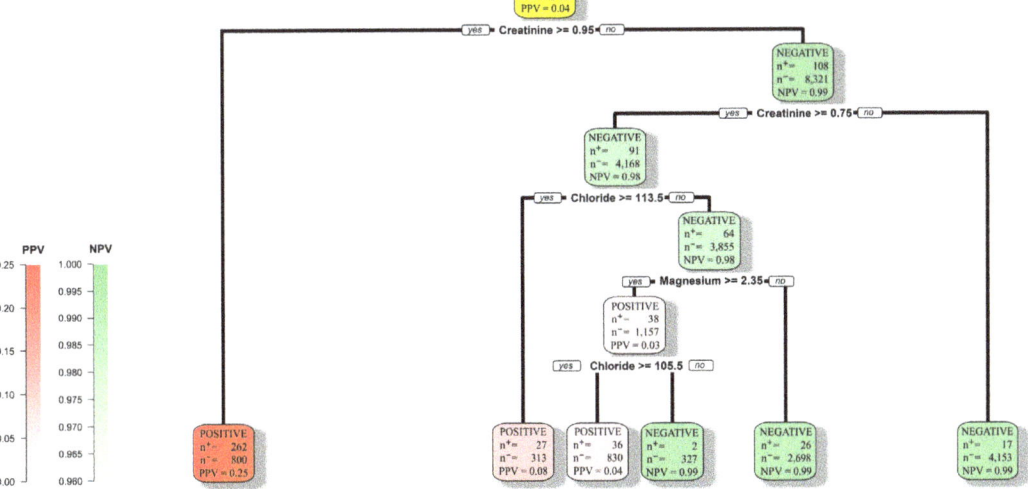

Figure 1. A DT structure that summarizes the main results of this study. The root node is colored yellow.

2. Materials and Methods

2.1. Study Cohort

Our study cohort was extracted from the Medical Information Mart for Intensive Care (MIMIC)-IV database, version 1.0, published in March 2021 [33,34]. The MIMIC database has been carefully de-identified to protect patient privacy. Its use for research purposes has been approved by the institutional review boards of the Massachusetts Institute of Technology (Protocol No. 0403000206) and Beth Israel Deaconess Medical Center (Protocol No. 2001-P-001699/14). These approvals indicate that the appropriate ethical considerations have been taken into account to ensure the responsible and lawful use of the database for research purposes.

Figure 2 shows the flow that we followed to generate our study cohort. Initially, the dataset contained 256,878 clinical records collected at the emergency department and the intensive care unit between 2008 and 2019. According to the 2012 Kidney Disease: Improving Global Outcomes (KDIGO) recommendation statements [35–38], AKI is defined by any of the following criteria: (1) an increase in the level of serum creatinine by 0.3 mg/dL (26.5 μmol/L) or more within 48 h or (2) an increase in the level of serum creatinine to 1.5 times the baseline level within 7 days. As the guideline requires two readings of the serum creatinine level and our study focused on patients in ICUs, 205,482 records in the database were excluded due to a lack of required information after admission into ICUs. As a result, only 51,396 records, all of which corresponded to the first available data after ICU admission, were included for subsequent analyses.

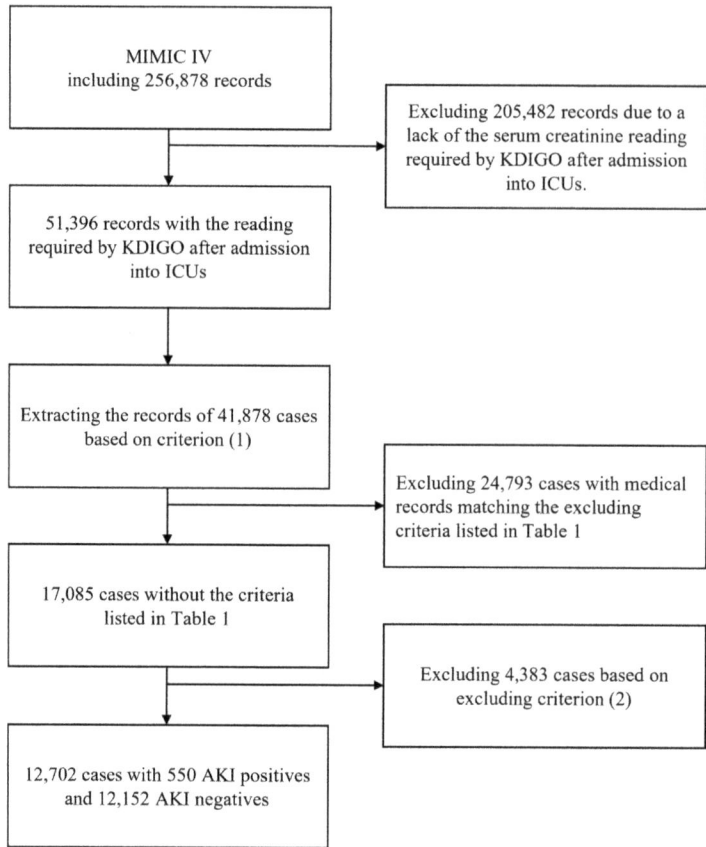

Figure 2. The flow for generating the study cohort. Table 1 lists the ICD-9 and ICD-10 codes employed to exclude the cases with AKI-related comorbidities/diseases. Criterion (1): (i) For a patient who had suffered from AKI, we included only the record corresponding to his/her stay in the ICU during which the patient suffered from AKI the first time. (ii) For a patient who had never suffered from AKI, we included only the record corresponding to his/her first stay in the ICU. Criterion (2): (i) the record of the case did not include all the readings listed in Table 2; (ii) one or more readings in the record were in the highest 0.1% or the lowest 0.1% of the distributions; or (iii) one or more readings in the record were not measured within 168 h of admission.

Table 1. Excluding criteria for the cases with AKI-related comorbidities/diseases.

Comorbidities/Diseases	ICD-9	ICD-10
Renal failure [1]	403.11, 403.91, 404.12, 404.92, 584.5–584.9, 585.1–585.9, 586, V42.0, V45.1, V56.0, V56.8	I12.0, I13.1, N17.0–N17.2, N17.8, N17.9, N18.1–N18.9, N19, N25.0, Z49.0–Z49.2, Z94.0, Z99.2
Congestive heart failure	398.91, 402.11, 402.91, 404.11, 404.13, 404.91, 404.93, 428.0–428.9	I09.9, I11.0, I13.0, I13.2, I25.5, I42.0, I42.5–I42.9, I50.0–I50.9, P29.0
Diabetes	250.0–250.7, 250.9	E10.0–E10.9, E11.0–E11.9, E12.0–E12.9, E13.0–E13.9, E14.0–E14.9
Fluid and electrolyte disorders	276.0–276.9	E22.2, E86.0, E86.1, E86.9, E87.0–E87.8

[1] Including end-stage renal disease, AKI, and chronic kidney disease.

Since one patient could be admitted into the ICU more than one time, for a patient who had suffered from AKI, we included only the record corresponding to his/her stay in the ICU during which the patient suffered from AKI the first time. On the other hand, for a patient who had never suffered from AKI, we included only the record corresponding to his/her first stay in the ICU. As a result, only 41,878 records corresponding to 41,878 individual cases remained. In the next step, we employed the criteria provided in Table 1 to exclude those patients whose medical records showed AKI-related comorbidities [39] so that the interferences from other factors such as renal impairment, cardiac failure, diabetes, and electrolyte imbalances would be avoided. After this step, only 17,085 cases remained in the dataset. Finally, we employed the following excluding criteria to further screen the dataset: (1) the record of the case did not include all the readings listed in Table 2; (2) one or more readings in the record were in the highest 0.1% or the lowest 0.1% of the distributions; and (3) one or more readings for the case were not made within 168 h of admission. In the end, our study cohort contained 550 AKI-positive cases and 12,152 AKI-negative cases. A demographic analysis of the study cohort is presented in Table 2.

Etiologically, the causes of AKI can be classified into three broad categories: pre-renal azotemia, intrinsic renal parenchymal damage, and post-renal obstruction. Tailoring treatment plans according to the specific causes of renal injury are crucial for improving patient outcomes. For instance, hypovolemia, often diagnosed by assessing a fluid status imbalance, insufficient renal perfusion, or inferior vena cava collapse, is a common clinical presentation associated with pre-renal azotemia. On the other hand, post-renal injury occurs when the urinary tract is partially or completely blocked due to functional or structural derangements anywhere from the renal pelvis to the tip of the urethra. Since the treatment plans for post-renal AKI patients are significantly different from the plans for non-post-renal AKI patients, we classified the AKI patients in our study cohort into two categories: post-renal AKI and non-post-renal AKI. According to several previous studies, the incidences of post-renal AKI accounted for less than 5% of all AKI cases [1,40,41]. In our study cohort, 24 out of 550 AKI cases, i.e., 4.4%, were post-renal, and the percentage was in line with the previous studies. Supplementary Table S1 shows the ICD-9 and ICD-10 codes employed to identify post-renal AKI cases. Table 3 shows the statistics of the post-renal AKI patents and non-post-renal AKI patients with respect to the features listed in Table 2.

Table 2. Demographic analysis of the study cohort.

Feature	550 Cases with AKI (Mean ± SD)	12,152 Cases without AKI (Mean ± SD)	p-Value
Age (years)	65.68 ± 14.69	60.34 ± 17.67	$p < 0.001$ *
Gender			$p < 0.001$ *
Male (%)	349 (63.45%)	6757 (55.60%)	
Female (%)	201 (36.55%)	5395 (44.40%)	
Serum			
BUN (mg/dL)	26.74 ± 15.39	18.06 ± 8.90	$p < 0.001$ *
Creatinine (mg/dL)	1.36 ± 0.64	0.86 ± 0.26	$p < 0.001$ *
Chloride (mEq/L)	110.37 ± 6.60	107.39 ± 5.28	$p < 0.001$ *
Potassium (mEq/L)	4.79 ± 0.75	4.47 ± 0.63	$p < 0.001$ *
Sodium (mEq/L)	142.81 ± 5.77	141.23 ± 4.59	$p < 0.001$ *
Magnesium (mg/dL)	2.53 ± 0.52	2.28 ± 0.44	$p < 0.001$ *
Phosphorus (mg/dL)	4.40 ± 1.34	3.80 ± 0.93	$p < 0.001$ *
Non-ionized calcium (mg/dL)	8.76 ± 0.73	8.73 ± 0.71	0.346

The symbol * indicates statistical significance. For categorical variables, the p-values were calculated based on the χ^2 test [42,43]. For continuous variables, the p-values were calculated based on the t-test [42,43]. SD represents standard deviation.

Table 3. Statistical analysis of the characteristics of the post-renal AKI patients and the non-post-renal AKI patients in our study cohort.

Feature	24 Cases with Post-Renal AKI (Mean ± SD)	526 Cases with Non-Post-Renal AKI (Mean ± SD)	p-Value
Age (years)	74.16 ± 12.54	65.30 ± 14.66	0.0037 *
Gender			0.0007 *
Male (%)	23 (95.66%)	326 (61.98%)	
Female (%)	1 (4.34%)	200 (38.02%)	
Serum			
BUN (mg/dL)	27.54 ± 10.72	26.70 ± 15.55	0.7944
Creatinine (mg/dL)	1.40 ± 0.57	1.36 ± 0.64	0.7459
Chloride (mEq/L)	110.08 ± 7.30	110.38 ± 6.57	0.5228
Potassium (mEq/L)	4.58 ± 0.56	4.80 ± 0.76	0.2258
Sodium (mEq/L)	142.81 ± 5.28	142.84 ± 5.79	0.9599
Magnesium (mg/dL)	2.54 ± 0.38	2.53 ± 0.53	0.1666
Phosphorus (mg/dL)	4.07 ± 0.93	4.41 ± 1.36	0.5254
Non-ionized calcium (mg/dL)	8.66 ± 0.54	8.76 ± 0.74	0.8278

The symbol * denotes statistical significance. The p-values were calculated based on the two-sample t-test. SD stands for standard deviation.

2.2. Machine Learning Models

As mentioned earlier, we used DT and RF models in order to investigate the compound impacts of two or more factors and provide a clear picture of how these factors interact with each other. In particular, we focused on the compound effects of serum creatinine, BUN, and the 6 serum electrolytes listed in Table 2. The serum creatinine and BUN were included because in medical practice the levels of serum creatinine and BUN as well as the BUN-to-creatinine ratio are measured to clarify different types of renal function impairment, including pre-renal azotemia, intrinsic renal parenchymal disease, and post-renal obstruction. The 6 serum electrolytes listed in Table 2 were included because previous studies had reported their associations with the development of AKI.

In order to address the needs in different clinical scenarios, we generated prediction models with varying levels of sensitivity and examined the prediction rules embedded in these models. In this respect, we set the parameters of the machine learning packages to various combinations and then employed a 5-fold cross-validation [22] to evaluate the levels of sensitivity delivered by the prediction models generated with these alternative parameter settings. In the 5-fold cross-validation process, the study cohort was randomly and evenly partitioned into 5 subsets. For each combination of parameter settings, every subset was employed to evaluate the prediction models generated with the other 4 subsets. Then, the evaluation results of these 5 subsets were collected to calculate the performance data, i.e., the sensitivity, specificity, positive predictive value (PPV), etc., corresponding to this particular parameter combination. Supplementary Table S2 shows the software packages employed to generate the DT and RF models as well as the alternative parameter settings employed to generate the prediction models in the 5-fold cross-validation process. In this respect, we tried a large number of possible parameter combinations in order to generate prediction models that delivered sensitivity at the levels of 0.95 and 0.80. Furthermore, as we had only 550 positive cases in our study cohort, we employed the 5-fold cross-validation process instead of the 10-fold cross-validation process, which may be more commonly used in machine learning research, so that each partition would contain a good number of positive cases.

3. Results

As mentioned above, in order to address the needs in different clinical scenarios, we generated prediction models with varying levels of sensitivity. In the subsequent discussions, we will focus on the prediction models with sensitivity at the levels of 0.95 and 0.80. Table 4 summarizes the performances of the DT, RF, and LR models observed during the 5-fold cross-validation procedure. The performances of the LR models were included to provide a reference because LR models are widely employed in biomedical research communities. Detailed performance data are presented in Supplementary Table S3.

Table 4. Summary of the performances observed during the 5-fold cross-validation process.

Level of Sensitivity	Model	Sensitivity	Specificity	PPV	AUC	Relative Risk
0.95	DT	0.949	0.479	0.076	0.767	16.893
	LR	0.949	0.414	0.068	0.855	13.872
	RF	0.949	0.382	0.065	0.666	13.012
0.80	DT	0.798	0.721	0.116	0.823	9.84
	LR	0.799	0.773	0.137	0.857	11.982
	RF	0.799	0.732	0.119	0.766	10.141

PPV stands for positive predictive value, also known as precision. AUC stands for the area under the receiver operating characteristic curve.

The performance data in Table 4 reveal that with respect to the specificity, the positive predictive value (PPV), the relative risk, and the area under the receiver operating characteristic curve (AUC), the DT model that delivered sensitivity at the level of 0.95 performed significantly superior to the RF model that delivered the same level of sensitivity. It was also observed that the RF model that delivered sensitivity at the level of 0.80 performed marginally superior to the rival DT model in terms of specificity, PPV, and relative risk but performed inferior to the rival DT model in terms of AUC. Based on these observations, we concluded that the overall performance of the DT models was superior to that of the RF models. Therefore, in the subsequent discussions, we will focus on the DT models and the decision rules embedded in the models.

Figure 3a,b show the DT models generated by feeding the entire study cohort into the decision tree package with the combinations of parameters cp and prior set to (0.005 and 0.5835) and (0.01 and 0.744), respectively. According to the 5-fold cross-validation addressed above, with cp and prior set to these two combinations, the generated DT models should deliver sensitivity at the levels of 0.80 and 0.95, respectively. One interesting observation regarding the DT model shown in Figure 3a is that the model predicts a patient with a serum creatinine level higher than 1.25 mg/dL to be at high risk. This prediction rule comes very close to the serum creatinine level of 1.3 mg/dL commonly used by physicians to determine whether a patient is at high risk of progression to AKI. It is also observed that the DT model shown in Figure 3b predicts a patient with a serum creatinine level higher than 0.95 mg/dL to be at high risk. This observation implies that 0.95 mg/dL can be employed as an alternative threshold if the physician wants to increase the sensitivity of his/her medical judgment.

The DT model shown in Figure 3a further reveals that for a patient with a serum creatinine level between 0.95 and 1.25 mg/dL, his/her level of serum magnesium can be used as a warning sign. If the reading is higher than 2.45 mg/dL, the patient is at high risk. If not, we should further examine his/her level of serum chloride. If the patient's level of serum chloride is over 106.5 mEq/L, the patient is at high risk.

The blue polygons in Figure 3a,b encircle the structure shared by these two DT models. According to the shared structure, for a patient with a serum creatinine level between 0.75 and 0.95 mg/dL, we should further examine his/her levels of serum magnesium and chloride. A patient is at high risk if (1) his/her level of serum chloride is higher than 113.5 mEq/L or (2) his/her level of serum chloride is between 105.5 and 113.5 mEq/L and his/her level of serum magnesium is higher than 2.35 mg/dL. Finally, since only a very limited number of positive cases in our study cohort met the criteria defined by the lower right parts of the tree structures in Figure 3a,b, we should be able to ignore the corresponding decision rules. In summary, the structures of the two DT models shown in Figure 3 illustrate that the levels of serum creatinine, chloride, and magnesium are the three major factors associated with the development of AKI. Though the level of serum phosphorus is present in these DT models, the nodes corresponding to the level of serum phosphorus are located in the lower parts of the structures, which implies that these nodes play less significant roles in the decision rules.

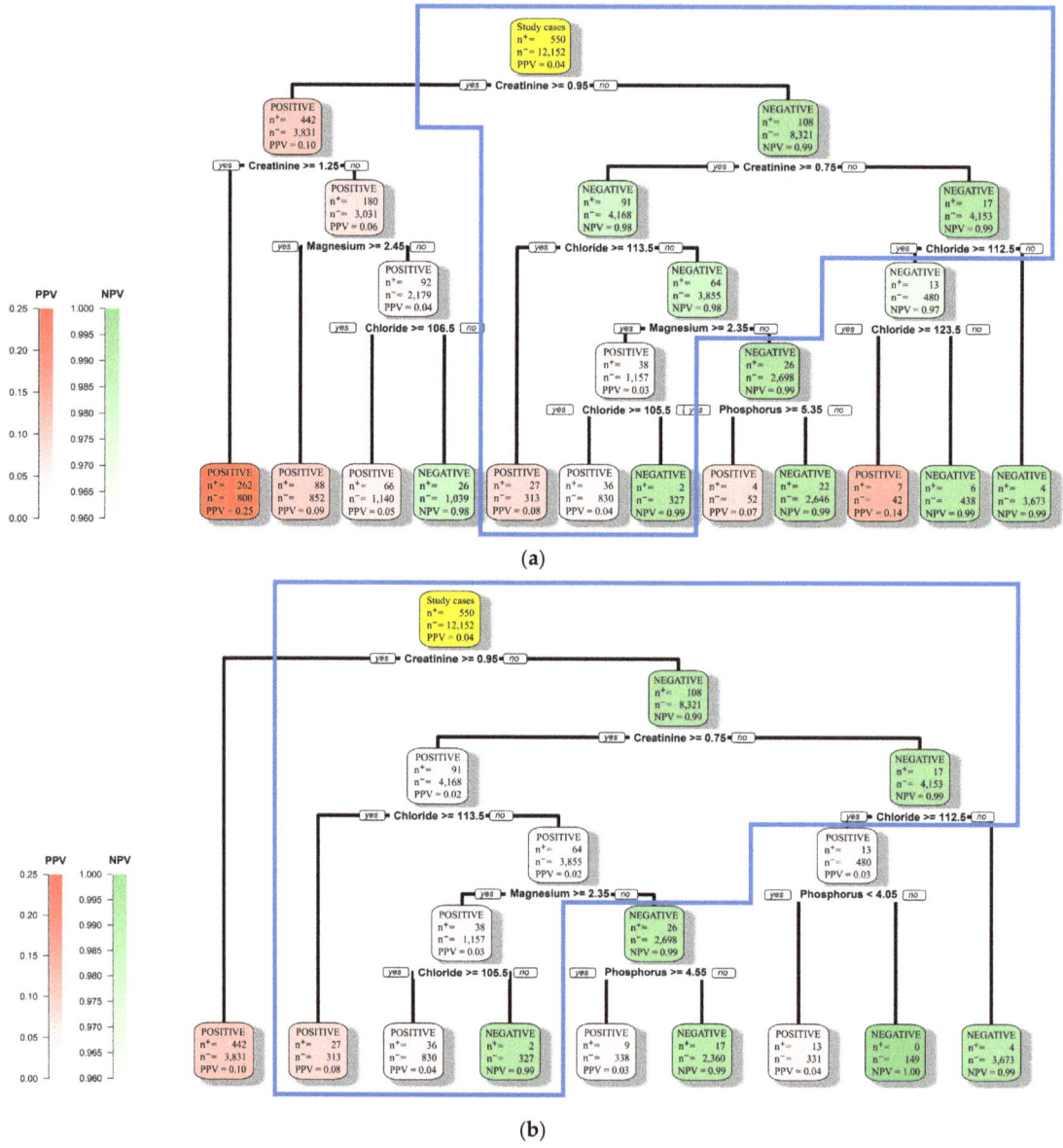

Figure 3. DT models with two different levels of sensitivity. (**a**) The DT model with sensitivity at the level of 0.80. (**b**) The DT model with sensitivity at the level of 0.95. The blue polygons encircle the structure shared by these 2 DT models. The root node is colored yellow.

4. Discussion

As of today, the clinical practice to assess the risk of AKI is based on the 2012 KDIGO Clinical Practice Guideline for Acute Kidney Injury, which monitors only the level of serum creatinine and the volume of urine output. Since AKI could lead to many complications and even fatality, identifying the risk factors of AKI and exploiting machine learning technologies to predict AKI incidences have attracted a lot of attention in biomedical research communities. In this respect, several serum electrolytes have been reported to be associated with the development of AKI. Nevertheless, the compound effects of serum creatinine, BUN, and clinically relevant serum electrolytes have yet to be thoroughly investigated. With this observation, we initiated this study aiming not only to illustrate how these factors interact with each other but also to provide new insights for developing new clinical practices for assessing AKI risk. In particular, we focused on ICU patients who had no prior history of AKI and were free of AKI-related comorbidities. By focusing on this specific group of patients, we were able to eliminate the confounding influences of these conditions and examine the associations between the levels of serum electrolytes and renal function in a more controlled manner. Furthermore, our results can provide valuable insights for developing early intervention and effective management strategies as well as for investigating the pathophysiology of AKI.

The performance data in Table 4 show that for those patients without a prior history of AKI or AKI-related comorbidities, the relative risks with these alternative prediction models were fairly high, ranging from 9.84 to 16.89. This implies that the group of patients predicted to be positive suffered significantly higher risk than the groups of patients predicted to be negative. However, the low PPVs suggest that there would be a large number of false positives if these prediction models were put into practical use. Nevertheless, according to the numbers shown in Figure 3a, this particular DT model, if put into practical use, should predict around 57% of the patients to be negative and deliver a sensitivity around 80%. Meanwhile, according to the numbers shown in Figure 3b, this particular DT model, if put into practical use, should predict around 51% of the patients to be negative and deliver a sensitivity around 95%. Therefore, a physician who employs the DT models developed in this study to assess the risks of AKI for his/her patients only needs to focus on about 50% of the patients, while the physician can expect this group of patients to suffer about 10 times the risk of the group of patients predicted to be at low risk.

Among the 10 variables listed in Table 2, only serum creatinine, chloride, magnesium, and phosphorus are present in the DT models shown in Figure 3a,b. It must be noted that this observation does not imply that serum potassium, sodium, and non-ionized calcium are not associated with the development of AKI. In fact, as mentioned earlier, previous studies have reported that serum potassium, sodium, and non-ionized calcium are all associated with the development of AKI. What happened must be that when building the prediction model, the DT algorithm figured out that the levels of serum chloride, magnesium, and phosphorus provided more information than the levels of serum potassium, sodium, and non-ionized calcium. The DT algorithm further figured out that the additional information provided by the levels of serum potassium, sodium, and non-ionized calcium after the levels of serum chloride, magnesium, and phosphorus had been incorporated was insignificant.

The DT models shown in Figure 3a,b identify the levels of serum creatinine, chloride, and magnesium as the three major factors associated with the development of AKI. Though the level of serum phosphorus is present in these two figures, all three nodes corresponding to the level of serum phosphorus are located in the lower levels of the structures. Furthermore, only a very limited number of positive cases in our study cohort met the criteria defined by these low-level structures. Therefore, in practice, we can ignore the role of serum phosphorus.

Since the level of serum creatinine is one of the major factors monitored in the current clinical practice, our study suggests that for those patients without a prior history of AKI or AKI-related comorbidities, the levels of serum chloride and magnesium should be taken into consideration in order to enhance the clinical guidelines. In this respect, the current clinical guideline, which monitors only the level of serum creatinine and the volume of urine output, may lead to misdiagnoses and/or delayed treatments in some cases because the level of serum creatinine generally reflects the degree of renal damage and should be considered as a delayed indicator of AKI. Furthermore, decreased urine output is a non-specific symptom and may only be evident once the AKI has progressed. Therefore, by incorporating the assessments of the serum chloride and magnesium levels into the enhanced clinical guideline, healthcare professionals can obtain a more comprehensive understanding of a patient's renal function and the risk of AKI. Furthermore, the numbers shown in Table 2 reveal that the distributions of the levels of serum creatinine for patients with AKI and patients without AKI must overlap to a large degree because the standard deviation of the level of serum creatinine for patients with AKI, which is 0.64, is larger than the difference between the means of these two groups of patients, which is 0.5. This implies that additional assessments must be incorporated if we would like to evaluate the risk of AKI of a patient more accurately. Finally, with respect to the decrease in urine output among AKI patients, it is a non-specific symptom and may only be evident once the AKI has progressed. Together, these observations imply that for an ICU patient without a prior history of AKI or AKI-related comorbidities, healthcare professionals can obtain a more comprehensive understanding of the patient's renal function and risk of AKI by incorporating assessments of serum chloride and magnesium levels into the enhanced clinical guideline. Accordingly, healthcare professionals will be able to evaluate and manage treatments more precisely and ultimately prevent disease progression and deterioration.

It must be noted that our results can only be immediately applied to ICU patients without a prior history of AKI or AKI-related comorbidities. For ICU patients with AKI-related comorbidities, further studies are needed. In this respect, we can partition the patients into several groups depending on the types of comorbidities that they suffer from so that patients in the same group have similar pathophysiological mechanisms. Then, we can apply the procedure presented in this article to each group of patients in order to develop a specific prediction model for each group and identify the critical factors accordingly.

One of the major limitations of our study is due to the different causes of AKI. As the causes of AKI are essential for physicians to develop effective treatment plans, in-depth subgroup analyses based on different categories of renal injury should be conducted to gain valuable insights into the different pathophysiological mechanisms involved and guide appropriate treatment strategies tailored to each subgroup. In this study, based on the information available in the MIMIC-IV dataset, we classified the AKI patients into two categories: post-renal and non-post-renal. The statistics in Table 3 reveal that there were no statistical differences between the levels of the eight serum ingredients for the post-renal and non-post-renal AKI patients. Therefore, our prediction models should be generally applicable to both post-renal and non-post-renal AKI patients. Nevertheless, in-depth subgroup analyses should be conducted in the future.

In addition to the limitation addressed above, this is a retrospective study based on data extracted from the MIMIC-IV database. Therefore, the results derived from this study should not be extensively applied in the decision process without taking into consideration the ethnic composition of the patients and the medical interventions that these patients may have received. Furthermore, our study was based on clinical records collected in ICUs. This implies that the patients involved had serious health conditions. The data in Table 2 also show that these patients were relatively old. Therefore, the results observed in our analyses should not be generalized to patients with different health conditions and in different age groups. Finally, our results only illustrate the associations between the investigated risk factors and the incidences of AKI. In other words, causal inferences have yet to be studied.

5. Conclusions

This study has led to an in-depth understanding of the compound effects of serum creatinine, chloride, and magnesium with respect to the development of AKI in ICUs. As we focused on patients who had no prior history of AKI and were free of AKI-related comorbidities, our study provides valuable insights for developing early intervention and effective management strategies. Furthermore, this understanding provides crucial clues not only for future enhancement of clinical practices but also for future investigation of the pathophysiological mechanisms that are involved.

Supplementary Materials: The following supporting information can be downloaded at https://www.mdpi.com/article/10.3390/diagnostics13152551/s1, Table S1: The ICD-9 and ICD-10 codes employed to identify post-renal AKI cases. Table S2: Summary of the software packages employed and parameter ranges. Table S3: The detailed performance data observed in the 5-fold cross-validation process.

Author Contributions: H.-H.L. initiated the study, and all authors contributed to the development of the methods. Software development and data analysis were performed by Y.-T.W., W.-S.K.L. and Y.-J.O. supervised the study and wrote the first version of the manuscript. All authors have read and agreed to the published version of the manuscript.

Funding: This work was partially supported by National Taiwan University grant #FD107016.

Institutional Review Board Statement: The study was conducted in accordance with the Declaration of Helsinki, and approved by the Institutional Review Boards of the Massachusetts Institute of Technology (Protocol No. 0403000206) and Beth Israel Deaconess Medical Center (Protocol No. 2001-P-001699/14).

Informed Consent Statement: Not applicable because the MIMIC-IV database has been carefully de-identified to protect patient privacy.

Data Availability Statement: MIMIC-IV ver. 1.0 was provided by physionet.

Acknowledgments: The authors would like to acknowledge Albert Li for his professional comments and advice.

Conflicts of Interest: The authors declare no conflict of interest in this work.

References

1. Loscalzo, J.; Fauci, A.S.; Kasper, D.L.; Hauser, S.L.; Longo, D.L.; Jameson, J.L.; Harrison, T.R. *Harrison's Principles of Internal Medicine*, 21st ed.; International edition; Loscalzo, J., Fauci, A.S., Kasper, D.L., Hauser, S.L., Longo, D.L., Jameson, J.L., Eds.; McGraw-Hill: New York, NY, USA, 2022.
2. Hoste, E.A.J.; Kellum, J.A.; Selby, N.M.; Zarbock, A.; Palevsky, P.M.; Bagshaw, S.M.; Goldstein, S.L.; Cerda, J.; Chawla, L.S. Global epidemiology and outcomes of acute kidney injury. *Nat. Rev. Nephrol.* **2018**, *14*, 607–625. [CrossRef]
3. Case, J.; Khan, S.; Khalid, R.; Khan, A. Epidemiology of acute kidney injury in the intensive care unit. *Crit. Care Res. Pract.* **2013**, *2013*, 479730. [CrossRef] [PubMed]
4. Huang, C.T.; Liu, K.D. Exciting developments in the field of acute kidney injury. *Nat. Rev. Nephrol.* **2020**, *16*, 69–70. [CrossRef]
5. Mercado, M.G.; Smith, D.K.; Guard, E.L. Acute Kidney Injury: Diagnosis and Management. *Am. Fam. Physician* **2019**, *100*, 687–694. [PubMed]
6. Koyner, J.L. Subclinical Acute Kidney Injury Is Acute Kidney Injury and Should Not Be Ignored. *Am. J. Respir. Crit. Care Med.* **2020**, *202*, 786–787. [CrossRef]
7. Leaf, D.E.; Christov, M. Dysregulated Mineral Metabolism in AKI. *Semin. Nephrol.* **2019**, *39*, 41–56. [CrossRef] [PubMed]
8. Yokota, L.G.; Sampaio, B.M.; Rocha, E.P.; Balbi, A.L.; Sousa Prado, I.R.; Ponce, D. Acute kidney injury in elderly patients: Narrative review on incidence, risk factors, and mortality. *Int. J. Nephrol. Renovasc Dis.* **2018**, *11*, 217–224. [CrossRef]
9. Blaine, J.; Chonchol, M.; Levi, M. Renal control of calcium, phosphate, and magnesium homeostasis. *Clin. J. Am. Soc. Nephrol.* **2015**, *10*, 1257–1272. [CrossRef]
10. Bellomo, R.; Kellum, J.A.; Ronco, C. Acute kidney injury. *Lancet* **2012**, *380*, 756–766. [CrossRef]
11. Kellum, J.A.; Romagnani, P.; Ashuntantang, G.; Ronco, C.; Zarbock, A.; Anders, H.J. Acute kidney injury. *Nat. Rev. Dis. Primers* **2021**, *7*, 52. [CrossRef]
12. Lv, Q.; Li, D.; Wang, Y.; Yu, P.; Zhao, L.; Chen, S.; Wang, M.; Fu, G.; Zhang, W. Admission electrolyte and osmotic pressure levels are associated with the incidence of contrast-associated acute kidney injury. *Sci. Rep.* **2022**, *12*, 4714. [CrossRef]
13. Suetrong, B.; Pisitsak, C.; Boyd, J.H.; Russell, J.A.; Walley, K.R. Hyperchloremia and moderate increase in serum chloride are associated with acute kidney injury in severe sepsis and septic shock patients. *Crit. Care* **2016**, *20*, 315. [CrossRef]
14. Marttinen, M.; Wilkman, E.; Petaja, L.; Suojaranta-Ylinen, R.; Pettila, V.; Vaara, S.T. Association of plasma chloride values with acute kidney injury in the critically ill—A prospective observational study. *Acta Anaesthesiol. Scand.* **2016**, *60*, 790–799. [CrossRef]
15. Moon, H.; Chin, H.J.; Na, K.Y.; Joo, K.W.; Kim, Y.S.; Kim, S.; Han, S.S. Hyperphosphatemia and risks of acute kidney injury, end-stage renal disease, and mortality in hospitalized patients. *BMC Nephrol.* **2019**, *20*, 362. [CrossRef]

16. Cheungpasitporn, W.; Thongprayoon, C.; Erickson, S.B. Admission hypomagnesemia and hypermagnesemia increase the risk of acute kidney injury. *Ren. Fail.* **2015**, *37*, 1175–1179. [CrossRef]
17. Thongprayoon, C.; Cheungpasitporn, W.; Mao, M.A.; Sakhuja, A.; Erickson, S.B. Admission calcium levels and risk of acute kidney injury in hospitalised patients. *Int. J. Clin. Pract.* **2018**, *72*, e13057. [CrossRef]
18. Thongprayoon, C.; Cheungpasitporn, W.; Chewcharat, A.; Mao, M.A.; Bathini, T.; Vallabhajosyula, S.; Thirunavukkarasu, S.; Kashani, K.B. Impact of admission serum ionized calcium levels on risk of acute kidney injury in hospitalized patients. *Sci. Rep.* **2020**, *10*, 12316. [CrossRef] [PubMed]
19. Chen, D.N.; Du, J.; Xie, Y.; Li, M.; Wang, R.L.; Tian, R. Relationship between early serum sodium and potassium levels and AKI severity and prognosis in oliguric AKI patients. *Int. Urol. Nephrol.* **2021**, *53*, 1171–1187. [CrossRef] [PubMed]
20. Yessayan, L.; Neyra, J.A.; Canepa-Escaro, F.; Vasquez-Rios, G.; Heung, M.; Yee, J.; Acute Kidney Injury in Critical Illness Study, G. Effect of hyperchloremia on acute kidney injury in critically ill septic patients: A retrospective cohort study. *BMC Nephrol.* **2017**, *18*, 346. [CrossRef] [PubMed]
21. Morooka, H.; Tanaka, A.; Kasugai, D.; Ozaki, M.; Numaguchi, A.; Maruyama, S. Abnormal magnesium levels and their impact on death and acute kidney injury in critically ill children. *Pediatr. Nephrol.* **2022**, *37*, 1157–1165. [CrossRef] [PubMed]
22. James, G.; Witten, D.; Hastie, T.; Tibshirani, R. *An Introduction to Statistical Learning: With Applications in R*; Springer: New York, NY, USA, 2013.
23. Cortes, C.; Vapnik, V. Support-Vector Networks. *Mach. Learn.* **1995**, *20*, 273–297. [CrossRef]
24. Koller, D.; Friedman, N. *Probabilistic Graphical Models: Principles and Techniques/Daphne Koller, Nir Friedman*; MIT Press: Cambridge, MA, USA, 2009.
25. Breiman, L. Random forests. *Mach. Learn.* **2001**, *45*, 5–32. [CrossRef]
26. Song, X.; Liu, X.; Liu, F.; Wang, C. Comparison of machine learning and logistic regression models in predicting acute kidney injury: A systematic review and meta-analysis. *Int. J. Med. Inform.* **2021**, *151*, 104484. [CrossRef]
27. Tomasev, N.; Glorot, X.; Rae, J.W.; Zielinski, M.; Askham, H.; Saraiva, A.; Mottram, A.; Meyer, C.; Ravuri, S.; Protsyuk, I.; et al. A clinically applicable approach to continuous prediction of future acute kidney injury. *Nature* **2019**, *572*, 116–119. [CrossRef]
28. Therneau, T.; Atkinson, B. Rpart: Recursive Partitioning and Regression Trees. Available online: https://CRAN.R-project.org/package=rpart (accessed on 21 March 2022).
29. Rokach, L.; Maimon, O. *Data Mining with Decision Trees Theory and Applications/Lior Rokach, Oded Maimon*, 2nd ed.; World Scientific: Hackensack, NJ, USA, 2015.
30. Cho, S.; Hong, H.; Ha, B.C. A hybrid approach based on the combination of variable selection using decision trees and case-based reasoning using the Mahalanobis distance: For bankruptcy prediction. *Expert. Syst. Appl.* **2010**, *37*, 3482–3488. [CrossRef]
31. Gao, W.; Wang, J.; Zhou, L.; Luo, Q.; Lao, Y.; Lyu, H.; Guo, S. Prediction of acute kidney injury in ICU with gradient boosting decision tree algorithms. *Comput. Biol. Med.* **2021**, *140*, 105097. [CrossRef]
32. Chen, T.; Guestrin, C. XGBoost. In Proceedings of the 22nd ACM SIGKDD International Conference on Knowledge Discovery and Data Mining, San Francisco, CA, USA, 13 August 2016; pp. 785–794.
33. Johnson, A.; Bulgarelli, L.; Pollard, T.; Horng, S.; Celi, L.A.; Mark, R. *MIMIC-IV*, Version 1.0; PhysioNet: Cambridge, MA, USA, 2021. [CrossRef]
34. Goldberger, A.L.; Amaral, L.A.; Glass, L.; Hausdorff, J.M.; Ivanov, P.C.; Mark, R.G.; Mietus, J.E.; Moody, G.B.; Peng, C.K.; Stanley, H.E. PhysioBank, PhysioToolkit, and PhysioNet: Components of a new research resource for complex physiologic signals. *Circulation* **2000**, *101*, E215–E220. [CrossRef] [PubMed]
35. Khwaja, A. KDIGO Clinical Practice Guidelines for Acute Kidney Injury. *Nephron Clin. Pract.* **2012**, *120*, c179–c184. [CrossRef]
36. Acute Kidney Injury Work Group. Section 2: AKI Definition. *Kidney Int. Suppl.* **2012**, *2*, 19–36. [CrossRef] [PubMed]
37. Kidney International Work Group. Summary of Recommendation Statements. *Kidney Int. Suppl.* **2012**, *2*, 8–12. [CrossRef]
38. Palevsky, P.M.; Liu, K.D.; Brophy, P.D.; Chawla, L.S.; Parikh, C.R.; Thakar, C.V.; Tolwani, A.J.; Waikar, S.S.; Weisbord, S.D. KDOQI US commentary on the 2012 KDIGO clinical practice guideline for acute kidney injury. *Am. J. Kidney Dis.* **2013**, *61*, 649–672. [CrossRef]
39. Quan, H.; Sundararajan, V.; Halfon, P.; Fong, A.; Burnand, B.; Luthi, J.C.; Saunders, L.D.; Beck, C.A.; Feasby, T.E.; Ghali, W.A. Coding algorithms for defining comorbidities in ICD-9-CM and ICD-10 administrative data. *Med. Care* **2005**, *43*, 1130–1139. [CrossRef] [PubMed]
40. Liano, F.; Pascual, J. Epidemiology of acute renal failure: A prospective, multicenter, community-based study. Madrid Acute Renal Failure Study Group. *Kidney Int.* **1996**, *50*, 811–818. [CrossRef] [PubMed]
41. Basile, D.P.; Anderson, M.D.; Sutton, T.A. Pathophysiology of acute kidney injury. *Compr. Physiol.* **2012**, *2*, 1303–1353. [CrossRef]
42. Dowdy, S.; Wearden, S.; Chilko, D. *Statistics for Research*; John Wiley & Sons, Incorporated: Hoboken, NJ, USA, 2004.
43. MacFarland, T.W.; Yates, J.M. *Introduction to Nonparametric Statistics for the Biological Sciences Using R*; Springer International Publishing AG: Cham, Switzerland, 2016.

Disclaimer/Publisher's Note: The statements, opinions and data contained in all publications are solely those of the individual author(s) and contributor(s) and not of MDPI and/or the editor(s). MDPI and/or the editor(s) disclaim responsibility for any injury to people or property resulting from any ideas, methods, instructions or products referred to in the content.

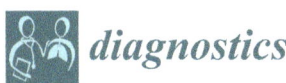

Article

Applicability of American College of Radiology Appropriateness Criteria Decision-Making Model for Acute Appendicitis Diagnosis in Children

Ozum Tuncyurek [1,2], Koray Kadam [3], Berna Uzun [4,5] and Dilber Uzun Ozsahin [6,7,*]

1. Kolan British Hospital, TRNC Mersin 10, Nicosia 99138, Turkey
2. Department of Radiology, Cyprus International University, TRNC Mersin 10, Nicosia 99138, Turkey
3. Department of Emergency, Faculty of Medicine, Near East University, TRNC Mersin 10, Nicosia 99138, Turkey
4. Department of Statistics, Carlos III de Madrid University, 28903 Madrid, Spain
5. Department of Mathematics, Faculty of Arts and Sciences, Near East University, TRNC Mersin 10, Nicosia 99138, Turkey
6. Medical Diagnostic Imaging Department, College of Health Science, University of Sharjah, Sharjah 27272, United Arab Emirates
7. Operational Research Center in Healthcare, Near East University, TRNC Mersin 10, Nicosia 99138, Turkey
* Correspondence: dozsahin@sharjah.ac.ae

Abstract: Acute appendicitis is one of the most common causes of abdominal pain in the emergency department and the most common surgical emergency reason for children younger than 15 years of age, which could be enormously dangerous when ruptured. The choice of radiological approach is very important for the diagnosis. In this way, unnecessary surgery is avoided. The aim of this study was to examine the validity of the American College of Radiology appropriateness criteria for radiological imaging in diagnosing acute appendicitis with multivariate decision criteria. In our study, pediatric patients who presented to the emergency department with abdominal pain were grouped according to the Appendicitis Inflammatory Response (AIR) score and the choice of radiological examinations was evaluated with fuzzy-based Preference Ranking Organization Method for Enrichment Evaluation (PROMETHEE) and with the fuzzy-based Technique for Order of Preference by Similarity to Ideal Solution (TOPSIS) model for the validation of the results. As a result of this study, non-contrast computed tomography (CT) was recommended as the first choice for patients with low AIR score (where $\Phi^{net} = 0.0733$) and with high AIR scores (where $\Phi^{net} = 0.0702$) while ultrasound (US) examination was ranked third in patients with high scores. While computed tomography is at the forefront with many criteria used in the study, it is still a remarkable practice that US examination is in the first place in daily routine. Even though there are studies showing the strengths of these tools, this study is unique in that it provides analytical ranking results for this complex decision-making issue and shows the strengths and weaknesses of each alternative for different scenarios, even considering vague information for the acute appendicitis diagnosis in children for different scenarios.

Keywords: appendicitis; diagnosis; fuzzy logic; decision making

1. Introduction

Acute appendicitis is the most common indication reason requiring emergency abdominal surgery [1–3]. Acute appendicitis (AA) is the most common surgical emergency in younger than 15 years old children [4]. Surgical treatment is the first option for this diagnosis. Although the treatment options are improved, there are 510 morbidity and 1–5% mortality rates, while there is a 5–42% negative appendectomy rate [2,3,5]. This causes 3 billion dollars of annual hospital spending according to USA data. Many biomarkers such as blood or urine analysis have been defined for diagnosis, but they are not definitive methods [6,7]. It can benefit from ultrasound, CT, and MRI in the diagnosis of appendicitis.

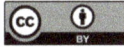

Diagnosing acute appendicitis (AA) in children remains challenging for physicians due to atypical presentations [8–10]. Proper diagnosis of AA can prevent complications such as perforation and abscess [11]. Ultrasound is an imaging technique with high specificity in diagnosis in the pediatric group. However, it is operator-dependent [12]. However, CT, which has higher specificity, has a narrow area of use due to X-ray exposure [13] and MRI for claustrophobia. US scanning was used initially, but CT scanning has become increasingly used as a diagnostic tool in adults as well as children to make a more accurate diagnosis and rule out appendicitis [14]. However, it is a controversial issue, as it is known that exposure to CT scanning increases the risk of cancer in the long term, especially in children [15]. There are many scoring systems for appropriate diagnostic techniques and surgical decisions in the management of right lower quadrant pain in pediatric patients in the emergency department [16]. The Appendicitis Inflammatory Response (AIR) score is AUROC 0.96 in the widest age range and enables us to avoid CT application [17]. The AIR score is one of the two scores (the other one is 'Adult Appendicitis Score', AAS) recommended by the 2020 World Society of Emergency Surgery clinical practice guidelines for the diagnosis and treatment of acute appendicitis [18]. The parameters of the AIR score are vomiting, right lower quadrant (RLQ) pain, rebound tenderness, body temperature, polymorphonuclear leukocytes (PNL), WBC count, and C-reactive protein (CRP) level [19] (Table 1). However, literature information on the applicability of these scores and their compatibility with the ACR eligibility criteria in the field is limited.

Table 1. Appendicitis Inflammatory Response (AIR) score.

Diagnosis	Score
Vomit	1
Pain in RLQ	1
Rebound tenderness low	1
Rebound tenderness mild	2
Rebound tenderness severe	3
Temperature > 38.5 °C	1
PNL 70–84%	1
PNL > 85%	2
Leukocytes (WBC) > 10.0–14.9 × 10⁹/L	1
Leukocytes (WBC) > 15.0 × 10⁹/L	2
CRP 10–49 g/L	1
CRP > 50 g/L	2

AIR: if sum 0–4 = low probability; if sum 5–8 = mild probability; if sum 9–12 = high probability.

Many multivariate decision criteria have been developed in medical studies for many machine learning algorithms and approaches. For diagnostic and classification purposes, conceptual decision-making models are most often used. Decision trees provide a useful and effective decision-making technique with high classification precision and these models are easy to compare to most classification algorithms. For the diagnosis of acute appendicitis, the sensitivity and specificity values of ultrasound are 78% and 83%, respectively [18], 100% and 94.8% for contrast-enhanced CT, and 90.5% and 100% for non-contrast CT, respectively [19]. The sensitivity and specificity values for 1.5 T MRI are 96.6% and 95.8%, respectively [20], and 100% and 98% for 3T MRI, respectively. Tseng et al. [21] showed that ultrasound was the cause of the highest rate of negative appendectomy. When CT imaging was added, there was a 0.6% reduction. Data from the National Surgical Quality Improvement Program (NSQIP) were used in this recent study. We wanted to test the ACR eligibility criteria with a new model that has not been studied in the literature before, in order to minimize the confusion in the diagnostic process. The purpose of this study is to determine which examination is the most appropriate for patients with low/high AIR score in the diagnosis of acute appendicitis.

Table 1 displays the score of the appendicitis inflammatory response for various diagnosis occurrence conditions.

In order to achieve our aim, we applied multi-criteria decision-making analysis approaches, specifically the fuzzy-based Preference Ranking Organization Method for Enrichment Evaluation (PROMETHEE) and the fuzzy-based Technique for Order of Preference by Similarity to an Ideal Solution (TOPSIS), to discover the strengths and weaknesses of each diagnosis technique for the acute appendicitis diagnosis in children using the multi-parameters assigned with the alternative's medical tools for the diagnosis.

2. Material and Method

2.1. Study Design

After Institutional Review Board approval was obtained (YDU/2020/85-1186), data of all cases under 16 years of age admitted 2019–2020 with diagnosis of the acute abdominal pain were collected. The diagnosis of the patients was confirmed by two researchers through analysis of all records of the patients. All patients were free of tumor, infection, and hematological diseases. As data for the analysis, the examinations were assessed by two expert observers (O.T., K.K.) in terms of imaging time, easy applicability of the examination, duration of the examination, specificity, sensitivity, user dependency, fee, diagnostic precision, request duration, and radiation exposure, and with their joint decision. Their answers were defined as five scale linguistic triangular fuzzy scales. The model made an examination selection ranking according to the AIR score data. This analysis was made for US, non-contrast CT, contrast-enhanced CT, 1.5 T MRI, and 3T MRI. Furthermore, the PROMETHEE and the TOPSIS techniques were applied for this evaluation. The Gaussian preference function was used for the PROMETHEE analysis for each criterion. Linguistic fuzzy scale was applied for the determination of the importance weights of the criteria and selected criteria and Yager index was used for the defuzzification of the defined triangular fuzzy values.

Figure 1 shows the linguistic fuzzy sets and their assigned fuzzy numbers used for the expression of the fuzzy parameters. VH: Very high; H: High; M: Medium; L: Low; and VL: Very low are defined as the linguistic expressions used for determination of the data. Each linguistic expression and the importance given to parameters selected by experts are assigned to triangular fuzzy values as shown in detail at Table 2 below.

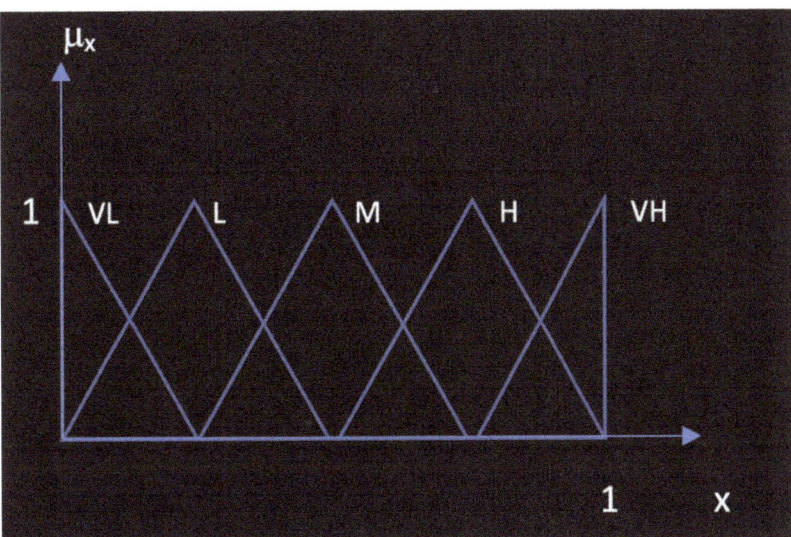

Figure 1. Linguistic fuzzy sets.

Table 2. Linguistic fuzzy scale.

Linguistic Scale for Evaluation	Triangular Fuzzy Scale	Criteria of the Decision Alternatives
VH	(0.75, 1, 1)	specificity, diagnostic precision, time of imaging, user dependency, radiation dose, comfortability
H	(0.50, 0.75, 1)	sensitivity, air score, disposition
M	(0.25, 0.50, 0.75)	time of order, result time, cost
L	(0, 0.25, 0.50)	-
VL	(0, 0, 0.25)	-

VH: Very high; H: High; M: Medium; L: Low; VL: Very low.

Using the fuzzy scale enables the expert to determine the weights or degrees of importance of the parameters used for the comparison of the medical diagnosis tools for acute appendicitis in pediatric patients. Then, after the defuzzification process, the decision matrix is constructed for use in MCDM approaches. Yager index is a value that provides the defuzzified point for the triangular fuzzy numbers, proposed by Ronald Yager as one of the most important ranking methods for fuzzy sets.

Data: Data included demographics, preoperative clinical findings for AIR score such as vomiting, pain in RLQ, rebound tenderness or muscular defense, body temperature, polymorphonuclear leukocytes rate, white blood cell count, and C-reactive protein concentration. Radiological data were not included in generator operator-independent data. Parental consent was obtained both of surgical approach and publication of the data. Diagnosis and management of appendicitis were determined through clinical, laboratory, radiological, and surgical findings.

Statistical analysis: Statistical analysis was performed with IBM SPSS Statistics 26.0.0 (Chicago, IL, USA). The characteristics of the study sample were analyzed by descriptive statistics, with dichotomous or ordinal data presented as percentage, and continuous data as means with SD. The Kolmogorov–Smirnov test was used to demonstrate normal distribution. One-way ANOVA was used for homogeneity of variables, while Student's t test was used. Statistical associations were considered significant if the p value was <0.05. In our daily life, we face many problems in different fields, the most common ones are the problems related to choosing or evaluating something included in groups of other choices. In some cases, the evaluation of the situations could be complex and needs to consider many factors with different weights or levels of importance for these factors for the evaluation. To solve this problem, multi criteria decision making (MCDM) is used and this principle refers to making decisions in the presence of multiple, usually conflicting, criteria [21]. Although MCDM problems are very common and popular, MCDM as a discipline has a short history of about 30 years. It developed relatively to computer advancements and development and because of this relation, computers gave us the ability to conduct complex and big MCDM problems which expands the applications of MCDM.

On the other hand, the popularity of computers and mobiles generated an enormous amount of data in several fields which makes MCDM more important and dominant in supporting design makers in different sectors with usable data [21]. The MCDM problems have three main components which are the decision maker/s (DMs), alternatives, and criteria. In general, the classification of MCDA problems depends on types of these three elements. Decision maker/s (DMs): in problems, we may have one decision maker which is responsible for determining what to do or multiple decision makers such as several people or organizations who are involved in the processes of MCDM. In case of multiple decision making, many different preferences, goals, criteria, and objectives appear so the results might not satisfy every DM [22]. In this case, obtaining usable outcomes depends mainly on the range of cooperation between the DMs. In case of the presence of multiple DMs with different preferences and priorities, the problem of their presence could be included in MCDM problems to be solved [23]. Alternatives: these are the things or possibilities that the decision maker/s should choose from. These possibilities could be identified previously or could be created through process. It is important to know that the decision space is the definition of the set of all possible alternatives [22]. Criteria: the specifications or requirements that each element of decision space should have or possess and depending on these requirements, each element is rated and evaluated by how well it possesses one of the process criteria [22].

There are many ways to classify the methods of multi criteria decision making. One of these ways is to classify according to decision makers which could be one decision maker or group of decision makers; the methods could also be classified according to the type of data used in the process, such as deterministic data which are accurate and clear data, stochastic which means the data are random and the opposite of deterministic data, and in some cases the data presented as fuzzy information which are not clear or vague. There are some subsidiary classifications such as in case of a deterministic, single decision maker. The classification problem considers the type of information and the number of decision makers [24]. Multi criteria decision making has many techniques such as Analytic Hierarchy Process (AHP) method, Preference Ranking Organization Method for Enrichment Evaluation (PROMETHEE), Technique for Order of Preference by Similarity to Ideal Solution (TOPSIS), Analytical Network Process (ANP), Compromise ranking method (VIKOR), Elimination Et Choix Traduisant la Realité (ELECTRE) [25,26], etc. In this study, two types of analytical methods were used, specifically F-PROMETHEE and F-TOPSIS.

2.2. Fuzzy PROMETHEE (F-PROMETHEE)

This definition or technique contains two main parts, fuzzy and PROMETHEE. With the fuzzy logic process, the vague and linguistic data could be defined and with the PROMETHEE process, the ranking of the alternatives under the fuzzy conditions can be obtained. The PROMETHEE method was created by Brans et al. (1984) in order to present a rational and clear method to rank alternatives [27,28]. The first part of the technique is the fuzzy process, which refers to mathematical means used to explain the non-numerical data or uncertain information mathematically. Distinguishing the real value depends on if it is completely true or false. This manner facilitates the utilizing, interpreting, and manipulating the data when there is a lack of certainty or clearance [29]. The second part is PROMETHEE and this method is used for evaluating and arranging the alternatives with different criteria to get a specific aim. This technique has two parts, PROMETHEE I and II; the first one used for obtaining the partial raking results and the second one used to get the net ranking results between the alternatives [9]. PROMETHEE is one of the outranking methods, which is well understood and has a lot of applications in many fields. There are mainly six steps of this method as shown below [30,31] after the decision matrix, the matrix that contains alternatives and the criterion, is constructed:

Step 1. Determination of the preference function for each criterion (p_k).
Step 2. Determination of the importance weights for each criterion (w_k).
Step 3. Calculation of the outranking relation/preference index $\pi(.)$ for each pair of alternatives with the Equation (1):

$$\pi(a_t, a_{t'}) = \sum_{k=1}^{K} w_k \cdot [p_k(f_k(a_t) - f_k(a_{t'}))], \quad AXA \to [0,1] \tag{1}$$

$\pi(a_t, a_{t'})$ stands for the preference index of the alternative a_t compared to alternative $a_{t'}$ by considering each criterion simultaneously and $f_k(a_i)$ denotes the value of the k-th criterion of i-th alternative.

Step 4. Calculations of the entering/negative outranking flow and leaving/positive outranking flow for each alternative using the Equations (2) and (3), respectively.

$$\Phi^-(a_t) = \frac{1}{n-1} \sum_{\substack{t'=1 \\ t' \neq t}}^{n} \pi(a_{t'}, a_t) \tag{2}$$

$$\Phi^+(a_t) = \frac{1}{n-1} \sum_{\substack{t'=1 \\ t' \neq t}}^{n} \pi(a_t, a_{t'}) \qquad (3)$$

where n denotes the number of alternatives.

The leaving flow indicates how good the alternative a_t is over other alternatives, while the entering flow indicates how much all other alternatives are better or more preferred than alternative a_t and it shows how weak the alternative a_t is.

Step 5. Generating the partial order of the alternatives based on the following statements: a_t should be preferred to $a_{t'}$ $(a_t P a_{t'})$ if

$$\{\Phi^+(a_t) > \Phi^+(a_{t'}) \text{ and } \Phi^-(a_t) \leq \Phi^-(a_{t'}) \; \Phi^+(a_t) = \Phi^+(a_{t'}) \text{ and } \Phi^-(a_t) < \Phi^-(a_{t'}) \qquad (4)$$

a_t is equally preferred to $a_{t'}$ $(a_t I a_{t'})$ if

$$(a_t I a_{t'}) \text{if} : \; \Phi^+(a_t) = \Phi^+(a_{t'}) \text{ and } \Phi^-(a_t) = \Phi^-(a_{t'}) \qquad (5)$$

a_t is incomparable to $a_{t'}$ $(a_t R a_{t'})$ if

$$\{\Phi^+(a_t) > \Phi^+(a_{t'}) \text{ and } \Phi^-(a_t) > \Phi^-(a_{t'}) \; \Phi^+(a_t) < \Phi^+(a_{t'}) \text{ and } \Phi^-(a_t) < \Phi^-(a_{t'}) \qquad (6)$$

The last statement occurring in this PROMETHEE I process the total ranking can be obtained by applying to PROMETHEE II method.

Step 6. The net ranking results should be determined by using Equation (7)

$$\Phi^{net}(a_t) = \Phi^+(a_t) - \Phi^-(a_t) \qquad (7)$$

Total ranking results can be obtained with the following statements.

$$(a_t P a_{t'}) \text{ if } \Phi^{net}(a_t) > \Phi^{net}(a_{t'}) \qquad (8)$$

$$(a_t I a_{t'}) \text{ if } \Phi^{net}(a_t) = \Phi^{net}(a_{t'}) \qquad (9)$$

The higher net flow ($\Phi^{net}(.)$ means a better alternative and that demonstrates the aim of PROMETHEE II (10).

2.3. TOPSIS

The TOPSIS method was created as an alternative to the ELECTRE method by Yoon and Hwang 1979 [11,32]. This method is based on the principle of when the alternative has the shortest distance to the ideal solution, that indicates that it is the best choice.

In the classical TOPSIS method, in the presence of one decision maker, the assumption is that the ratings and the weights are well represented by numerical data. The assumption differs and is more complex if there are many decision makers, because the preferences and vision differ. There are mainly 5 steps for the TOPSIS process as follows [12]:

Step 1: Creation of decision matrix $X = [x_{ij}]_{mxn}$ and the importance weights (w_j) where

$$\sum_{1}^{n} w_j = 1 \qquad (10)$$

Step 2. Calculate the normalized decision matrix; the commonly used normalization data can be calculated by using the Equation (11):

$$n_{ij} = \frac{X_{ij}}{\sqrt{\sum_{i=1}^{m} X_{ij}^2}} \qquad (11)$$

Step 3. Calculate the weighted normalized decision values (v_{ij}) to obtain the weighted normalized matrix using the Equation (12).

$$v_{ij} = w_j n_{ij} \qquad (12)$$

where $i = 1, \ldots, m; j = 1, \ldots, n$.

Step 4. Determine the positive ideal solution (PIS/A^+) and negative ideal solution (NIS/A^-). In this step, two extreme sides (negative and positive) are identified as given in Equations (13) and (14).

$$A^+ = (v_1^+, v_2^+, \ldots, v_n^+) = [[v_{ij} \,|\, j \in I], [v_{ij} \,|\, j \in J]] \tag{13}$$

$$A^- = (v_1^-, v_2^-, \ldots, v_n^-) = [[v_{ij} \,|\, j \in I], [v_{ij} \,|\, j \in J]] \tag{14}$$

where $i = 1, \ldots, m; j = 1, \ldots, n$, I denotes the beneficial criteria and J denotes the non-beneficial criteria.

Step 5. Calculate the distance measures from the positive ideal solution (d_i^+) and the negative ideal solution (d_i^-) for each alternative by using the n dimensional Euclidean metric using the following equations:

$$d_i^+ = \sqrt{\sum_{j=1}^{n} (v_{ij} - v_j^+)^2}, \; i = 1, 2, \ldots, m \tag{15}$$

$$d_i^- = \sqrt{\sum_{j=1}^{n} (v_{ij} - v_j^-)^2}, \; i = 1, 2, \ldots, m \tag{16}$$

Step 6. Rank the alternatives based on the relative closeness to the positive ideal solution (R_i) in descending order where:

$$R_i = \frac{d_i^-}{d_i^- + d_i^+} \tag{17}$$

3. Results

Of 51 patients, who were admitted in 2019–2020 to the Emergency Department with abdominal pain, ultrasound (US) was performed in 96% (n: 49) patients. Computed tomography (CT) was performed in 0.7% (n: 4) patients. In 69% (n: 34) of the patients, the US result was acute appendicitis. In 31% (n: 15) patients, appendicitis was not detected on ultrasound. The mean AIR score of patients diagnosed with acute appendicitis by US (n: 34) was 6 ± 1.8 (mean ± SD), and the patients not diagnosed with appendicitis (n: 15) were 4.6 ± 2.3 (mean ± SD) ($p = 0.03$). The mean AIR score of patients diagnosed with acute appendicitis with CT was 7.5 ± 1.3 (mean ± SD), and the patients without CT were 5.5 ± 2 (mean ± SD) ($p = 0.04$). 72% ($n = 37$) of the patients had undergone surgery. The AIR score was 6.3 ± 1.6 (mean ± SD), and the 14 patients who did not undergo appendectomy were 3.9 ± 2.2 (mean ± SD) ($p = 0.00$). For the cost of 51 patients, it was an average of 752.3 ± 549 USD (mean ± SD), while the AIR score value of 52% ($n = 27$) patients costing more than 750 USD was 6.37 ± 1.6, the mean AIR score value of the remaining 24 patients was found to be 4.96 ± 2.3 ($p = 0.01$). The mean duration of hospital stay was 1.92 ± 2.1 days for 51 patients, while the mean AIR score value of 30 patients staying more than two days was 6.43 ± 1.7, and the mean AIR score value of 21 patients staying one day was 4.67 ± 2.1 ($p = 0.00$). In addition, four patients without any findings of appendicitis in the US were operated on. One of them was diagnosed with appendicitis on CT and the air score was 6. The other three patients were operated on due to an increase in AIR score (mean AIR score: 7) without additional cross-sectional imaging. In two patients, patients who did not accept surgery (mean AIR score: 5.5) even though the US diagnosis was appendicitis were discharged with medical treatment.

Multi Criteria Decision Making Theory Results (MCDM)

If the patient's AIR score is below 6, non-contrast CT ($\Phi^{net} = 0.0733$) should be selected as the first display option. The second option was contrast enhanced CT ($\Phi^{net} = 0.0535$), then US ($\Phi^{net} = 0.1305$) and MRI ($\Phi^{net} = -0.0432$), in that order, based on the fuzzy-PROMETHEE ranking result as displayed in Table 3.

Table 3. Ranking of the acute appendicitis diagnosis for low AIR score by F-PROMETHEE approach.

Rank	Alternatives	Φ^{net}
1	CT non-contrast	0.0733
2	CT contrast	0.0535
3	US	0.1305
4	MRI	−0.0432

The graphic in Figure 2 shows which test to choose for the patient group with low AIR score based on the F-PROMETHEE approach.

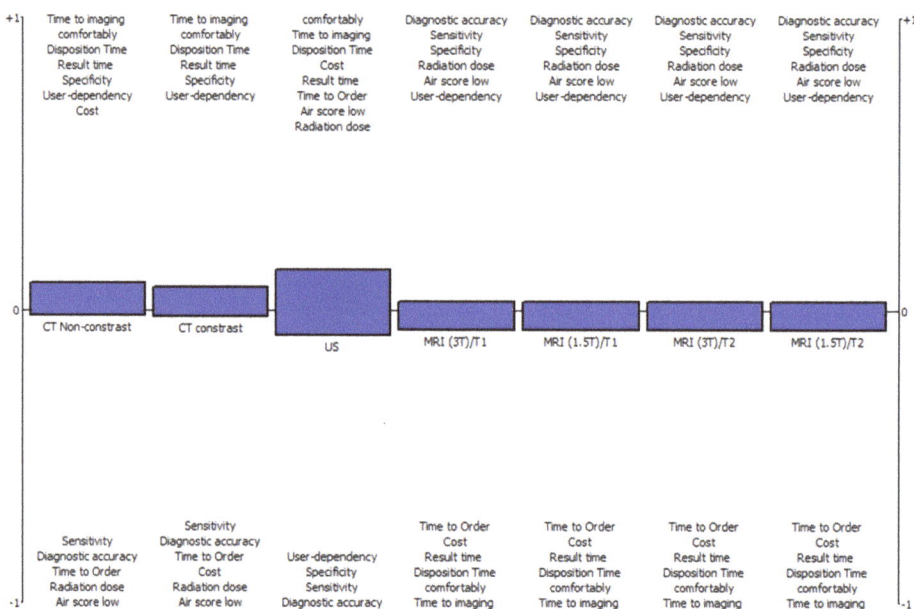

Figure 2. Evaluation of the acute appendicitis diagnosis for low AIR score with F-PROMETHEE.

The detailed ranking results by the F-TOPSIS method are shown in Table 4, where the patients' air score is low. Using the F-TOPSIS technique, we obtained the ranking results, where the air score is low, as the best option is CT-non-contrast ($R_i = 0.6315$), and the last option is MRI ($R_i = 0.5217$) as similar to F-PROMETHEE results.

Table 4. Ranking of the acute appendicitis diagnosis for low AIR score by F-TOPSIS approach.

Rank	Alternatives	d_i^+	d_i^-	R_i
1	CT non-contrast	0.0927	0.1588	0.6315
2	CT contrast	0.0946	0.1561	0.6227
3	US	0.1210	0.1435	0.5425
4	MRI	0.1288	0.1405	0.5217

If the patient's AIR score is above 6, F-PROMETHEE results shows that non-contrast CT ($\Phi^{net} = 0.0702$) should be chosen as the first imaging option. The second option was US ($\Phi^{net} = 0.0617$), contrast-enhanced CT ($\Phi^{net} = 0.0503$), or MRI ($\Phi^{net} = 0.0456$), in that order, as displayed in Table 5.

Table 5. Ranking of the acute appendicitis diagnosis for high AIR score by F-PROMETHEE approach.

Rank	Alternatives	Φ^{net}
1	CT non-contrast	0.0702
2	US	0.0617
3	CT contrast	0.0503
4	MRI	0.0456

The graphic in Figure 3 shows which test to choose for the patient group with high AIR score based on the F-PROMETHEE approach.

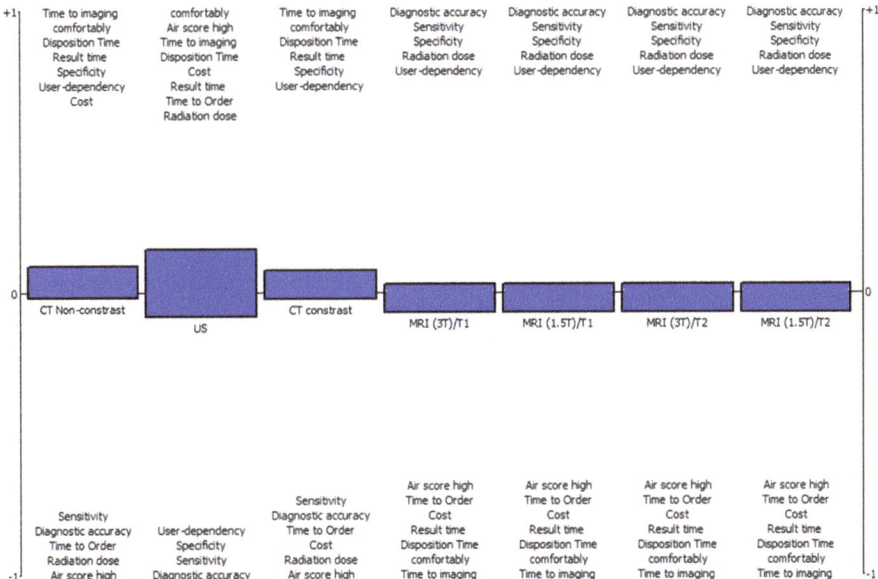

Figure 3. Evaluation of the acute appendicitis diagnosis for high AIR score patients with F-PROMETHEE.

As seen in Table 6. using the F-TOPSIS technique, we obtained the ranking results, where the air score is high, as the best option is CT-non-contrast ($R_i = 0.6191$), and the last option is MRI ($R_i = 0.5153$) as similar to the F-PROMETHEE results.

Table 6. Ranking of the acute appendicitis diagnosis for high AIR score by F-TOPSIS approach.

Ranking	Alternatives	d_i^+	d_i^-	R_i
1	CT non-contrast	0.0977	0.1588	0.6191
2	CT contrast	0.0995	0.1561	0.6107
3	US	0.1210	0.1468	0.5481
4	MRI	0.1316	0.1399	0.5153

4. Discussion

The result we found in the appendicitis diagnosis algorithm matches the pediatric patient group of our sample group. With this study, mathematical modeling was used for the first time in the literature for the diagnosis of acute appendicitis in pediatric patients. There are no similar studies in the literature. The method is a support system with which imaging will be more appropriate when pediatric patients suffer from appendicitis. In this study, a radiology and an emergency medicine specialist entered the MCDM program in line with the ACR appropriateness criteria. Consistent with the result in the study group, if ultrasound is preferred in the group with low AIR score, treatment can be performed quickly. The use of a cross-sectional imaging method, CT or MRI, is seen as a method that will facilitate diagnosis and treatment in patients with high AIR scores for whom US examination may be insufficient. This model is a decision support system that allows for which examination to choose for diagnosis in the emergency department. In this model, the weight of importance can be updated according to the expert doctor. According to the literature update, the criteria for this decision support system can be expanded, new imaging technologies can be added and easily renewed.

The criteria chosen in our study were imaging time, easy applicability of the examination, duration of the examination, time to result, specificity, sensitivity, user dependency, cost, diagnostic precision, request time, and radiation exposure level. Benabbas [4] et al. showed that while testing the superiority of ED point-of-care US over MR and CT, they did not use such factors as treatment cost, applicability of imaging method, and length of hospital stay, but we also included these factors in our study. Results depend on the observer. The advantage of this is that it enables experienced people to share their clinical practice approach. Thus, data can be globalized. Local differences are important. However, it is easy to update the program for these as well.

Aydın et al. [33] used blood tests decision trees for acute appendicitis diagnosis. We compared imaging techniques for diagnosis. With a similar thought, we tested which of the imaging methods used for diagnosis was more helpful in our study.

We did not use only one model in our study. We proved the accuracy of the results with the second model. In this way, we had an objective approach. It has been observed that the criteria of MRI devices for abdominal imaging are identical. Therefore, no difference was observed in the order of these devices. The first limitation of the study is the limited number of observers. We aimed to convey the experiences of both the emergency service and the radiology specialist in our own sample group. The second limitation is the retrospective analysis of the sample group. In conclusion, while computed tomography is at the forefront with many criteria used in the study, it is still a remarkable practice that US examination is in the first place in daily routine.

In conclusion, CT is the most reliable method for diagnosis with our model. Although it contains radiation that reduces the use of this examination, it is superior to the US examination in daily practice in order to minimize the damage that the patients may experience during the treatment process.

Author Contributions: Conceptualization, D.U.O. and O.T.; methodology, D.U.O. and B.U.; software, D.U.O. and B.U.; validation, D.U.O. and O.T.; formal analysis, D.U.O. and B.U.; investigation, D.U.O., K.K., O.T. and B.U.; resources, K.K. and O.T.; data curation, O.T., K.K. and D.U.O.; writing—original draft preparation, B.U., O.T., K.K. and D.U.O.; writing—review and editing, B.U., K.K., O.T. and D.U.O.; visualization, B.U. and D.U.O.; supervision, O.T. and D.U.O.; project administration, D.U.O. and O.T. All authors have read and agreed to the published version of the manuscript.

Funding: This research received no external funding.

Institutional Review Board Statement: This study was conducted according to the guidelines of the Declaration of Cyprus and approved by the Institutional Review Board (or Ethics Committee) of Near East University Hospital (YDU/2020/85-1186).

Informed Consent Statement: Not applicable.

Data Availability Statement: The data used to support the findings of this study can be provided upon the request from the authors.

Conflicts of Interest: There is no conflict of interest between the authors.

References

1. Omari, A.H.; Khammash, M.R.; Qasaimeh, G.R.; Shammari, A.K.; Yaseen, M.K.B.; Hammori, S.K. Acute appendicitis in the elderly: Risk factors for perforation. *World J. Emerg. Surg.* **2014**, *9*, 6. [CrossRef] [PubMed]
2. Ashdown, H.F.; D'Souza, N.; Karim, D.; Stevens, R.J.; Huang, A.; Harnden, A. Pain over speed bumps in diagnosis of acute appendicitis: Diagnostic accuracy study. *BMJ* **2012**, *345*, e8012. [CrossRef] [PubMed]
3. Andersson, R.E. The magic of an appendicitis score. *World J. Surg.* **2015**, *39*, 110–111. [CrossRef]
4. Benabbas, R.; Hanna, M.; Shah, J.; Sinert, R. Diagnostic Accuracy of History, Physical Examination, Laboratory Tests, and Point-of-care Ultrasound for Paediatric Acute Appendicitis in the Emergency Department: A Systematic Review and Meta-analysis. *Acad. Emerg. Med.* **2017**, *24*, 523–551. [CrossRef] [PubMed]
5. Atema, J.J.; Van Rossem, C.C.; Leeuwenburgh, M.M.; Stoker, J.; A Boermeester, M. Scoring system to distinguish uncomplicated from complicated acute appendicitis. *Br. J. Surg.* **2015**, *102*, 979–990. [CrossRef] [PubMed]
6. Yu, C.W.; Juan, L.I.; Wu, M.H.; Shen, C.; Wu, J.; Lee, C. Systematic review and meta-analysis of the diagnostic accuracy of procalcitonin, C-reactive protein and white blood cell count for suspected acute appendicitis. *Br. J. Surg.* **2013**, *100*, 322–329. [CrossRef]
7. Acharya, A.; Markar, S.R.; Ni, M.; Hanna, G.B. Biomarkers of acute appendicitis: Systematic review and cost–benefit trade-off analysis. *Surg. Endosc.* **2017**, *31*, 1022–1031. [CrossRef]
8. Becker, T.; Kharbanda, A.; Bachur, R. Atypical clinical features of paediatric appendicitis. *Acad. Emerg. Med.* **2007**, *14*, 124–129. [CrossRef]
9. Nance, M.L.; Adamson, W.T.; Hedrick, H.L. Appendicitis in the young child: A continuing diagnostic challenge. *Pediatr. Emerg. Care* **2000**, *16*, 160–162. [CrossRef]
10. Davenport, M. Acute abdominal pain in children. *BMJ* **1996**, *312*, 498–501. [CrossRef]
11. Narsule, C.K.; Kahle, E.J.; Kim, D.S.; Anderson, A.C.; Luks, F.I. Effect of delay in presentation on rate of perforation in children with appendicitis. *Am. J. Emerg. Med.* **2011**, *29*, 890–893. [CrossRef] [PubMed]
12. Kharbanda, A.B.; Taylor, G.A.; Fishman, S.J.; Bachur, R.G. A clinical decision rule to identify children at low risk for appendicitis. *Paediatrics* **2005**, *116*, 709–716. [CrossRef]
13. Martin, A.E.; Vollman, D.; Adler, B.; Caniano, D.A. CT scans may not reduce the negative appendectomy rate in children. *J. Pediatr. Surg.* **2004**, *39*, 886–890, discussion 886–890. [CrossRef]
14. Partrick, D.A.; Janik, J.E.; Janik, J.S.; Bensard, D.D.; Karrer, F.M. Increased CT scan utilization does not improve the diagnostic accuracy of appendicitis in children. *J. Paediatr. Surg.* **2003**, *38*, 659–662. [CrossRef] [PubMed]
15. Miglioretti, D.L.; Johnson, E.; Williams, A.; Greenlee, R.T.; Weinmann, S.; Solberg, L.I.; Feigelson, H.S.; Roblin, D.; Flynn, M.J.; Vanneman, N.; et al. The use of computed tomography in paediatrics and the associated radiation exposure and estimated cancer risk. *JAMA Paediatr.* **2013**, *167*, 700–707. [CrossRef]
16. Alvarado, A. Diagnostic Scores in Acute Appendicitis. In *Current Issues in the Diagnostics and Treatment of Acute Appendicitis*; IntechOpen: London, UK, 2018; 43p. [CrossRef]
17. de Castro, S.M.M.; Unlu, C.; Ph Steller, E.; van Wangensveld, A.; Vrouenraets, B.C. Evaluation of the appendicitis inflammatory response score for patients with acute appendicitis. *World J. Surg.* **2012**, *36*, 1540–1545. [CrossRef]
18. Di Saverio, S.; Podda, M.; De Simone, B.; Ceresoli, M.; Augustin, G.; Gori, A.; Boermeester, M.; Sartelli, M.; Coccolini, F.; Tarasconi, A.; et al. Diagnosis and treatment of acute appendicitis: 2020 update of the WSES Jerusalem guidelines. *World J. Emerg. Surg.* **2020**, *15*, 27. [CrossRef]
19. Andersson, M.; Kolodziej, B.; Andersson, R.E. Validation of the Appendicitis Inflammatory Response (AIR) Score. *World J. Surg.* **2021**, *45*, 2081–2091. [CrossRef]
20. Cartwright, S.L.; Knudson, M.P. Diagnostic imaging of acute abdominal pain in adults. *Am. Fam. Physician* **2015**, *91*, 452–459.
21. Tseng, J.; Cohen, T.; Melo, N.; Alban, R.F. Imaging utilization affects negative appendectomy rates in appendicitis: An ACS-NSQIP study. *Am. J. Surg.* **2019**, *217*, 1094–1098. [CrossRef]
22. Chiu, Y.H.; Chen, J.D.; Wang, S.H.; Tiu, C.M.; How, C.K.; Lai, J.I.; Chou, Y.H.; Chen, R.J. Whether intravenous contrast is necessary for CT diagnosis of acute appendicitis in adult ED patients? *Acad. Radiol.* **2013**, *20*, 73–78. [CrossRef] [PubMed]
23. Repplinger, M.D.; Levy, J.F.; Peethumnongsin, E.; Gussick, M.E.; Svenson, J.E.; Golden, S.K.; Ehlenbach, W.J.; Westergaard, R.P.; Reeder, S.B.; Vanness, D.J. Systematic review and meta-analysis of the accuracy of MRI to diagnose appendicitis in the general population. *J. Magn. Reason. Imaging* **2016**, *43*, 1346–1354. [CrossRef] [PubMed]
24. Xu, L.; Yang, J.-B. *Introduction to Multi-Criteria Decision Making and the Evidential Reasoning Approach*; Manchester School of Management: Manchester, UK, 2001; ISBN 186115111X.
25. Zarghami, M.; Szidarovszky, F. *Multicriteria Analysis: Applications to Water and Environment Management*; Springer: Berlin/Heidelberg, Germany, 2011.
26. Karamouz, M.; Szidarovszky, F.; Zahraie, B. *Water Resources Systems Analysis*; Lewis Publishers: Boca Raton, FL, USA, 2003.
27. Pardalos, P.M.; Hearn, D. Multi-Criteria Decision Making Methods: A Comparative Study. In *Multi-Criteria Decision Making Methods: A Comparative Study*; Springer: Boston, MA, USA, 2000.
28. Kittur, J. Using the PROMETHEE and TOPSIS multi-criteria decision making methods to evaluate optimal generation. In Proceedings of the 2015 International Conference on Power and Advanced Control Engineering (ICPACE), Bengaluru, India, 12–14 August 2015; pp. 80–85. [CrossRef]

29. El Hachami, K.; Alaoui, Y.L.; Tkiouat, M. Sectorial evaluation of islamic banking contracts: A fuzzy multi-criteria-decision-making approach. *Invest. Manag. Financ. Innov.* **2019**, *16*, 370–382. [CrossRef]
30. Brans, J.P.; Mareschal, B.; Vincke, P. Promethee: A New Family of Outranking Methods in Multicriteria Analysis. *ULB Inst. Repos.* **1984**, 477–490.
31. Uzun, B.; Yıldırım, F.S.; Sayan, M.; Şanlıdağ, T.; Ozsahin, D.U. The Use of Fuzzy PROMETHEE Technique in Antiretroviral Combination Decision in Paediatric HIV Treatments. In Proceedings of the 2019 Advances in Science and Engineering Technology International Conferences (ASET), Dubai, United Arab Emirates, 26 March–10 April 2019. [CrossRef]
32. Uzun, B.; Ozsahin, I.; Oru Agbor, V.; Uzun Ozsahin, D. Chapter 2—Theoretical aspects of multi-criteria decision-making (MCDM) methods. In *Applications of Multi-Criteria Decision-Making Theories in Healthcare and Biomedical Engineering*; Ozsahin, I., Ozsahin, D.U., Uzun, B., Eds.; Academic Press: London, UK, 2021; pp. 3–40. ISBN 9780128240861.
33. Aydin, E.; Turkmen, I.U.; Namlı, G.; Ozturk, C.; Esen, A.B.; Eray, Y.N.; Eroglu, E.; Akova, F. A novel and simple machine learning algorithm for preoperative diagnosis of acute appendicitis in children. *Pediatr. Surg. Int.* **2020**, *36*, 735–742. [CrossRef]

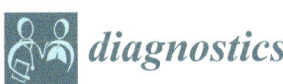

Article

Prognostic Model of ICU Admission Risk in Patients with COVID-19 Infection Using Machine Learning

Khandaker Reajul Islam [1], Jaya Kumar [1,*], Toh Leong Tan [2], Mamun Bin Ibne Reaz [3], Tawsifur Rahman [4], Amith Khandakar [4], Tariq Abbas [5], Md. Sakib Abrar Hossain [4], Susu M. Zughaier [6] and Muhammad E. H. Chowdhury [4,*]

1. Department of Physiology, Faculty of Medicine, University Kebangsaan Malaysia, Kuala Lumpur 56000, Malaysia
2. Department of Emergency Medicine, Faculty of Medicine, Universiti Kebangsaan Malaysia, Kuala Lumpur 56000, Malaysia
3. Department of Electrical, Electronics and Systems Engineering, Universiti Kebangsaan Malaysia, Bangi 43600, Malaysia
4. Department of Electrical Engineering, Qatar University, Doha P.O. Box 2713, Qatar
5. Urology Division, Surgery Department, Sidra Medicine, Doha P.O. Box 26999, Qatar
6. Department of Basic Medical Sciences, College of Medicine, QU Health, Qatar University, Doha P.O. Box 2713, Qatar
* Correspondence: jayakumar@ukm.edu.my (J.K.); mchowdhury@qu.edu.qa (M.E.H.C.)

Citation: Islam, K.R.; Kumar, J.; Tan, T.L.; Reaz, M.B.I.; Rahman, T.; Khandakar, A.; Abbas, T.; Hossain, M.S.A.; Zughaier, S.M.; Chowdhury, M.E.H. Prognostic Model of ICU Admission Risk in Patients with COVID-19 Infection Using Machine Learning. *Diagnostics* **2022**, *12*, 2144. https://doi.org/10.3390/diagnostics12092144

Academic Editor: Zhongheng Zhang

Received: 5 August 2022
Accepted: 26 August 2022
Published: 3 September 2022

Publisher's Note: MDPI stays neutral with regard to jurisdictional claims in published maps and institutional affiliations.

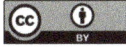

Copyright: © 2022 by the authors. Licensee MDPI, Basel, Switzerland. This article is an open access article distributed under the terms and conditions of the Creative Commons Attribution (CC BY) license (https:// creativecommons.org/licenses/by/ 4.0/).

Abstract: With the onset of the COVID-19 pandemic, the number of critically sick patients in intensive care units (ICUs) has increased worldwide, putting a burden on ICUs. Early prediction of ICU requirement is crucial for efficient resource management and distribution. Early-prediction scoring systems for critically ill patients using mathematical models are available, but are not generalized for COVID-19 and Non-COVID patients. This study aims to develop a generalized and reliable prognostic model for ICU admission for both COVID-19 and non-COVID-19 patients using best feature combination from the patient data at admission. A retrospective cohort study was conducted on a dataset collected from the pulmonology department of Moscow City State Hospital between 20 April 2020 and 5 June 2020. The dataset contains ten clinical features for 231 patients, of whom 100 patients were transferred to ICU and 131 were stable (non-ICU) patients. There were 156 COVID positive patients and 75 non-COVID patients. Different feature selection techniques were investigated, and a stacking machine learning model was proposed and compared with eight different classification algorithms to detect risk of need for ICU admission for both COVID-19 and non-COVID patients combined and COVID patients alone. C-reactive protein (CRP), chest computed tomography (CT), lung tissue affected (%), age, admission to hospital, and fibrinogen parameters at hospital admission were found to be important features for ICU-requirement risk prediction. The best performance was produced by the stacking approach, with weighted precision, sensitivity, F1-score, specificity, and overall accuracy of 84.45%, 84.48%, 83.64%, 84.47%, and 84.48%, respectively, for both types of patients, and 85.34%, 85.35%, 85.11%, 85.34%, and 85.35%, respectively, for COVID-19 patients only. The proposed work can help doctors to improve management through early prediction of the risk of need for ICU admission of patients during the COVID-19 pandemic, as the model can be used for both types of patients.

Keywords: intensive care unit; COVID-19; early prediction; machine learning; clinical biomarkers

1. Introduction

The COVID-19 pandemic began in Wuhan, China at the end of 2019, and spread quickly throughout the world [1]. Some countries experienced more than one wave of the pandemic. As of 11 July 2022, globally there have been around 560 M confirmed cases and around 6.3 M deaths caused by COVID-19 [2]. This novel coronavirus mostly affects a patient's lungs, resulting in pneumonia [3]. The majority of individuals have a mild form of the illness, with typical respiratory symptoms [4]. The most frequent clinical signs are fever and cough; however, some patients develop severe illness, which results in intensive care unit (ICU) admission and even death [5]. During the pandemic, along with the non-COVID critically ill patients, COVID-19 patients were also transferred to ICU [6], which resulted in the demand for ICU resources substantially increasing, exceeding the capacity in many healthcare systems [7]. ICUs are costly and time-sensitive resources, and if their capacity is challenged, it can have a major consequence for healthcare services [8]. In addition, as the number of critically ill patients continues to increase, their stays in the ICU have become even longer [9,10], especially during the COVID-19 situation. To solve this issue, some scoring systems have been used for the early identification of ICU requirements. Scoring techniques rely on the identification of prognostic markers associated with the severity of the disease [11]. Similar scoring systems are available for ICU admission risk prediction among non-COVID patients. Analysis of coagulation parameters has been very useful in identifying the severity of non-COVID-related pneumonia [12]. The severity of COVID-19 can also be identified from a similar analysis of blood-profile deviations, including lymphopenia, thrombocytopenia, and coagulopathies, such as prolonged prothrombin time [13–16]. However, these studies could be improved further by increasing their robustness by training on a larger dataset, and also by providing an approach that could be used for both COVID and non-COVID patients [17]. A model that can be generalized for both types of patients is not available in the literature, to the best of the authors' knowledge.

The research implication of this study is the development of a novel framework that reliably and accurately helps in calculating the risk of ICU admission among two types (COVID and non-COVID) of patients. The severity scoring systems can be used to predict adverse outcomes for initial triage and treatment [18]. This can help in the efficient management of ICU resources for timely intervention. During the peak of the pandemic, it may even be crucial to predict and manage the ICU requirement beforehand so that potential capacity challenges can be managed.

The rest of the paper is organized in the following manner: Section 1 is the introduction outlining the motivation for the study, along with the potential research implication. Section 2 summarizes the relevant works in this domain and also summarizes the contribution of this work. Section 3 provides the methodology, which includes the details of the dataset description, statistical analysis, data preprocessing, feature ranking techniques, machine learning (ML) techniques, and performance metrics used in this study. Section 4 provides the results of the investigations followed by a detailed discussion. Finally, the conclusion is provided in Section 5.

2. Related Work

Radiological images, such as chest X-rays (CXR) and computed tomography (CT) images, have been extensively used in the stratification of COVID-19 patients [19–24]. Poly et al. [25] have performed a systematic review with a meta-analysis of relevant studies to quantify the performance of deep learning algorithms in the automatic stratification of COVID-19 patients using CXR images. It is reported that the deep learning models provided satisfactory results and can be used in the fast screening of COVID-19 patients. However, these models should be further validated using independent unknown test sets. Several studies have reported the usefulness of CT images for COVID-19 detection and severity stratification and in follow-on studies. CXR- or CT-based approaches cannot be used as prognostic models.

Clinical biomarkers from electronic health records have shown great promise in developing a prognostic model and scoring technique as an early predictor of severity or mortality for COVID-19 patients [26–28]. Thus, clinical biomarkers can be used as reliable predictors for COVID-19 stratification, severity detection, and mortality risk prediction. Most importantly, these prognostic models can make reliable predictions based on the data at admission. Electronic health records have been utilized in developing machine learning models for predicting the length of stay (LOS) in patients suffering from sepsis and COVID-19 in ICU [29–32]. Alabbad et al. [33] used a random forest classifier to predict the ICU requirement of COVID-19 patients and estimated their LOS in ICU with an accuracy of 94.16%, using data from King Fahad University Hospital, Saudi Arabia. The Kuwait Progression Indicator (KPI) Score is an ICU admission risk prediction scheme for COVID-19 patients [34], which uses three biomarkers—lactic dehydrogenase (LDH), lymphocytes, and high-sensitivity C-reactive protein (hs-CRP). Yan et al. [35] were able to predict a patient's mortality with over 90% accuracy 10 days in advance. It was reported that a high LDH level is a crucial indicator for the vast majority of patients who require urgent medical care. However, it does not include any scoring system that could help doctors to objectively stratify individuals at risk. Chowdhury et al. [36] proposed a nomogram scoring system for early mortality prediction for COVID-19 patients using five biomarkers. The proposed model provided the area under the curve (AUC) of 0.961 and 0.991 for the derivation and validation cohort, respectively. However, the model requires some bio-markers that are not routinely monitored in a resource-limited setup [37]. This can pose a restriction on the wide usage of the proposed scoring system. Moreover, this is a mortality prediction system and cannot be used for ICU-admission risk prediction. Similarly, Lorenzoni et al. [38] used data from 25 ICUs from the Veneto ICU network between 28 February 2020 to 4 April 2021 to predict ICU mortality risk among COVID-19 patients. The reported performance was 0.72–0.90 on the test set, while scores of 0.75–0.85 were observed on an external validation set. Magunia et al. [39] developed a model to stratify patient risk and predict ICU survival and outcomes using data collected in a retrospective and prospective manner from different parts of Germany for COVID-19 ICU patients. Age, inflammatory and thrombotic activity, and severity of acute respiratory distress syndrome (ARDS) at ICU admission were reported as strong contributing factors.

Although machine learning approaches have been utilized for ICU admission risk prediction using clinical biomarkers [40–45], to the best of our knowledge, no machine learning model has been developed that can be applied for both COVID-19 and non-COVID patients. Identification and prioritization of the patients at high risk are essential for resource planning as well as treatment planning. Patients can be continuously monitored for ICU admission risk during their hospital stay using an easy-to-use and reliable scoring system. This proposed study can help clinicians make early predictions regarding patients at risk of ICU admission; for patients at risk of organ dysfunction, providing early treatment could save their lives. This study proposed a machine-learning-based model that can reliably predict ICU admission risk among both COVID-19 and non-COVID patients using patient data at hospital admission. This work may help in the development of a framework of prognostic models using machine learning approaches, adding to the body of knowledge.

3. Materials and Methods

The methodology adopted in the study is presented in this section. The study attempted to investigate ICU admission risk prediction for (i) both COVID-19 and non-COVID-19 patients and (ii) COVID-19 patients only. For both experiments, the impacts of combined features and individual features were investigated in terms of ICU prediction. Firstly, different imputation techniques were used in a preprocessing step to impute the missing data. This missing data imputation technique is very common in clinical studies.

After preprocessing the dataset, three different feature selection methods (Pearson correlation coefficient, chi-square test, and recursive feature elimination) were used for ranking all the parameters in the dataset. Later on, these three techniques were combined to rank the features using the combined scores from three models. A stacking ML model was proposed and compared with the different ML classifiers to predict ICU-requirement risk among COVID-19 and Non-COVID patients. The dataset was divided into training, validation, and testing sets, where the training and validation sets were used to determine the best-performing combination of (i) imputation technique, (ii) combination of features using the feature ranking techniques, and (iii) machine learning model. The testing set was used to state the classification performance. The details of the complete methodology are provided below and can also be referred to in Figure 1.

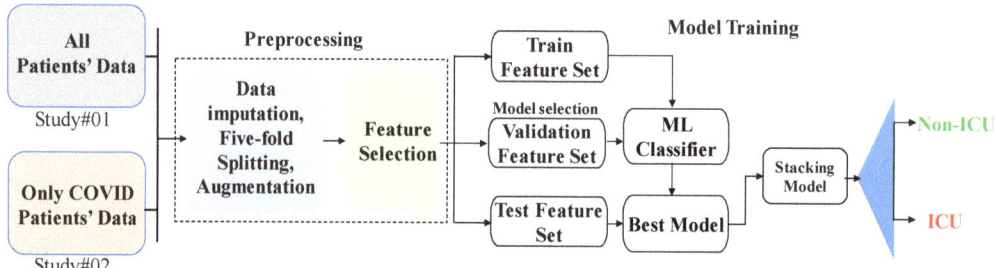

Figure 1. Methodology of the study.

3.1. Study Population

In this study, we used a dataset that contained COVID-19 and non-COVID-19 patients' data collected from the pulmonology department of Moscow City State Hospital between 20 April 2020 and 5 June 2020 [46]. The dataset contained data from 231 patients; among them, 100 patients were transferred to ICU and 131 patients were non-ICU patients. Of the 231 patients, 156 patients were COVID-19-positive and 75 patients were COVID-19-negative.

Among the COVID-19 patients, confirmed by real-time reverse-transcriptase–polymerase-chain-reaction (RT-PCR) assay of nasal and pharyngeal swab probes, 82 developed refractory respiratory failure (RRF) or severe acute respiratory distress syndrome (SARDS) and were transferred to ICU, and 74 patients had a stable course of the disease and were not transferred to ICU, as shown in Figure 2. Clinical, radiological, and laboratory parameters present upon admission were extracted from electronic health records (EHR). Some of the parameters were present for longitudinal evaluation. However, since all the parameters were not collected longitudinally, longitudinal data could not be considered for the investigation. Only data present at hospital admission were considered. Patients who regularly received anticoagulant therapy before admission, as well as patients with pregnancy (or in lactation period), oncological diseases (in the last 5 years), chronic liver diseases, human immunodeficiency virus (HIV) infection, syphilis, or hepatitis, were excluded from the study.

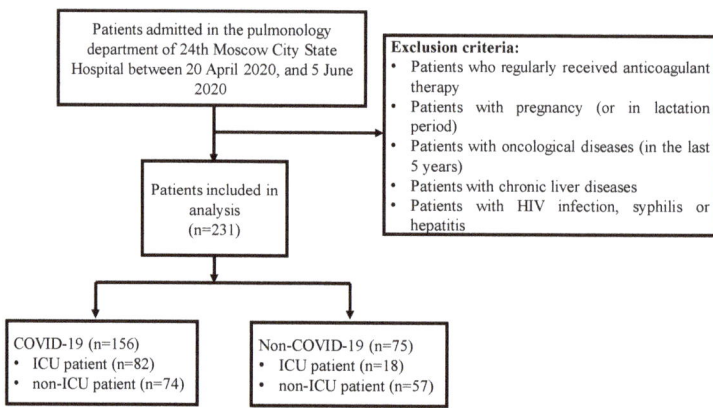

Figure 2. Population details of the study.

Figure 3 shows the distribution of nine features in the dataset: (i) Gender; (ii) Age; (iii) Admission2Hosp (admission to hospital); (iv) CRP (C-Reactive Protein); (v) INR (international normalized ratio); (vi) PT (Prothrombin Time); (vii) Fibrinogen; (viii) Chest CT lung tissue affected, and (ix) Platelet count for ICU and non-ICU patients. The distribution plots confirm that the values for the features were well distributed. For example, the dataset contained patients of all ages, with a higher number of patients in ICU being over 70 years of age while for non-ICU, the average was 60 years. Similarly, CRP among the ICU-patients showed a significantly different distribution compared to that for non-ICU patients. Prothrombin time for the patients varied from 10 to 20 s, with most of the patients having a prothrombin time of around 13 s for both ICU and non-ICU patients. Figure 4 shows the details of demographic variations (age and gender) between the ICU and non-ICU patients. Patients from both categories (ICU and non-ICU patients) are normally distributed among males and females.

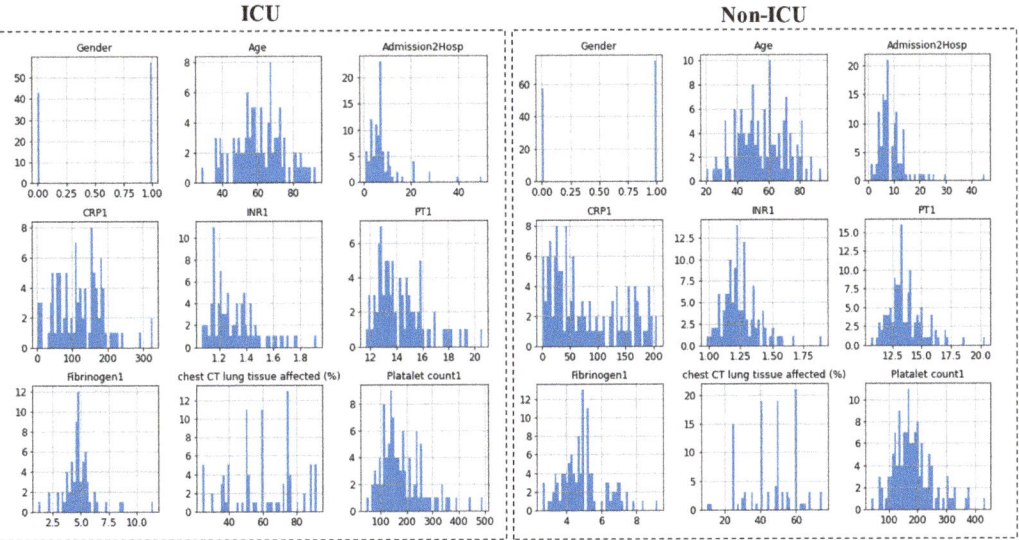

Figure 3. Histogram plots depicting the distributions of nine features at admission among the ICU and non-ICU patients. Here, '0' represents 'female' and '1' represents 'male'.

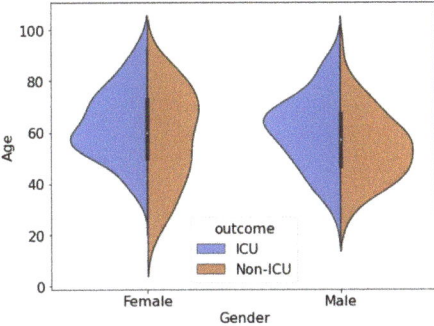

Figure 4. Demographic feature (gender and age) distributions for ICU and non-ICU cases. The blue and orange areas correspond to negative and positive cases, respectively.

3.2. Statistical Analysis

Statistical analysis was performed using Python programming language (version 3.7, Creator-Guido van Rossum, The Netherland), where the chi-square univariate test and rank-sum test were conducted to identify the statistically significantly different features among the ICU and Non-ICU (stable) groups. The difference was considered significant if the *p*-value was <0.05. Table 1 summarizes continuous variables, age, and other clinical data reported with a mean and standard deviation of the data, and frequency for each biomarker among the ICU and Non-ICU groups.

Table 1. Statistical characteristic analysis of all patients in ICU and Non-ICU groups using the dataset.

Item	ICU	Non-ICU	Total	Method	χ^2 = 17.5	*p* Value
Gender						
Male (%)	57 (57%)	74 (56.5%)	131 (57%)	Chi-square test	χ^2 = 17.5	<0.05 *
Female (%)	43 (43%)	57 (43.5%)	100 (43%)			
Age (years)						
N(missing)	100 (0)	131 (0)	231 (0)			
Mean ± SD	61.6 ± 13.8	55.9 ± 15.7	58.4 ± 15.1	Rank-sum test	Z = −6.2	<0.05 *
Q1, Q3	53, 70.2	44, 68.5	48.0, 69.0			
Min, Max	28, 93	20, 94	20, 94			
The time between the disease and admission to hospital (Admission 2Hospital) (Days)						
N(missing)	99 (1)	128 (3)	227 (4)	Rank-sum test	Z = −6.2	<0.05 *
Mean ± SD	7.9 ± 7.45	9.1 ± 5.68	8.6 ± 6.53			
Q1, Q3	4, 8	6, 11	5.0, 10.0			
Min, Max	1, 50	1, 45	1, 50			
C-reactive protein 1(CRP1) (mg/L)						
N(missing)	97 (3)	128 (3)	225 (6)			
Mean ± SD	123 ± 67.1	78 ± 61.7	97 ± 67.9	Rank-sum test	Z = −4.34	<0.05 *
Q1, Q3	64, 166	26, 134	40, 157			
Min, Max	4, 328	1, 207	1, 328			
International normalized ratio (INR)						
N(missing)	86 (14)	122 (9)	208 (23)			
Mean ± SD	1.32 ± 0.18	1.25 ± 0.14	1.28 ± 0.16	Rank-sum test	Z = 6.53	0.78
Q1, Q3	1.17, 1.4	1.16, 1.3	1.17, 1.36			
Min, max	1.07, 1.92	0.98, 1.9	0.98, 1.92			
Prothrombin time 1 (PT1) (s)						
N(missing)	86 (14)	122 (9)	208 (23)			
Mean ± SD	14.39 ± 1.91	13.63 ± 1.52	13.95 ± 1.73	Rank-sum test	Z = 3.27	<0.05 *
Q1, Q3	12.9, 15.3	12.7, 14.2	12.8, 14.9			
Min, max	11.7, 20.6	10.7, 20.4	10.7, 20.6			
Fibrinogen 1 (mg/L)						
N(missing)	68 (32)	113 (18)	181 (50)			
Mean ± SD	4.9 ± 1.44	4.99 ± 1.25	4.9 ± 1.32	Rank-sum test	Z = −5.89	<0.05 *
Q1, Q3	4.2, 5.3	4.18, 5.45	4.2, 5.4			
Min, max	1.2, 11.5	2.68, 9.21	1.2, 11.5			
Chest CT lung tissue affected (%)						
N(missing)	88 (12)	110 (21)	198 (33)			
Mean ± SD	59.9 ± 19	46.1 ± 14.1	52.2 ± 17.8	Rank-sum test	Z = −1.11	<0.05 *
Q1, Q3	49.5, 75	40, 60	40, 60			
Min, max	24, 92	10, 75	10, 92			
Platelet count 1 (10^9/L)						
N(missing)	100 (0)	131 (0)	231 (0)			
Mean ± SD	182 ± 83.2	183 ± 68.8	183 ± 75.2	Rank-sum test	Z = 4.74	0.44
Q1, Q3	126, 233	138, 216	129, 219			
Min, max	47, 493	38, 436	38, 493			
Outcome	100 (43%)	131 (57%)	231 (100%)			

* *p* value less than 0.05 is significant.

3.3. Data Preprocessing

3.3.1. Missing Data Imputation

Only the first-day data were used for model training and validation in identifying the primary predictors for ICU admission. Figure 5 shows the count of different features in the dataset, and it can be seen that some parameters were missing for some patients, such as the time between the disease onset and admission to the hospital (days), CRP1, prothrombin time upon admission (PT1 in second), fibrinogen upon admission (Fibrinogen1), and lung tissue affected (%) from chest computed tomography (CT).

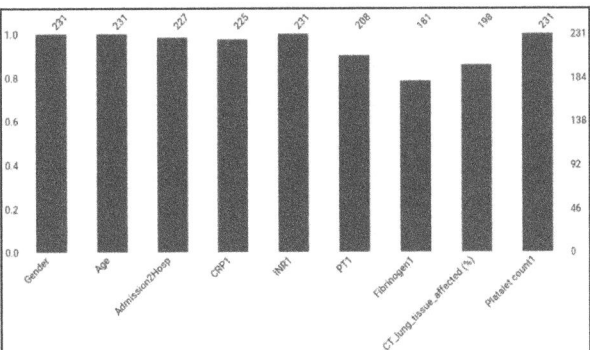

Figure 5. Count of different features in the dataset.

Missing data issues are a constant challenge in clinical data analysis, and this can lead to biased models or degraded model performance. Similarly, a model can produce a biased result if the rows of the missing data are deleted from the study [47]. In this study, three common imputation techniques to tackle the missing data problem were investigated: (i) multiple imputations using the chained equations (MICE) [45], (ii) random forest [48,49], and (iii) nearest neighbor [50] imputation techniques. One of the most common techniques for clinical data imputation is the MICE data imputation technique, which uses logistic regression for binary variables and statistical mean matching for continuous variables. On the other hand, the random forest algorithm has a built-in routine to handle the values that are missing by weighing the frequency of values with the proximity of a random forest after the training of an initially imputed mean dataset. This approach requires a response variable that is useful for random forest training. K-nearest neighbor can predict both discrete attributes (the most frequent value among the k-nearest neighbors) and continuous attributes (the mean among the k-nearest neighbors). The k-nearest neighbor can be easily adapted to work with any attribute as a class, by just modifying which attributes will be considered in the distance metric.

3.3.2. Balancing the Dataset

An imbalanced dataset can result in a biased model, and therefore, the dataset needs to be balanced. The synthetic minority oversampling technique (SMOTE) is a powerful approach to tackling the imbalance problem [51]. This study investigated two different phases. Firstly, all data were used to predict ICU-admission-risk patients, where ICU and non-ICU patients were 100 and 131, respectively. For the investigation with only COVID-19 patients, ICU and non-ICU patients numbered 82 and 74, respectively. SMOTE technique was used to balance the dataset for different investigations. Rather than using simple replication of minor class data using an over-sampling technique, SMOTE was used to create synthetic data to avoid data imbalance among the classes.

3.4. Feature Reduction

Nine different features were present in the dataset. After preprocessing, the correlation among different features was checked to identify and remove highly correlated features, as removing them has always helped in improving the classifier performance in the author's previous works [52,53]. As seen in Figure 6, there was no high correlation between the features, and all the features could be used in this study.

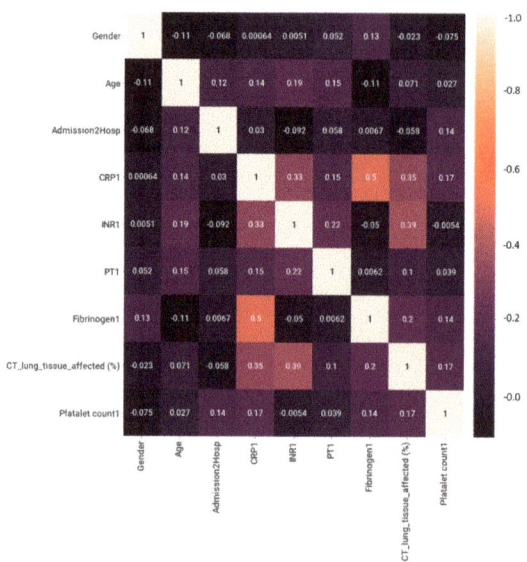

Figure 6. Color map of correlation among different features.

3.5. Feature Selection

In this study, three different feature selection techniques, namely the chi-square test [54], Pearson correlation coefficient [55], and recursive feature elimination (RFE) [56], were used for detecting ICU admission risk. Additionally, we utilized an average of the feature importance score as a threshold for choosing the features for each technique, after calculating the feature importance score for each feature using each of the three feature selection techniques. Finally, we chose the features for the classification model that exceeded the threshold (feature importance score ≥ 3) for all three feature selection procedures.

3.6. Stacking-Based Machine Learning Model

The study proposed a stacking-based approach and compared the performance with conventional ML classifiers. This approach consisted of a two-step learner comprising a base learner and meta learner; this approach has produced good results in the author's previous works [20,53,57]. Eight different ML classifiers were investigated in this study, namely random forest [45], support vector machine (SVM) [46], K-nearest neighbor (KNN) [47], XGBoost [48], extra trees [43], gradient boosting [49], MLP [50], and logistic regression [50]. Three feature selection strategies were used to choose the top features, which were then used to compare the different classifiers' performance. The stacking architecture was used on the three top-performing classifiers (C_1, C_2, C_3) as the base-learner model, and logistic regression was used as the meta-learner model (C_f) in the second phase of the stacking model to provide the best performance. Figure 7 shows the architecture of the proposed stacking model, which combines n numbers of best-performing classifiers $C, \ldots, C_n$ using an input dataset D, which had a feature vector (x_i) and corresponding label (y_i). In the first step, N base level ML classifier produced the prediction probabilities $y_1, \ldots, y_p$.

Finally, the prediction probabilities of the best performing base learners fed to a logistic regression-based meta-learner classifier (C_f) for the final prediction.

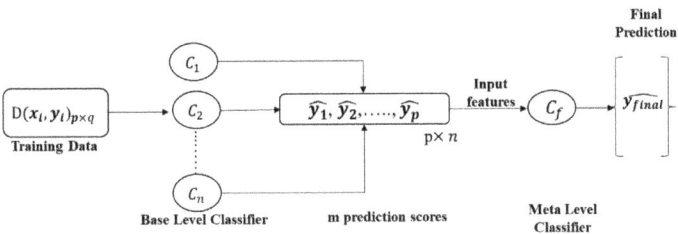

Figure 7. Proposed stacking model architecture.

3.7. Development and Validation of Classification Model

In this study, various machine learning models were examined using 5-fold cross-validation, where 80% of the subjects' data were used in training and validation and 20% were used in the testing set for a single fold. This was repeated 5-fold, with a new test set on each fold. Several performance criteria, such as sensitivity, specificity, precision, accuracy, and F1-score, were used to assess the performance of several models on the test dataset. Mathematical representations of the different metrics are shown in Equations (1)–(5). The areas under the curve (AUC) for individual predictors, as well as combinations of them, were assessed to ascertain how well-ranked parameters performed in stratifying ICU and non-ICU patients. The performances of unseen (test) folds were combined to create the overall confusion matrix for the 5-fold cross-validation. It is worth noting that leave-one-out cross-validation (LOOCV) was also investigated, where all the subjects apart from one were used for training and validation while one subject's data were used in testing, and the procedure was repeated based on the number of subjects in the experiment.

$$\text{Accuracy} = \frac{(TP + TN)}{(TP + FN) + (FP + TN)} \qquad (1)$$

$$\text{Sensitivity} = \frac{(TP)}{(TP + FN)} \qquad (2)$$

$$\text{Specificity} = \frac{(TN)}{(FP + TN)} \qquad (3)$$

$$\text{Precision} = \frac{(TP)}{(TP + FP)} \qquad (4)$$

$$\text{F1 Score} = \frac{(2*TP)}{(2*TP + FN + FP)} \qquad (5)$$

The number of patients with ICU outcomes classified as ICU is denoted as True Positive (TP), the number of non-ICU patients identified as Non-ICU is denoted as True Negative (TN), the number of non-ICU patients incorrectly identified as ICU is denoted as False Positive (FP), and the number of ICU patients incorrectly identified as Non-ICU is denoted as False Negative (FN). The performance of the ML classifier was assessed using different evaluation metrics with 95% confidence intervals (CIs), calculated using Equation (6).

$$r = z\sqrt{metric(1 - metric)/N} \qquad (6)$$

where, N is the number of test samples and z is the level of significance that is 1.96 for 95% CI.

4. Results

4.1. Characteristics and Outcomes

Two different investigations were conducted in this study: (i) an investigation of the ICU admission risk of all patients (n = 231), where 156 patients were COVID-19-positive and 75 were COVID-19-negative, and (ii) an investigation of the ICU admission risk of COVID-19-positive (n = 156) patients alone. Each investigation was used to identify the best feature combination and individual best feature for detecting ICU admission risk using eight different machine learning classifiers. Three different imputation techniques were used in this study, where the MICE data imputation technique outperformed KNN and random forest for identifying the best feature combination from the ranked features in both investigations. It was found that age, gender, admission-to-hospital time, CRP, fibrinogen, chest CT lung tissue affected (%), and PT had statistically significant differences between ICU and non-ICU groups, while differences between INR and platelet count were statistically insignificant across the groups (Table 1).

4.2. Best Feature Combination for Early Prediction of ICU

In both experiments, three different feature selection approaches were used to select a feature combination supported by all these techniques. All of the three feature selection techniques selected five features—CRP, chest CT lung tissue affected (%), age, admission to hospital, and fibrinogen to classify ICU and non-ICU patients, as shown in Table 2.

Table 2. Ranked Features by different algorithms.

Features	Pearson Correlation Coefficient	Chi-Square Test	Recursive Feature Elimination	Total
CRP	✓	✓	✓	3
Chest CT lung tissue affected (%)	✓	✓	✓	3
Age	✓	✓	✓	3
Admission2Hospital	✓	✓	✓	3
Fibrinogen	✓	✓	✓	3
Platelet Count	✓	✓		2
Gender		✓	✓	2
PT	✓		✓	2
INR	✓		✓	2

4.3. Development and Validation of the Stacking Model

The five selected features were used in both the investigations using the eight different ML classifiers, and then the stacking approach was implemented to boost the performance further. A logistic regression model was used as a meta-learner in the stacking model. The top three performing classifiers were random forest, gradient boosting, and extra trees. The accuracies obtained from these models were 82.33%, 81.03%, and 79.74% respectively, as shown in Table 3. These three models were used to train the meta-learners logistic regression classifier, which boosted the performance and provided weighted precision, sensitivity, F1-score, specificity, and accuracy of about 84.45%, 84.48%, 83.64%, 84.47%, and 84.48%, respectively. It is evident from Table 3 that the stacking approach improved the accuracy by more than 2%. With 90% AUC, the stacking approach clearly outperforms other ML classifiers, as can be seen in Figure 8.

Table 3. Performance comparison between different ML classifiers using all (both COVID-19 and non-COVID-19) patients' data.

Classifier	Overall	Weighted with 95% CI			
	Accuracy	Precision	Sensitivity	Specificity	F1-Score
Support Vector Machine (SVM)	61.21 ± 1.99	63.17 ± 1.97	61.21 ± 1.99	63.09 ± 1.97	61.29 ± 1.99
XGBoost (XGB)	65.52 ± 1.94	65.92 ± 1.93	65.52 ± 1.94	65.15 ± 1.94	65.64 ± 1.94
MLP	71.12 ± 1.85	70.98 ± 1.85	71.12 ± 1.85	69.4 ± 1.88	71.02 ± 1.85
Logistic Regression (LR)	71.12 ± 1.85	70.92 ± 1.85	71.12 ± 1.85	68.67 ± 1.89	70.86 ± 1.85
K-Nearest Neighbors (KNN)	71.55 ± 1.84	71.55 ± 1.84	71.55 ± 1.84	70.45 ± 1.86	71.55 ± 1.84
Extra Trees (ET)	79.74 ± 1.64	79.68 ± 1.64	79.74 ± 1.64	78.11 ± 1.69	79.64 ± 1.64
Gradient Boosting (GB)	81.03 ± 1.6	80.98 ± 1.6	81.04 ± 1.6	79.81 ± 1.64	80.98 ± 1.6
Random Forest (RF)	82.33 ± 1.56	82.33 ± 1.56	82.33 ± 1.56	80.55 ± 1.61	82.2 ± 1.56
Stacking model (RF+ GB+ ET)	**84.48 ± 1.48**	**84.45 ± 1.48**	**84.48 ± 1.48**	**83.64 ± 1.51**	**84.47 ± 1.48**

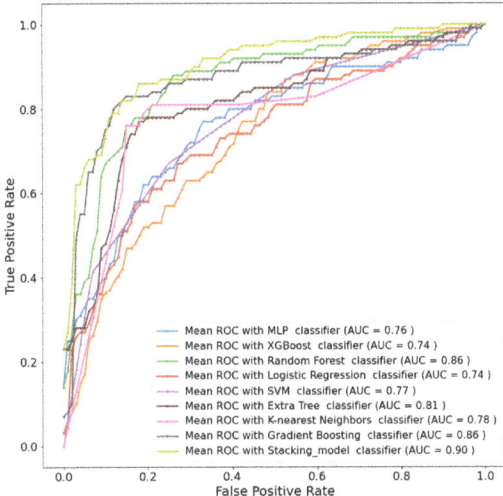

Figure 8. ROC curves using all (both COVID-19 and non-COVID-19) patients' data.

Similarly, for COVID-19 patients only, random forest, extra trees, and K-nearest neighbors were the top three performing classifiers. The accuracies obtained from these models were 83.44%, 82.8%, and 82.17%, as shown in Table 4. The stacking model employed a logistic regression model as a meta-learner. This approach boosted the performance to weighted precision, sensitivity, F1-score, specificity, and overall accuracy of 85.34%, 85.35%, 85.11%, 85.34%, and 85.35%, respectively. Table 4 shows an overall improvement in accuracy of 2% using the stacking model. With 91% AUC, the stacking approach clearly outperforms other ML classifiers, as can be seen in Figure 9.

Figure 10 shows the confusion matrix for the best-performing stacking model to identify ICU risk patients using all (both COVID-19 and non-COVID-19) patients' data and using only COVID-19 patients' data. In Figure 10A it is clearly shown that the stacking model correctly identified 81 out of 100 ICU patients from both COVID-19 and non-COVID-19 patients, while the stacking model correctly identified 71 out of 82 COVID-19 ICU patients (Figure 10B).

Table 4. Performance comparison between different ML classifiers using only COVID-19 patient data.

Classifier	Overall		Weighted with 95% CI		
	Accuracy	Precision	Sensitivity	Specificity	F1-Score
XGBoost (XGB)	67.52 ± 2.32	67.86 ± 2.32	67.52 ± 2.32	67.82 ± 2.32	67.56 ± 2.32
Support Vector Machine (SVM)	71.97 ± 2.23	72.4 ± 2.22	71.97 ± 2.23	72.42 ± 2.22	72 ± 2.23
MLP	77.71 ± 2.07	77.92 ± 2.06	77.71 ± 2.07	77.93 ± 2.06	77.73 ± 2.06
Gradient Boosting (GB)	78.98 ± 2.02	79.34 ± 2.01	78.98 ± 2.02	79.4 ± 2.01	79 ± 2.02
Logistic Regression (LR)	80.25 ± 1.98	80.25 ± 1.98	80.25 ± 1.98	79.97 ± 1.99	80.25 ± 1.98
K-Nearest Neighbors (KNN)	82.17 ± 1.9	82.26 ± 1.9	82.16 ± 1.9	81.45 ± 1.93	82.09 ± 1.9
Extra Tree (ET)	82.80 ± 1.87	82.90 ± 1.87	82.80 ± 1.87	82.90 ± 1.87	82.82 ± 1.87
Random Forest (RF)	83.44 ± 1.84	83.49 ± 1.84	83.44 ± 1.84	83.45 ± 1.84	83.45 ± 1.84
Stacking model (RF + ET + KNN)	**85.35 ± 1.75**	**85.34 ± 1.76**	**85.35 ± 1.75**	**85.11 ± 1.77**	**85.34 ± 1.76**

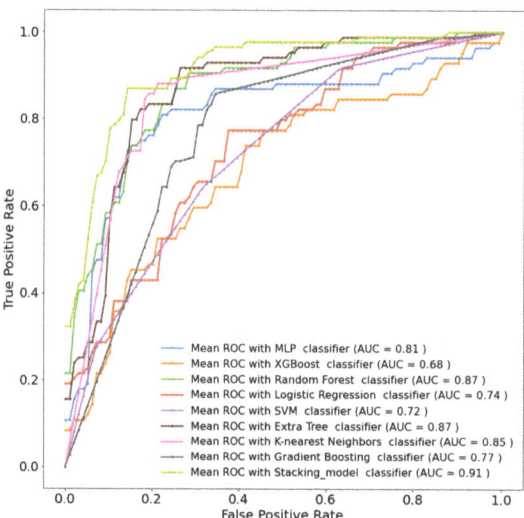

Figure 9. ROC curves using only COVID-19 patient data.

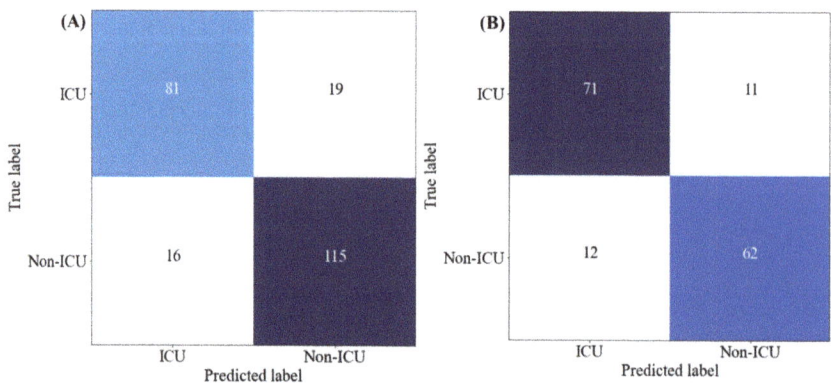

Figure 10. Confusion matrix for ICU and Non-ICU classification using the best performing stacking model for (**A**) all (both COVID-19 and non-COVID-19) patients' data, and (**B**) only COVID-19 patient data.

4.4. Individual Feature as ICU Admission Predictor

The study also investigated individual feature performance with the best-performing stacking classification model to ascertain the top individual feature simultaneously for all (both COVID-19 and non-COVID-19) patients and only COVID-19 patients.

For both COVID-19 and non-COVID-19 patients, chest CT lung tissue affected (%) is the most important feature for the stacking classifier. Table 5A provides the performance metrics with a 95% confidence interval to identify the contribution of the individual features. Chest CT lung tissue affected (%) produced the best performance with overall accuracy and weighted precision, sensitivity, specificity, and F1-score of 74.43%, 77.65%, 74.43%, 74.43%, and 71.75%, respectively.

Table 5. Comparison of performance evaluation parameters to identify the best classifier for individual feature impact to predict ICU admission risk patients using (**A**) both COVID-19 and non-COVID-19 patients' data, and (**B**) only COVID-19 patients' data.

(A)					
	95% Confidence Interval Results				
Feature	Overall Accuracy	Weighted Precision	Weighted Recall	Weighted Specificity	Weighted F1-Score
CRP	71.11 ± 1.85	70.56 ± 1.86	71.11 ± 1.85	71.11 ± 1.85	70.58 ± 1.86
Chest CT lung tissue affected (%)	**74.43 ± 1.78**	**77.65 ± 1.7**	**74.43 ± 1.78**	**74.43 ± 1.78**	**71.75 ± 1.84**
Age	61.01 ± 1.99	36.46 ± 1.96	61.01 ± 1.99	61.01 ± 1.99	45.34 ± 2.03
Admission2Hospital	62.41 ± 1.98	37.86 ± 1.98	62.41 ± 1.98	62.41 ± 1.98	46.74 ± 2.03
Fibrinogen	65.31 ± 1.98	65.62 ± 1.97	65.31 ± 1.98	65.31 ± 1.98	65.47 ± 2.04
Platelet Count	67.01 ± 1.92	42.46 ± 2.02	67.01 ± 1.92	67.01 ± 1.92	51.34 ± 2.04
Gender	64.21 ± 1.95	61.51 ± 1.98	64.21 ± 1.95	64.21 ± 1.95	62.65 ± 2.04
PT	57.91 ± 1.9	43.36 ± 2.02	57.91 ± 1.9	57.91 ± 1.9	52.24 ± 2.04
INR	59.81 ± 2	35.26 ± 1.95	59.81 ± 2	59.81 ± 2	44.14 ± 2.02
(B)					
	95% Confidence Interval Results				
Feature	Overall Accuracy	Weighted Precision	Weighted Recall	Weighted Specificity	Weighted F1-Score
CRP	64.29 ± 2.38	64.6 ± 2.37	64.29 ± 2.38	64.29 ± 2.38	64.29 ± 2.38
Chest CT lung tissue affected (%)	68.77 ± 2.3	71.79 ± 2.23	68.77 ± 2.3	68.77 ± 2.3	67.88 ± 2.32
Age	55.95 ± 2.46	56.51 ± 2.46	55.95 ± 2.46	55.95 ± 2.46	55.75 ± 2.46
Admission2Hospital	**73.9 ± 2.18**	**73.99 ± 2.18**	**73.9 ± 2.18**	**73.9 ± 2.18**	**73.92 ± 2.18**
Fibrinogen	57.24 ± 2.46	57.15 ± 2.46	57.24 ± 2.46	57.24 ± 2.46	57.17 ± 2.46
Platelet Count	47.62 ± 2.48	47.96 ± 2.48	47.62 ± 2.48	47.62 ± 2.48	47.2 ± 2.48
Gender	52.75 ± 2.48	53.19 ± 2.48	52.75 ± 2.48	52.75 ± 2.48	52.57 ± 2.48
PT	51.47 ± 2.48	50.64 ± 2.48	51.47 ± 2.48	51.47 ± 2.48	50.43 ± 2.48
INR	53.39 ± 2.48	53.68 ± 2.47	53.39 ± 2.48	53.39 ± 2.48	53.37 ± 2.48

By contrast, for COVID-19 patients, the time between the disease onset and admission to the hospital (days) was the most important feature for the stacking classifier. Table 5B shows the overall accuracies and weighted average performance with a 95% confidence interval for the other matrices to identify the contribution of individual features using all features for five-fold cross-validation with the best performing classifier. The time between the disease onset and admission to the hospital (days) produced the best performance, with overall accuracy, weighted precision, sensitivity, specificity, and F1-score of 73.9%, 73.99%, 73.9%, 73.9%, and 73.92%, respectively. We also developed and validated all ML models and stacking approaches with the leave-one-out cross-validation (LOOCV) approach, and compared the performances. Supplementary Tables S1 and S2 represent the performances of all models for the two different studies using the LOOCV approach. The stacking approach produced the best performance for both studies, which was comparable with the five-fold CV (see Tables 3 and 4 for five-fold CV results). However, the experimental time for the stacking model with the LOOCV technique was 25–30 times longer than the five-fold CV technique.

5. Discussion

The primary goal of the present study was to accurately identify the ICU admission risk of the hospital patients on the first day of hospital admission using a few clinical parameters. In addition to this, the correlation between ICU admission risk and clinical data for both COVID-19-positive and negative patients and COVID-19-positive patients alone was also investigated. Based on all patients' data, it was found that five important features (chest CT lung tissue affected (%), CRP, fibrinogen, age, and admission-to-hospital time) in combination performed better than others, and produced 84.48% sensitivity using the stacking model. Similarly, for COVID-19-positive patients alone, it was found that these five features combined using the stacking model outperformed other ML classifiers and produced 85.35% sensitivity. It is evident from this study that for all data or data from COVID patients alone, carefully selected multiple parameters can provide better sensitivity in predicting the ICU admission risk.

In addition, the most important individual feature for detecting ICU admission risk using combined and COVID-19 patients' data was also investigated. Based on all patients' data, it was found that the most impactful feature was the chest CT lung tissue affected (%) which individually can predict ICU patients with 74.43% sensitivity. In [46], it was reported that prothrombin time is a good predictor of ICU admission risk; however, in this study, it was found that PT was a weak predictor, with 57.91% prediction sensitivity for the combined data. For COVID-19-positive patients alone, the time between the disease onset and admission to the hospital (days) was the most impactful feature, individually predicting ICU admission risk with 73.9% sensitivity, while CRP predicted with 64.29% sensitivity. As reported in [46], PT is a good predictor, but this was not observed in this study. Therefore, it is evident that machine-learning-based study can provide better prediction accuracy in comparison to standard statistical analysis. Moreover, the parameters found to be strong contributors in this machine-learning-based study were also reported in other recent studies as strong contributors for COVID mortality prediction, which is highly related to ICU admission risk prediction.

Age is one of the most commonly agreed risk factors for predicting the outcomes and severity of COVID-19, where patients older than 60 years of age have the highest fatality rates [58]. This is related to the associated risk factors in this particular age group, including renal disease, coronary heart disease/cerebrovascular disease, hypertension, diabetes, low immunity, and previous respiratory disease. Likewise, patients with older age (>60 years) and comorbidity had worse outcomes in severe acute respiratory syndrome (SARS) [59]. However, in this dataset, this trend was not evident, which could be because this dataset was small and the ICU patient group had a widely distributed age range. If this model can be validated on a large population, the effect of age will be pronounced, and the model performance could be further enhanced.

Several reports have shown a trend toward abnormal hemostasis and coagulation profile in patients with COVID-19 [5]. Hospitalized patients with particularly higher levels of fibrinogen and D-dimer typically develop disseminated intravascular coagulation and lung embolism, and also have worse outcomes [14,60]. Higher serum fibrinogen levels were noted in patients in the early stages of acute respiratory distress syndrome (ARDS). However, these factors were typically explored after hospitalization and were not used as early predictors to determine the patients with potentially severe forms of COVID-19 based on their initial presentation [61]. Hospitalized patients with severe COVID 19 show a trend toward hyperfibrinolysis and loss of coagulation factor (fibrinogen). Furthermore, fibrinogen is an acute phase reactant that increases during infection and provokes hypercoagulation. It is a glycoprotein that covers fibrin when exposed to thrombin leads to clot formation to stop bleeding. Zou et al. [30] concluded that fibrinogen greater than 7.0 g/L is more prevalent in patients with severe COVID-19 disease (around 19.1%) compared to patients with mild COVID-19 disease (around 5.7%). At later stages of the disease, fibrinogen levels decrease, and fibrinogen less than 2.0 g/L is considered an indicator of thromboprophylaxis and cause for hospital admission [62]. In the current study, since we used the data at admission, most of the patients were not severe at that time, and therefore, while fibrinogen was found to be a useful predictor, it was not the best predictor. However, if we had had longitudinal data, we could have evaluated the model performance when the patients were admitted to ICU.

Serum C-reactive protein (CRP) is a critical indicator that changes considerably in patients with severe COVID-19 [30]. CRP is an early marker of inflammation and infection and is produced by the liver [63]. CRP binds to phosphocholine, which is expressed on the surfaces of damaged cells and which modulates phagocytic activities [64]. It was found that CRP changes significantly at the early stages of the disease in patients with COVID-19, as reported previously [15], and patients who died from the disease had levels of serum CRP 10 times greater in comparison to those who recovered [16]. This is in line with the finding of this study. In both of the investigations, CRP was found to be an important biomarker.

Chest CT is a widely available and noninvasive modality for pneumonia detection and monitoring. When RT-PCR was utilized as the gold standard tool, CT chest was shown to have 97% sensitivity and 68% accuracy in diagnosing COVID-19 [14]. Furthermore, follow-up CT chest showed that 42% of the patients had their lung abnormalities resolved before RT-PCR became negative [14]. Furthermore, CT chest is effective in diagnosing COVID in the absence of symptoms, and is considered an early marker for possible worsening of disease severity [65]. Likewise, changes in CT findings were shown to be an early predictor for speeding up the diagnostic workup in symptomatic patients [66]. The typical findings include bilateral, multi-lobe, posterior peripheral ground-glass opacities, as defined by the Radiological Society of North America (RSNA) Consensus statement [67]. Several CT severity scoring systems are valid for evaluating disease severity and burden [68,69]. It is evident from the above discussion that lung infection manifestation is a vital parameter for later-stage COVID-19 infection detection and quantification. However, in the early infection stage, it could be a good predictor for COVID-19 patients, but not the best predictor.

Predicting the ICU risk for patients when they are admitted to the hospital can greatly aid the hospital management team in allocating the proper resources to the appropriate patient during a crisis. Ineffective management of resources and distribution during the early stages of the pandemic in many countries has led to extremely high patient mortality rates as no ML-based prediction tool was used. In contrast, patients who do not require ICU admission but who are at risk can receive care in the special ward, lessening the strain on hospitals and healthcare facilities. The proposed model is deployed as a web application that can be used by clinicians. The details of the deployment are outside of the scope of this work; however, the link (https://qu-mlg.com/projects/qu-ukm-icucare, accessed on 1 March 2022) is shared here, so that clinicians and interested readers can use it.

The limitation of the proposed tool is that it takes into consideration several clinical and biological parameters and does not integrate symptoms, vitals, and treatments, and therefore, has a risk of bias. The model presented in this work utilizes several clinical variables that can be acquired in most clinics and hospitals, making this work potentially suitable for deployment in a wide range of patient evaluations. However, some further useful biomarkers (e.g., procalcitonin, D-dimers, neutrophils, lymphocytes, etc.) could be investigated, as these were not present in this dataset. Lastly, the number of patients studied was not high, which may cause the developed model to be less generalizable. The

6. Conclusions

In conclusion, the proposed model in this study can predict the ICU admission risk for patients with good discrimination for COVID-19 or non-COVID patients, with 90% AUC, and with 91% AUC for COVID-19 cases alone. Five predictors (chest CT lung tissue affected (%), CRP, fibrinogen, age, and admission-to-hospital time) were required for both studies. The model can predict the risk of admission to ICU based on the hospital admission data; i.e., predicting it much earlier than the real clinical outcome. This study evaluated the various combinations of feature selection approaches, features, and machine learning classifiers. Classical machine learning classifiers are computationally inexpensive and easy to deploy [52], while they can provide better performance in tabular values, such as the data from electronic health records (EHRs). Thus, the proposed study can help physicians in patient stratification in the early stages, which will ultimately facilitate better and more efficient resource management and thereby lessen strain on healthcare resources, reducing mortality risk by supporting seriously ill patients earlier. The proposed framework is deployed as a web application, which can be easily used by clinicians. Considering the potential of this application for pandemic/non-pandemic situations, the authors plan to collect more patient data from the Hamad General Hospital (HGH) to make the model more generalized, and to externally validate the model on a larger dataset. The authors will also continue to work on making the model robust and suitable for a different population.

Supplementary Materials: The following supporting information can be downloaded at: https://www.mdpi.com/article/10.3390/diagnostics12092144/s1, Table S1: Performance comparison between different ML classifiers using all (both COVID-19 and non-COVID-19) patients' data with LOOCV. Table S2: Performance comparison between different ML classifiers using only COVID-19 patient data with LOOCV.

Author Contributions: Conceptualization, K.R.I., J.K., T.L.T., M.B.I.R., T.R., A.K., S.M.Z. and M.E.H.C.; Data curation, K.R.I., T.R. and M.E.H.C.; Formal analysis, K.R.I., T.R. and A.K.; Funding acquisition, M.E.H.C.; Investigation, K.R.I., T.R. and M.E.H.C.; Methodology, K.R.I., T.A., M.S.A.H. and M.E.H.C.; Project administration, J.K., T.L.T., M.B.I.R., T.R. and M.E.H.C.; Software, M.S.A.H.; Supervision, J.K., T.L.T. and M.E.H.C.; Validation, K.R.I., T.R., T.A. and M.E.H.C.; Visualization, K.R.I. and T.R.; Writing—original draft, K.R.I., J.K., T.L.T., M.B.I.R., T.R., A.K., T.A. and M.E.H.C.; Writing—review & editing, K.R.I., J.K., T.L.T., M.B.I.R., T.R., A.K., T.A., M.S.A.H. and M.E.H.C. All authors have read and agreed to the published version of the manuscript.

Funding: This work was supported by the Faculty of Medicine, Universiti Kebangsaan Malaysia (UKM), and UKM Grant Number DIP-2020-004, Grant Number GP-2020-K017701, and by the Qatar National Research fund under Grant UREP28-144-3-046. The statements made herein are solely the responsibility of the authors.

Institutional Review Board Statement: Not applicable.

Informed Consent Statement: Not applicable.

Data Availability Statement: Data used in this study can be accessed from Baranovskii et al. [46].

Acknowledgments: The authors would like to thank Baranovskii et al. [46] for providing their study data.

Conflicts of Interest: Authors have no conflict of interest to declare.

References

1. Krit, B.; Kuvshinov, V.; Kukushkin, D.Y.; Morozova, N.; Omel'chuk, Y.A.; Revenok, T.; Sleptsov, V. The application of nanocluster coatngs for modification of image receiving surface of thermophotoelectric energy converters. *Surf. Eng. Appl. Electrochem.* **2020**, *56*, 100–104. [CrossRef]
2. COVID-19 Coronavirus Pandemic. Available online: https://www.worldometers.info/coronavirus/ (accessed on 1 July 2022).

3. Zhu, N.; Zhang, D.; Wang, W.; Li, X.; Yang, B.; Song, J.; Zhao, X.; Huang, B.; Shi, W.; Lu, R. A novel coronavirus from patients with pneumonia in China, 2019. *N. Engl. J. Med.* **2020**, *382*, 727–733. [CrossRef] [PubMed]
4. Huang, C.; Wang, Y.; Li, X.; Ren, L.; Zhao, J.; Hu, Y.; Zhang, L.; Fan, G.; Xu, J.; Gu, X. Clinical features of patients infected with 2019 novel coronavirus in Wuhan, China. *Lancet* **2020**, *395*, 497–506. [CrossRef]
5. Liu, Y.; Yan, L.-M.; Wan, L.; Xiang, T.-X.; Le, A.; Liu, J.-M.; Peiris, M.; Poon, L.L.; Zhang, W. Viral dynamics in mild and severe cases of COVID-19. *Lancet Infect. Dis.* **2020**, *20*, 656–657. [CrossRef]
6. Herring, A.A.; Ginde, A.A.; Fahimi, J.; Alter, H.J.; Maselli, J.H.; Espinola, J.A.; Sullivan, A.F.; Camargo, C.A., Jr. Increasing critical care admissions from US emergency departments, 2001–2009. *Crit. Care Med.* **2013**, *41*, 1197. [CrossRef] [PubMed]
7. Halpern, N.A.; Pastores, S.M. Critical care medicine in the United States 2000–2005: An analysis of bed numbers, occupancy rates, payer mix, and costs. *Crit. Care Med.* **2010**, *38*, 65–71. [CrossRef]
8. American College of Emergency Physicians. Boarding of Admitted and Intensive Care Patients in the Emergency Department. Available online: https://pubmed.ncbi.nlm.nih.gov/18655931/ (accessed on 1 February 2022).
9. Goldstein, R.S. Management of the critically ill patient in the emergency department: Focus on safety issues. *Crit. Care Clin.* **2005**, *21*, 81–89. [CrossRef]
10. Aslaner, M.A.; Akkaş, M.; Eroğlu, S.; Aksu, N.M.; Özmen, M.M. Admissions of critically ill patients to the ED intensive care unit. *Am. J. Emerg. Med.* **2015**, *33*, 501–505. [CrossRef]
11. Frater, J.L.; Zini, G.; d'Onofrio, G.; Rogers, H.J. COVID-19 and the clinical hematology laboratory. *Int. J. Lab. Hematol.* **2020**, *42*, 11–18. [CrossRef]
12. Agapakis, D.I.; Tsantilas, D.; Psarris, P.; Massa, E.V.; Kotsaftis, P.; Tziomalos, K.; Hatzitolios, A.I. Coagulation and inflammation biomarkers may help predict the severity of community-acquired pneumonia. *Respirology* **2010**, *15*, 796–803. [CrossRef]
13. Giannis, D.; Ziogas, I.A.; Gianni, P. Coagulation disorders in coronavirus infected patients: COVID-19, SARS-CoV-1, MERS-CoV and lessons from the past. *J. Clin. Virol.* **2020**, *127*, 104362. [PubMed]
14. Wang, D.; Yin, Y.; Hu, C.; Liu, X.; Zhang, X.; Zhou, S.; Jian, M.; Xu, H.; Prowle, J.; Hu, B. Clinical course and outcome of 107 patients infected with the novel coronavirus, SARS-CoV-2, discharged from two hospitals in Wuhan, China. *Crit. Care* **2020**, *24*, 1–9.
15. Tan, C.; Huang, Y.; Shi, F.; Tan, K.; Ma, Q.; Chen, Y.; Jiang, X.; Li, X. C-reactive protein correlates with computed tomographic findings and predicts severe COVID-19 early. *J. Med. Virol.* **2020**, *92*, 856–862. [CrossRef] [PubMed]
16. Luo, X.; Zhou, W.; Yan, X.; Guo, T.; Wang, B.; Xia, H.; Ye, L.; Xiong, J.; Jiang, Z.; Liu, Y. Prognostic value of C-reactive protein in patients with coronavirus 2019. *Clin. Infect. Dis.* **2020**, *71*, 2174–2179. [CrossRef] [PubMed]
17. Zhai, Q.; Lin, Z.; Ge, H.; Liang, Y.; Li, N.; Ma, Q.; Ye, C. Using machine learning tools to predict outcomes for emergency department intensive care unit patients. *Sci. Rep.* **2020**, *10*, 20919.
18. Hong, K.J.; Shin, S.D.; Ro, Y.S.; Song, K.J.; Singer, A.J. Development and validation of the excess mortality ratio–based Emergency Severity Index. *Am. J. Emerg. Med.* **2012**, *30*, 1491–1500. [PubMed]
19. Purohit, K.; Kesarwani, A.; Kisku, D.R.; Dalui, M. COVID-19 detection on chest X-ray and ct scan images using multi-image augmented deep learning model. In Proceedings of the Seventh International Conference on Mathematics and Computing, Chongqing, China, 18–20 March 2022; pp. 395–413.
20. Rahman, T.; Chowdhury, M.E.; Khandakar, A.; Mahbub, Z.B.; Hossain, M.S.A.; Alhatou, A.; Abdalla, E.; Muthiyal, S.; Islam, K.F.; Kashem, S.B.A. BIO-CXRNET: A Robust Multimodal Stacking Machine Learning Technique for Mortality Risk Prediction of COVID-19 Patients using Chest X-Ray Images and Clinical Data. *arXiv* **2022**, arXiv:2206.07595.
21. Tahir, A.M.; Qiblawey, Y.; Khandakar, A.; Rahman, T.; Khurshid, U.; Musharavati, F.; Islam, M.; Kiranyaz, S.; Al-Maadeed, S.; Chowdhury, M.E. Deep learning for reliable classification of COVID-19, MERS, and SARS from chest X-ray images. *Cogn. Comput.* **2022**, 1–21. [CrossRef]
22. Borghesi, A.; Golemi, S.; Scrimieri, A.; Nicosia, C.M.C.; Zigliani, A.; Farina, D.; Maroldi, R. Chest X-ray versus chest computed tomography for outcome prediction in hospitalized patients with COVID-19. *La Radiol. Med.* **2022**, *127*, 305–308. [CrossRef]
23. Rahman, T.; Khandakar, A.; Qiblawey, Y.; Tahir, A.; Kiranyaz, S.; Kashem, S.B.A.; Islam, M.T.; Al Maadeed, S.; Zughaier, S.M.; Khan, M.S. Exploring the effect of image enhancement techniques on COVID-19 detection using chest X-ray images. *Comput. Biol. Med.* **2021**, *132*, 104319. [CrossRef]
24. Qiblawey, Y.; Tahir, A.; Chowdhury, M.; Khandakar, A.; Kiranyaz, S.; Rahman, T.; Ibtehaz, N.; Mahmud, S.; Al Maadeed, S.; Musharavati, F. Detection and severity classification of COVID-19 in CT images using deep learning. *Diagnostics* **2021**, *11*, 893. [CrossRef] [PubMed]
25. Poly, T.N.; Islam, M.M.; Li, Y.-C.J.; Alsinglawi, B.; Hsu, M.-H.; Jian, W.S.; Yang, H.-C. Application of artificial intelligence for screening covid-19 patients using digital images: Meta-analysis. *JMIR Med. Inform.* **2021**, *9*, e21394. [CrossRef] [PubMed]
26. Feng, C.; Wang, L.; Chen, X.; Zhai, Y.; Zhu, F.; Chen, H.; Wang, Y.; Su, X.; Huang, S.; Tian, L. A novel artificial intelligence-assisted triage tool to aid in the diagnosis of suspected COVID-19 pneumonia cases in fever clinics. *Ann. Transl. Med.* **2021**, *9*, 201. [CrossRef] [PubMed]
27. Calvet, J.; Berenguer-Llergo, A.; Gay, M.; Massanella, M.; Domingo, P.; Llop, M.; Sánchez-Jiménez, E.; Arévalo, M.; Carrillo, J.; Albiñana, N. Biomarker candidates for progression and clinical management of COVID-19 associated pneumonia at time of admission. *Sci. Rep.* **2022**, *12*, 640. [CrossRef]

28. Halasz, G.; Sperti, M.; Villani, M.; Michelucci, U.; Agostoni, P.; Biagi, A.; Rossi, L.; Botti, A.; Mari, C.; Maccarini, M. A machine learning approach for mortality prediction in COVID-19 pneumonia: Development and evaluation of the Piacenza score. *J. Med. Internet Res.* **2021**, *23*, e29058.
29. Alsinglawi, B.; Alnajjar, F.; Mubin, O.; Novoa, M.; Karajeh, O.; Darwish, O. Benchmarking predictive models in electronic health records: Sepsis length of stay prediction. In Proceedings of the International Conference on Advanced Information Networking and Applications, Caserta, Italy, 15–17 April 2020; pp. 258–267.
30. Zou, Y.; Guo, H.; Zhang, Y.; Zhang, Z.; Liu, Y.; Wang, J.; Lu, H.; Qian, Z. Analysis of coagulation parameters in patients with COVID-19 in Shanghai, China. *Biosci. Trends* **2020**, *14*, 285–289. [CrossRef]
31. Weng, Z.; Chen, Q.; Li, S.; Li, H.; Zhang, Q.; Lu, S.; Wu, L.; Xiong, L.; Mi, B.; Liu, D. ANDC: An early warning score to predict mortality risk for patients with coronavirus disease 2019. *J. Transl. Med.* **2020**, *18*, 328. [CrossRef]
32. Gong, J.; Ou, J.; Qiu, X.; Jie, Y.; Chen, Y.; Yuan, L.; Cao, J.; Tan, M.; Xu, W.; Zheng, F. A tool for early prediction of severe coronavirus disease 2019 (COVID-19): A multicenter study using the risk nomogram in Wuhan and Guangdong, China. *Clin. Infect. Dis.* **2020**, *71*, 833–840. [CrossRef]
33. Alabbad, D.A.; Almuhaideb, A.M.; Alsunaidi, S.J.; Alqudaihi, K.S.; Alamoudi, F.A.; Alhobaishi, M.K.; Alaqeel, N.A.; Alshahrani, M.S. Machine learning model for predicting the length of stay in the intensive care unit for COVID-19 patients in the eastern province of Saudi Arabia. *Inform. Med. Unlocked* **2022**, *30*, 100937. [CrossRef] [PubMed]
34. Al Youha, S.; Doi, S.A.; Jamal, M.H.; Almazeedi, S.; Al Haddad, M.; AlSeaidan, M.; Al-Muhaini, A.; Al-Ghimlas, F.; Al-Sabah, S. Validation of the Kuwait Progression Indicator Score for predicting progression of severity in COVID19. *MedRxiv* **2020**. [CrossRef]
35. Ai, T.; Yang, Z.; Hou, H.; Zhan, C.; Chen, C.; Lv, W.; Tao, Q.; Sun, Z.; Xia, L. Correlation of chest CT and RT-PCR testing in coronavirus disease 2019 (COVID-19) in China: A report of 1014 cases. *Radiology* **2020**, *296*, E32–E40. [CrossRef]
36. Chowdhury, M.E.; Rahman, T.; Khandakar, A.; Al-Madeed, S.; Zughaier, S.M.; Hassen, H.; Islam, M.T. An early warning tool for predicting mortality risk of COVID-19 patients using machine learning. *Cogn. Comput.* **2021**, 1–16. [CrossRef]
37. Rahman, T.; Al-Ishaq, F.A.; Al-Mohannadi, F.S.; Mubarak, R.S.; Al-Hitmi, M.H.; Islam, K.R.; Khandakar, A.; Hssain, A.A.; Al-Madeed, S.; Zughaier, S.M. Mortality prediction utilizing blood biomarkers to predict the severity of COVID-19 using machine learning technique. *Diagnostics* **2021**, *11*, 1582. [PubMed]
38. Lorenzoni, G.; Sella, N.; Boscolo, A.; Azzolina, D.; Bartolotta, P.; Pasin, L.; Pettenuzzo, T.; De Cassai, A.; Baratto, F.; Toffoletto, F. COVID-19 ICU mortality prediction: A machine learning approach using SuperLearner algorithm. *J. Anesth. Analg. Crit. Care* **2021**, *1*, 3.
39. Magunia, H.; Lederer, S.; Verbuecheln, R.; Gilot, B.J.; Koeppen, M.; Haeberle, H.A.; Mirakaj, V.; Hofmann, P.; Marx, G.; Bickenbach, J. Machine learning identifies ICU outcome predictors in a multicenter COVID-19 cohort. *Crit. Care* **2021**, *25*, 295.
40. Liang, W.; Yao, J.; Chen, A.; Lv, Q.; Zanin, M.; Liu, J.; Wong, S.; Li, Y.; Lu, J.; Liang, H. Early triage of critically ill COVID-19 patients using deep learning. *Nat. Commun.* **2020**, *11*, 3543.
41. Wang, C.; Deng, R.; Gou, L.; Fu, Z.; Zhang, X.; Shao, F.; Wang, G.; Fu, W.; Xiao, J.; Ding, X. Preliminary study to identify severe from moderate cases of COVID-19 using combined hematology parameters. *Ann. Transl. Med.* **2020**, *8*, 593. [PubMed]
42. Cai, Y.-Q.; Zeng, H.-Q.; Zhang, X.-B.; Wei, X.-J.; Hu, L.; Zhang, Z.-Y.; Ming, Q.; Peng, Q.-P.; Chen, L.-D. Prognostic value of neutrophil-to-lymphocyte ratio, lactate dehydrogenase, D-Dimer and CT score in patients with COVID-19. *Aging* **2020**, *13*, 20896–20905. [CrossRef] [PubMed]
43. McRae, M.P.; Simmons, G.W.; Christodoulides, N.J.; Lu, Z.; Kang, S.K.; Fenyo, D.; Alcorn, T.; Dapkins, I.P.; Sharif, I.; Vurmaz, D. Clinical decision support tool and rapid point-of-care platform for determining disease severity in patients with COVID-19. *Lab Chip* **2020**, *20*, 2075–2085.
44. Wang, G.; Wu, C.; Zhang, Q.; Wu, F.; Yu, B.; Lv, J.; Li, Y.; Li, T.; Zhang, S.; Wu, C. C-reactive protein level may predict the risk of COVID-19 aggravation. In *Open Forum Infectious Diseases*; Oxford University Press: Oxford, MI, USA, 2020; p. ofaa153.
45. Hegde, H.; Shimpi, N.; Panny, A.; Glurich, I.; Christie, P.; Acharya, A. MICE vs. PPCA: Missing data imputation in healthcare. *Inform. Med. Unlocked* **2019**, *17*, 100275.
46. Baranovskii, D.S.; Klabukov, I.D.; Krasilnikova, O.A.; Nikogosov, D.A.; Polekhina, N.V.; Baranovskaia, D.R.; Laberko, L.A. Prolonged prothrombin time as an early prognostic indicator of severe acute respiratory distress syndrome in patients with COVID-19 related pneumonia. *Curr. Med. Res. Opin.* **2021**, *37*, 21–25. [CrossRef]
47. Rahman, T.; Khandakar, A.; Hoque, M.E.; Ibtehaz, N.; Kashem, S.B.; Masud, R.; Shampa, L.; Hasan, M.M.; Islam, M.T.; Al-Maadeed, S. Development and Validation of an Early Scoring System for Prediction of Disease Severity in COVID-19 Using Complete Blood Count Parameters. *IEEE Access* **2021**, *9*, 120422–120441. [CrossRef]
48. Stevens, J.R.; Suyundikov, A.; Slattery, M.L. Accounting for missing data in clinical research. *JAMA* **2016**, *315*, 517–518. [CrossRef]
49. Speiser, J.L.; Miller, M.E.; Tooze, J.; Ip, E. A comparison of random forest variable selection methods for classification prediction modeling. *Expert Syst. Appl.* **2019**, *134*, 93–101. [CrossRef]
50. Beretta, L.; Santaniello, A. Nearest neighbor imputation algorithms: A critical evaluation. *BMC Med. Inform. Decis. Mak.* **2016**, *16*, 74. [CrossRef]
51. Chawla, N.V.; Bowyer, K.W.; Hall, L.O.; Kegelmeyer, W.P. SMOTE: Synthetic minority over-sampling technique. *J. Artif. Intell. Res.* **2002**, *16*, 321–357. [CrossRef]

52. Khandakar, A.; Chowdhury, M.E.; Reaz, M.B.I.; Ali, S.H.M.; Hasan, M.A.; Kiranyaz, S.; Rahman, T.; Alfkey, R.; Bakar, A.A.A.; Malik, R.A. A machine learning model for early detection of diabetic foot using thermogram images. *Comput. Biol. Med.* **2021**, *137*, 104838.
53. Khandakar, A.; Chowdhury, M.E.; Reaz, M.B.I.; Ali, S.H.M.; Kiranyaz, S.; Rahman, T.; Chowdhury, M.H.; Ayari, M.A.; Alfkey, R.; Bakar, A.A.A. A Novel Machine Learning Approach for Severity Classification of Diabetic Foot Complications Using Thermogram Images. *Sensors* **2022**, *22*, 4249. [PubMed]
54. Tallarida, R.J.; Murray, R.B. Chi-square test. In *Manual of Pharmacologic Calculations*; Springer: Berlin/Heidelberg, Germany, 1987; pp. 140–142.
55. Saidi, R.; Bouaguel, W.; Essoussi, N. Hybrid feature selection method based on the genetic algorithm and pearson correlation coefficient. In *Machine Learning Paradigms: Theory and Application*; Springer: Berlin/Heidelberg, Germany, 2019; pp. 3–24.
56. Lin, X.; Yang, F.; Zhou, L.; Yin, P.; Kong, H.; Xing, W.; Lu, X.; Jia, L.; Wang, Q.; Xu, G. A support vector machine-recursive feature elimination feature selection method based on artificial contrast variables and mutual information. *J. Chromatogr. B* **2012**, *910*, 149–155. [CrossRef] [PubMed]
57. Hosseini, S.; Khandakar, A.; Chowdhury, M.E.; Ayari, M.A.; Rahman, T.; Chowdhury, M.H.; Vaferi, B. Novel and robust machine learning approach for estimating the fouling factor in heat exchangers. *Energy Rep.* **2022**, *8*, 8767–8776.
58. Romero Starke, K.; Petereit-Haack, G.; Schubert, M.; Kämpf, D.; Schliebner, A.; Hegewald, J.; Seidler, A. The age-related risk of severe outcomes due to COVID-19 infection: A rapid review, meta-analysis, and meta-regression. *Int. J. Environ. Res. Public Health* **2020**, *17*, 5974. [CrossRef] [PubMed]
59. Booth, C.M.; Matukas, L.M.; Tomlinson, G.A.; Rachlis, A.R.; Rose, D.B.; Dwosh, H.A.; Walmsley, S.L.; Mazzulli, T.; Avendano, M.; Derkach, P. Clinical features and short-term outcomes of 144 patients with SARS in the greater Toronto area. *JAMA* **2003**, *289*, 2801–2809. [CrossRef] [PubMed]
60. Scudiero, F.; Silverio, A.; Di Maio, M.; Russo, V.; Citro, R.; Personeni, D.; Cafro, A.; D'Andrea, A.; Attena, E.; Pezzullo, S. Pulmonary embolism in COVID-19 patients: Prevalence, predictors and clinical outcome. *Thromb. Res.* **2021**, *198*, 34–39. [CrossRef]
61. Iba, T.; Levi, M.; Levy, J.H. Sepsis-induced coagulopathy and disseminated intravascular coagulation. In *Seminars in Thrombosis and Hemostasis*; Thieme Medical: Stuttgart, Germany, 2020; pp. 089–095.
62. Thachil, J.; Tang, N.; Gando, S.; Falanga, A.; Cattaneo, M.; Levi, M.; Clark, C.; Iba, T. ISTH interim guidance on recognition and management of coagulopathy in COVID-19. *J. Thromb. Haemost.* **2020**, *18*, 1023–1026. [CrossRef]
63. Marnell, L.; Mold, C.; Clos, T.W.D. C-reactive protein: Ligands, receptors and role in inflammation. *Clin. Immunol.* **2005**, *117*, 104–111. [CrossRef] [PubMed]
64. Young, B.; Gleeson, M.; Cripps, A.W. C-reactive protein: A critical review. *Pathology* **1991**, *23*, 118–124. [CrossRef]
65. Wang, Y.; Dong, C.; Hu, Y.; Li, C.; Ren, Q.; Zhang, X.; Shi, H.; Zhou, M. Temporal changes of CT findings in 90 patients with COVID-19 pneumonia: A longitudinal study. *Radiology* **2020**, *296*, E55–E64. [CrossRef]
66. Francone, M.; Iafrate, F.; Masci, G.M.; Coco, S.; Cilia, F.; Manganaro, L.; Panebianco, V.; Andreoli, C.; Colaiacomo, M.C.; Zingaropoli, M.A. Chest CT score in COVID-19 patients: Correlation with disease severity and short-term prognosis. *Eur. Radiol.* **2020**, *30*, 6808–6817. [CrossRef]
67. Simpson, S.; Kay, F.U.; Abbara, S.; Bhalla, S.; Chung, J.H.; Chung, M.; Henry, T.S.; Kanne, J.P.; Kligerman, S.; Ko, J.P. Radiological society of north America expert consensus document on reporting chest CT findings related to COVID-19: Endorsed by the society of thoracic Radiology, the American college of Radiology, and RSNA. *Radiol. Cardiothorac. Imaging* **2020**, *2*, e200152. [CrossRef]
68. Sayeed, S.; Belqees, Y.F.; Aslam, S.; Masood, L.; Saeed, R. CT Chest Severity Score for COVID 19 Pneumonia: A Quantitative Imaging Tool for Severity Assessment of Disease. *J. Coll. Physicians Surg.—Pak. JCPSP* **2021**, *30*, 388–392.
69. Mruk, B.; Plucińska, D.; Walecki, J.; Półtorak-Szymczak, G.; Sklinda, K. Chest Computed Tomography (CT) Severity Scales in COVID-19 Disease: A Validation Study. *Med. Sci. Monit. Int. Med. J. Exp. Clin. Res.* **2021**, *27*, e931283-1. [CrossRef] [PubMed]

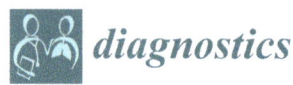

Article

Artificial Intelligence Based Pain Assessment Technology in Clinical Application of Real-World Neonatal Blood Sampling

Xiaoying Cheng [1,†], Huaiyu Zhu [2,†], Linli Mei [3], Feixiang Luo [4], Xiaofei Chen [5], Yisheng Zhao [2], Shuohui Chen [3,*] and Yun Pan [2,*]

1. Quality Improvement Office, The Children's Hospital, Zhejiang University School of Medicine, National Clinical Research Center for Child Health, Hangzhou 310052, China; cxynicu@163.com
2. College of Information Science and Electronic Engineering, Zhejiang University, Hangzhou 310027, China; zhuhuaiyu@zju.edu.cn (H.Z.); zhaoys@zju.edu.cn (Y.Z.)
3. Administration Department of Nosocomial Infection, The Children's Hospital, Zhejiang University School of Medicine, National Clinical Research Center for Child Health, Hangzhou 310052, China; 22018565@zju.edu.cn
4. Neonatal Intensive Care Unit, The Children's Hospital, Zhejiang University School of Medicine, National Clinical Research Center for Child Health, Hangzhou 310052, China; luofeixiang@zju.edu.cn
5. Gastroenterology Department, The Children's Hospital, Zhejiang University School of Medicine, National Clinical Research Center for Child Health, Hangzhou 310052, China; hzxiao0914@163.com
* Correspondence: chcsh2@zju.edu.cn (S.C.); panyun@zju.edu.cn (Y.P.)
† These authors contributed equally to this work.

Abstract: Background: Accurate neonatal pain assessment (NPA) is the key to neonatal pain management, yet it is a challenging task for medical staff. This study aimed to analyze the clinical practicability of the artificial intelligence based NPA (AI-NPA) tool for real-world blood sampling. Method: We performed a prospective study to analyze the consistency of the NPA results given by a self-developed automated NPA system and nurses' on-site NPAs (OS-NPAs) for 232 newborns during blood sampling in neonatal wards, where the neonatal infant pain scale (NIPS) was used for evaluation. Spearman correlation analysis and the degree of agreement of the pain score and pain grade derived by the NIPS were applied for statistical analysis. Results: Taking the OS-NPA results as the gold standard, the accuracies of the NIPS pain score and pain grade given by the automated NPA system were 88.79% and 95.25%, with kappa values of 0.92 and 0.90 ($p < 0.001$), respectively. Conclusion: The results of the automated NPA system for real-world neonatal blood sampling are highly consistent with the results of the OS-NPA. Considering the great advantages of automated NPA systems in repeatability, efficiency, and cost, it is worth popularizing the AI technique in NPA for precise and efficient neonatal pain management.

Keywords: neonatal pain; on-site assessment; artificial intelligence; blood sampling; real-world data

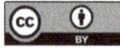

1. Introduction

Pain assessment and management is one of the research hotspots in the neonatal care field. Although premature and full-term infants usually experience a high frequency of painful stimuli during hospitalization, neonatal pain assessment (NPA) has not been given adequate attention in clinical practice, where painful clinical procedures with a severe degree of pain are prevalent [1]. The operations, such as blood sampling, sputum suction, and indwelling needle puncture, are the major procedures in neonatal care that occur most frequently [2]. These painful procedures are mostly performed on infants within the first 3 days of admission, and no pharmacological interventions are applied for them in most cases [3]. Assessments of continuous pain occurred in less than one-third of neonates, and daily in only 10% [4]. As neonatal pain has a great impact on the short-term and long-term development of newborns [5,6], more attention should be paid to pain management in routine neonatal care.

Accurate NPA is the key to effective pain management. In clinical NPA, the facial expression is considered to be the most explicit indicator, on which a number of pain-assessment scales have been designed, such as the neonatal facial coding system (NFCS) [7], children and infants postoperative pain scale (CHIPPS) [8], premature infant pain profile (PIPP) [9], and neonatal infant pain scale (NIPS) [10]. These NPA scales mainly consider the facial-expression characteristics of newborns, and some of them also integrate factors such as crying, limb movement, and vital signs. Traditional scale-based on-site NPA (OS-NPA) is a process that requires dynamic monitoring by nurses rather than an instantaneous operation. Therefore, regular OS-NPA for pain management is time consuming and laborious. Meanwhile, the results of the OS-NPA could be affected by many factors, including subjective differences in observers [2], interruption from other clinical procedures, a lack of time [11], the gender difference [12], the interference of neonatal activity, inadequate pain-assessment tools [1], and the loss of some transient behaviors.

With the rapid development of artificial intelligence (AI), deep learning has been integrated into neonatal pain-expression-recognition technology [13]. The automatic recognition of neonatal pain expressions has undergone a process from static images to dynamic videos, and from theoretical experiments to system development [14], which has enabled AI-based NPA (AI-NPA). On the one hand, AI-NPA could make up for the shortcomings of the OS-NPA performed by medical staff, and it has the advantages of convenience and efficiency. On the other hand, AI-NPA requires a large number of accurately labeled neonatal pain data to build a model with strong anti-interference ability and high robustness for real-world data.

Unfortunately, the current public reported neonatal pain-expression databases [15–18] still suffer from a limited number of newborns and samples, deficient population information, limited types of pain stimuli that have large differences with painful clinical procedures, the coarse labeling granularity of pain, etc. Moreover, these state-of-the-art databases and many AI-NPA methods [19–22] focus on ideal neonatal pain samples, which are samples with restrictions on the neonatal activities and facial posture in the data-collection stage, or with manual screening to avoid disturbed neonatal pain data. These methods make it difficult to meet the clinical requirements regarding accuracy, and they are not feasible for processing neonatal pain data collected in real-world clinical scenes. Hence, there is still a large gap between the current AI-NPA methods and the actual clinical needs in terms of the pain-analysis objectives and scenarios, which has resulted in limited clinical applications.

In order to realize an automated NPA system for actual clinical needs, we previously established a video database of neonatal facial expressions during painful clinical procedures in neonatal wards [23], and we developed an AI-NPA method for real-world data. Our AI-NPA method is robust to facial occlusion and pose variations. Concretely, the method applied generative adversarial networks (GANs) to learn how to recover ideal facial images from real-world facial images with variant poses and occlusion for obtaining modified facial features that enable subsequent interference-adaptive fine-grained neonatal pain assessment. Based on our AI-NPA method, we further completed the design of an automated NPA system for neonatal pain on a mobile platform with an in-hospital server.

In this paper, we propose a prospective study to analyze the consistency of the NPA results given by the automated NPA system and OS-NPA in a real-world clinical operation scenario, thus verifying the clinical practicability of automated NPA systems. A total of 232 newborns who underwent blood-sampling operations in the neonatal wards of the Children's Hospital of Zhejiang University School of Medicine were recruited and participated in this experiment. Both the OS-NPA performed by two nurses and the AI-NPA given by our automated NPA system were applied during the implementation of four types of blood-sampling operations (i.e., venous, arterial, heel, and fingertip blood sampling) to give their own NPA results in the form of a pain score and pain grade with reference to the NIPS. The correlation and consistency of the OS-NPA and AI-NPA results, as well as the performance of our automated NPA system on real-world clinical neonatal pain data, were derived and analyzed.

The experiment results show that, according to the OS-NPA results on 232 newborns, the accuracy of the automated NPA system was 88.79%, with kappa values of 0.92 and 95.25%, and a kappa value of 0.90 for the NIPS pain score and pain grade, both with $p < 0.001$. This indicates that the NPA results have a high consistency between the on-site evaluation and the AI inference, even in the neonatal pain data in the real-world blood-sampling scenario. This study could provide a performance baseline for the clinical application of automated NPA systems.

2. Materials and Methods

2.1. Study Design

This prospective study was approved by the ethics committee of the Children's Hospital of Zhejiang University School of Medicine (2018-IRB-051), and parental informed consent was obtained. Newborns who underwent blood-sampling operations in the Department of Neonatology between 1 July 2018 and 30 June 2019 were studied, and the duration of the blood-sampling operations were controlled within 1 min. As shown in Figure 1, when the neonates needed four types of blood sampling (i.e., venous, arterial, heel, and fingertip blood sampling) for clinical diagnosis and treatment, two nurses used the NIPS to perform the respective OS-NPA. Meanwhile, a third nurse used our automated NPA system to shoot the responses of the newborns during the procedure at the bedside, and to retrieve pain scores and pain grades with reference to the NIPS generated by the system. The NIPS pain scores and pain grades of the OS-NPA performed by the two nurses and the AI-NPA performed by the automated NPA system were collected for subsequent statistical analysis.

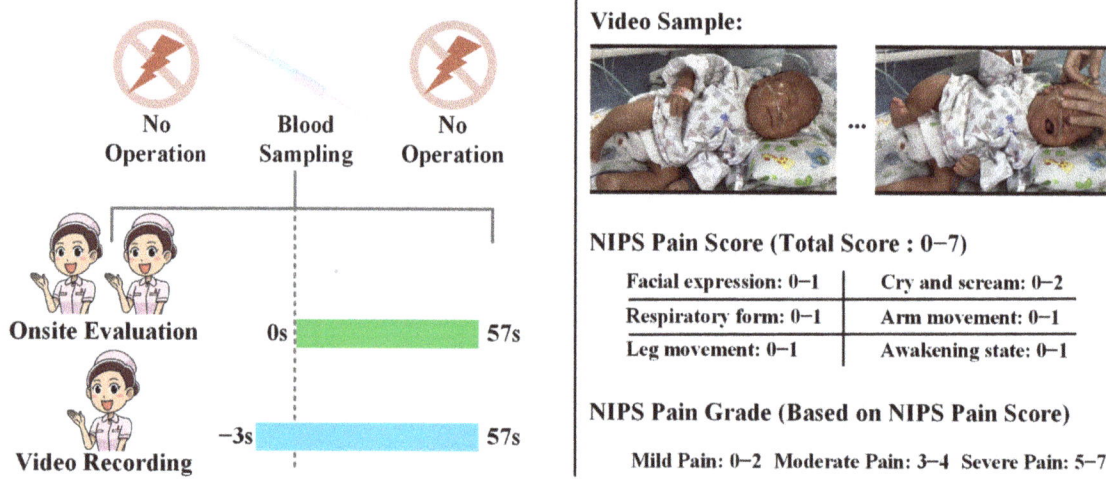

Figure 1. The study design of the clinical practicability of automated NPA systems.

2.2. Inclusion and Exclusion Criteria

Neonates who were hospitalized in the Department of Neonatology for more than 3 days and who underwent the abovementioned four types of blood sampling were included in this prospective study. Exclusion criteria included: serious illness conditions, such as serious birth injury, severe asphyxia, shock, metabolic encephalopathy, moderate and severe hypoxic-ischemic encephalopathy, and severe cardiopulmonary disease; newborns with conditions affecting facial-image acquisition, such as severe congenital malformations, facial malformations, facial nerve injury, and facial surgery. Neonates should not have used sedative or analgesic drugs within 72 h to avoid inaccurate NPA results in the experiment.

2.3. OS-NPA Performed by Nurses

Two experienced nurses were assigned to quantitatively assess the pain of the four types of blood sampling for newborns using the NIPS [10]. The pain indicators of the NIPS are defined by the following parameters, with a total score range from 0 to 7 points: facial expression (0–1 point), cry (0–2 points), breathing pattern (0–1 point), position of arms (0–1 point), position of legs (0–1 point), and state of arousal (0–1 point). This is suitable for acute pain assessment, and the pain severity can be classified into mild pain with a score of 0–2, moderate pain with a score of 3–4, and severe pain with a score of 5–7. The Spearman correlation analysis was used to analyze the independent pain-score results of the two nurses, and the correlation coefficient was 0.89 with $p < 0.001$, which indicates the high confidence of the OS-NPA results. Data with a difference in two independent pain scores were further reviewed by these two nurses. They checked the corresponding on-site video to obtain a consistently confirmed pain score as the final OS-NPA result.

2.4. AI-NPA Performed by the Automated NPA System

The automated NPA system was implemented with the client–server model. The application was designed to run on the mobile nursing personal digital assistant (MNPDA) device. When performing the AI-NPA, the nurse could use the application to record videos of the newborns' behavior during blood sampling. Specifically, the nurse pressed the shooting key 3 s before the blood-sampling operation and the end key 57 s after the operation to achieve a 60 s video for each operation. The heads and faces of the infants were required to be completely presented in the video frame during the whole process. Figure 2 presents the typical image sequence of the neonatal pain video. The video stream was then transmitted to the in-hospital server hosting the AI-NPA model for real-time NPA inference.

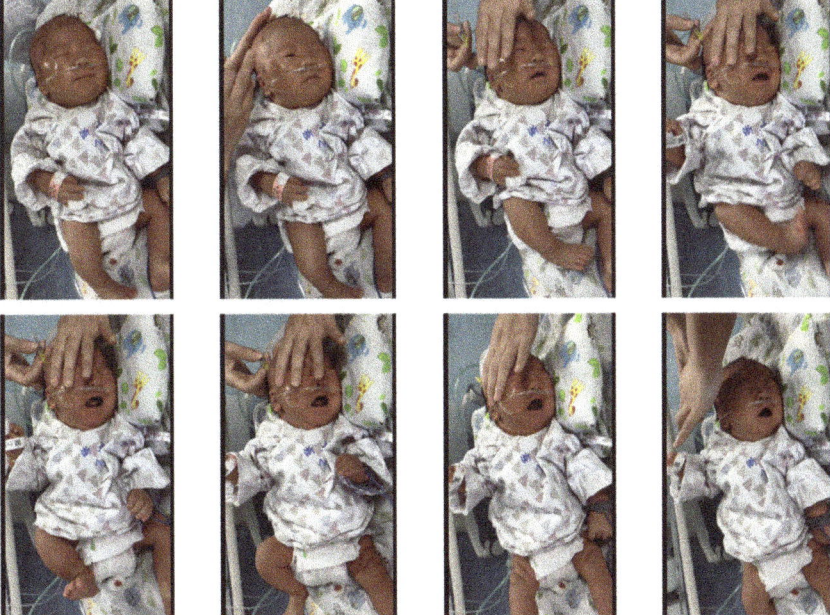

Figure 2. Samples of image sequence in a neonatal pain video.

The AI-NPA model of our automated NPA system in this study was pretrained on a larger expression-recognition database and was further modulated by a self-built neonatal facial-pain database based on our previous work [23]. Our AI-NPA method includes two parts: unsupervised feature modification and self-attention pain classification. In the unsupervised-feature-modification part, we apply a generative adversarial network (GAN) to modify the facial features toward the direction of face frontalization and deocclusion.

Specifically, we use the latent vector of the generator as the modified facial features. That is, we only need the encoder network of the generator to extract facial features during the testing phase. The generator of the GAN has two paths, focusing on the reasoning of the global shapes and the transformation of the local details [24]. The discriminator of the GAN is responsible for learning to distinguish between the output of the generator and the normal (frontal and nonoccluded) face images, which pushes the facial features into the manifold of a normal face. We further employed four loss functions: symmetry loss, adversarial loss, identity-preserving loss, and total variation regularization, to train the generator network and discriminator network jointly, as shown in Figure 3.

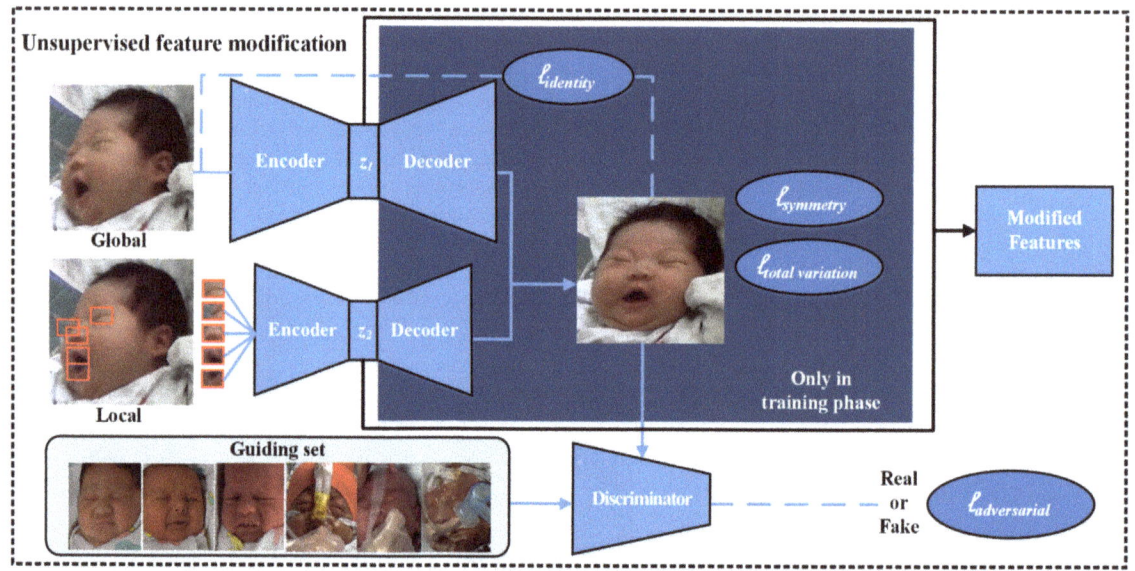

Figure 3. The framework of the unsupervised-feature-modification part in our AI-NPA model.

For the self-attention pain classification, considering that the modified facial features still contain many useless, redundant, and even wrong features, we choose the self-attention mechanism to further filter and enhance the modified features. Specifically, we build an attention branch parallel to the residual branch, which is based on the bottom-up top-down structure [25], and which can output the same size-attention mask that softly weights the facial features.

In the pretraining stage, a total of 12,271 basic expression images in the RAF-DB [26] were applied to obtain the initial model parameters. We then trained this model on 508 neonatal pain images from our real-world neonatal pain database, and we adjusted the parameters to the optimal through the backpropagation algorithm. The samples of our neonatal pain database are shown in Figure 4. The AI-NPA model is deployed on an in-hospital server. The software platform of the server is Ubuntu 16.4.7 with Python 3.6.8, and the hardware configuration is Intel® Xeon® CPU E5-2678 v3 (12/24 cores/threads, 2.5/3.1 GHz base/turbo), 112 GB 2400 MHz DDR4 RAM, and two Nvidia® GeForce® RTX 2080Ti GPUs (1350/1454 MHz base/boost with 11GB GDDR 6 VRAM).

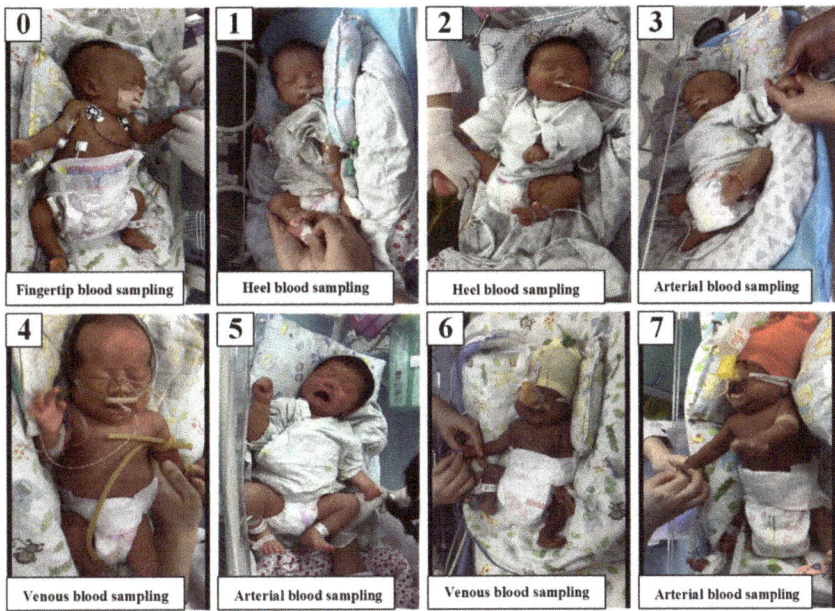

Figure 4. Samples of neonatal pain data with different blood-sampling operations and pain scores.

After the video is transmitted to the server, the AI-NPA model detects the face region of each frame of the image in the video by a built-in algorithm, and it crops the facial image with the size of 224 × 224. Based on the NIPS, the pain scores and pain grades are automatically generated, paired with the images, and stored on the server. The final AI-NPA results are determined as the highest pain score and the corresponding pain grade during one blood-sampling operation, which are used for the subsequent validation of the accuracy of the automated NPA system. The AI-NPA results could be pushed to the application on the MNPDA for on-site nurses or could be checked by the attending doctor for further neonatal pain management, as shown in Figure 5.

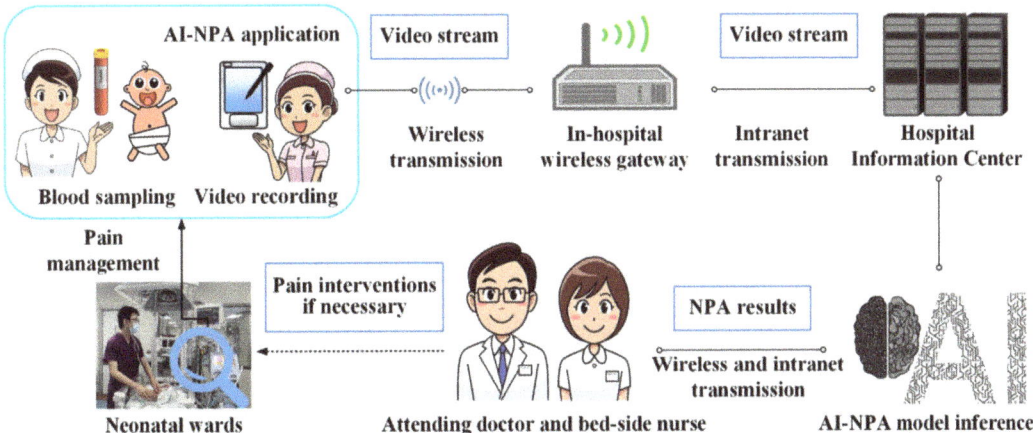

Figure 5. The framework of the automated NPA system and its application.

2.5. Statistical Analysis

Descriptive statistics for the categorical variables were reported as numbers and percentages, and a chi-square test was used for the comparison between groups; statistics were reported as means and standard deviations for continuous variables, and a *t*-test or nonparametric test was used for the group comparison. To analyze the correlation and consistency of the AI-NPA and OS-NPA results, the Spearman correlation analysis, receiver operating characteristic curve (ROC), and kappa coefficient test were used. SAS 9.4 statistical software was used for data analysis, and $p < 0.05$ was considered statistically significant. Because the NIPS pain scores are discrete-integer results, we used the confusion matrix to show the number of cases in which the results were different between the OS-NPA and AI-NPA in detail.

3. Results

3.1. Study Population

A total of 232 newborns were included in this study, with a mean gestational age of 33.93 ± 4.77 weeks, a mean age of 21 (8.5, 41) days, and a mean birth weight of 2250 ± 1010 g. The detailed demographic characteristics are listed in Table 1. Two nurses performed a total of 464 independent OS-NPAs during 232 neonatal blood-sampling operations for each newborn. As a result, one set of consensus NIPS pain scores and grades was given by the two nurses for every OS-NPA and was used as the gold standard.

Table 1. Demographic characteristics of newborns in this study.

Metrics		Number of Cases	Composition Ratio (%)
Sex	Male	86	37.07
	Female	146	62.93
Delivery mode	Spontaneous delivery	95	41.13
	Cesarean section	136	58.87
Main diagnosis	Respiratory disorders	113	48.71
	Digestive disorders	63	27.15
	Nervous-system disorders	22	9.48
	Infection disease	34	14.66
Operation type	Venous blood sampling	36	15.52
	Arterial blood sampling	75	32.33
	Heel blood sampling	75	32.33
	Fingertip blood sampling	46	19.82

3.2. Comparison of NIPS Pain Scores between OS-NPA and AI-NPA

The NIPS pain scores of the OS-NPA and AI-NPA were 5.06 ± 1.85 and 5.17 ± 1.84, respectively. The Spearman correlation analysis showed a correlation coefficient of 0.95 ($p < 0.001$) when comparing the NIPS pain scores of the OS-NPA and AI-NPA. The agreement between the two groups was compared, with a kappa value of 0.92 (0.88, 0.95) ($p < 0.001$). The accuracy of the pain score given by the automated NPA system was 88.79% (206/232), and the confusion matrix of the NIPS pain scores for the two methods is shown in Table 2.

Table 2. Confusion matrix of the NIPS pain scores for OS-NPA and AI-NPA.

OS-NPA	AI-NPA Given by the Automated NPA System							
	0	1	2	3	4	5	6	7
0	5	1	0	0	0	0	0	0
1	1	5	0	0	0	0	0	0
2	0	0	13	0	1	0	1	0	0
3	0	0	0	15	1	1	1	0
4	0	0	1	1	21	4	2	0
5	0	0	0	0	0	37	2	4
6	0	0	0	0	0	2	47	2
7	0	0	0	0	0	0	1	63

The background is highlighted for the diagonal of the confusion matrix.

3.3. Comparison of the NIPS Pain Grades between OS-NPA and AI-NPA

According to the pain-grade criteria of the NIPS, the OS-NPA showed mild pain in 27 patients (8.94%), moderate pain in 47 patients (20.26%), and severe pain in 158 patients (68.10%). The AI-NPA derived mild pain in 26 patients (11.21%), moderate pain in 39 patients (16.81%), and severe pain in 167 patients (71.98%). Compared with the on-site evaluation, the accuracy of the NIPS pain grade given by the AI-NPA was 95.25% (221/232), and the agreement between the two groups was compared, with a kappa value of 0.90 (0.84, 0.96) ($p < 0.001$). See Table 3 for details.

Table 3. Consistency analysis of NIPS pain grading by OS-NPA and AI-NPA.

OS-NPA	AI-NPA			Kappa Value and 95%CI	*p* Value
	Mild	Moderate	Severe		
Mild	25	1	1	0.90 [0.84, 0.96]	< 0.001
Moderate	1	38	8		
Severe	0	0	158		

The background is highlighted for the diagonal of the confusion matrix.

We further investigated the cases of the severe-pain grade. Using the results of the OS-NPA as the criterion, the sensitivity and specificity of the AI-NPA for identifying severe pain were 100% and 87.84%, respectively. The corresponding kappa values and areas under the ROC curve (AUC) of the AI-NPA for identifying severe pain were calculated with different types of blood-sampling operations, as listed in Table 4.

Table 4. Consistency analysis of AI-NPA and OS-NPA of severe pain.

Operation Type	Number of Subjects with Severe Pain (Proportion %)		Kappa Value and 95% CI	AUC and 95% CI	*p* Value
	OS-NPA	AI-NPA			
Venous blood sampling	32 (88.8)	32 (88.8)	1.00 [1.00, 1.00]	1.000 [1.000, 1.000]	<0.001
Arterial blood sampling	57 (76.0)	60 (80.0)	0.88 [0.76, 1.00]	0.967 [0.924, 1.000]	<0.001
Heel blood sampling	43 (57.3)	46 (61.3)	0.92 [0.83, 1.00]	0.984 [0.959, 1.000]	<0.001
Fingertip blood sampling	26 (56.5)	29 (63.3)	0.86 [0.72, 1.00]	0.957 [0.899, 1.000]	<0.001

4. Discussion

4.1. High Evaluation Consistency of the Automated NPA System

The kappa value was used to test the degree of agreement between the results of the different NPA methods. The kappa value ranged from −1 to U+1; the larger the value, the higher the degree of agreement between the two, where the kappa value of the consistency between the NIPS pain scores of the OS-NPA and AI-NPA was 0.92 (0.88, 0.95) ($p < 0.001$). Using the NIPS pain score of the OS-NPA as the gold standard, the accuracy of the pain score given by the automated NPA system was 88.79%. The comparison between the AI-NPA and OS-NPA showed that the correlation coefficient between the two was 0.95 ($p < 0.001$), which was highly positive. These results indicated that there was high consistency in the NIPS pain scores between the AI-NPA and OS-NPA.

Meanwhile, the accuracy of the NIPS pain grade given by the AI-NPA was 95.25%, with a kappa value of 0.90 (0.84, 0.96) ($p < 0.001$). The AI-NPA was also highly consistent with the OS-NPA regarding the evaluation of the degree of pain. Because the guidelines recommend a stepped approach for neonatal pain management, including environmental, nonpharmacological, and pharmacological interventions, provided that a standardized approach is used to assess the pain [27], in addition to judging the presence or absence of pain, it is also necessary to distinguish the pain grade.

4.2. AI-NPA of Severe Pain

The statistical results in Table 4 show that most of the four types of blood-sampling operations in this study were with severe pain, and especially for the venous sampling, of which 88.8% belongs to severe pain. The AI-NPA of severe pain showed an AUC of 0.974, with a 95% confidence interval (0.952, 0.995), and the kappa value was greater than 0.75. The sensitivity and specificity of the AI-NPA for identifying severe pain were 100% and 87.84%, respectively. The relatively low specificity of the AI-NPA of severe pain was due to the fact that the AI assessment mostly focused on the facial expression, while the assessment parameter "crying" of the NIPS varied the most, with corresponding scores of 0–2 assigned to "not crying", "sobbing", and "crying", respectively.

In real-world complex clinical operation scenarios, neonatal crying is easily interfered with by noisy environments, the alarms of monitors, and the occlusion of respiratory-support devices, and there was also an objective difference in the assessment of the "crying" by the nurses. Although the range of scores for "crying" is the largest of all the items in the NIPS, "facial expression" has been proven to be the most specific indicator of pain, and additional information such as "crying" and "physiological signals" could not provide stable performance increments for the AI-NPA methods [28–31]. The main bottleneck for highly accurate AI-NPAs is still the volume of the current training data.

While it is currently not possible to accurately assess pain scores or pain grades by AI technology, it is feasible to tune an AI model to make a tradeoff between the sensitivity and specificity of pain assessments according to the clinical requirements. Based on the views of our neonatal care experts, we prefer sensitivity so that as many neonates as possible who are suffering from pain can be screened for diagnosis and possible analgesia by physicians. Therefore, the overestimation of severe pain by our AI-NPA method is currently a purposeful choice driven by clinical needs. Although further improvement is required for our AI-NPA method, it is superior to those reported in the relevant literature [19–22,30,31], and especially in real-world scenarios. Nevertheless, the specificity of the automated NPA system for identifying severe pain in this study was completely acceptable in clinical practice.

4.3. Strengths and Limitations of the Automated AI-NPA System

The strengths of our automated AI-NPA system are threefold: It could enable 24 h real-time pain-status monitoring, saving laborious human assessment by medical staff; it is robust to occlusion and extreme facial-pose-change disturbance compared with other automated methods; recorded videos and their automated assessment results in the system could facilitate research and education related to clinical pain assessment.

The main limitation of our automated AI-NPA system is that the videos evaluated by the AI-NPA method are currently recorded by nurses using mobile nursing personal digital assistants. Considering that it is not feasible for medical staff to perform both the medical operation and video filming, the automated NPA system currently requires an additional nurse to record the video. This conflicts with our desire to significantly reduce the workload of medical staff through automated pain assessment, given the fact that healthcare resources are valuable and limited. Therefore, as the AI technology further matures and works with automatic face-tracking algorithms, we will automate the entire process by recording video with bedside cameras in the future.

5. Conclusions

Accurate NPA is the premise of standardized neonatal pain management. The AI technique in NPA based on facial recognition can provide convenience for medical staff. This study showed that the automated NPA system could obtain real-time dynamic pain-evaluation results for blood sampling in a real-world neonatal ward scene, which is helpful to implementing the stepped analgesia program for neonatal pain management. Combined with the concept of closed-loop management, the AI technology embedded in the electronic-medical-record (EMR) system in the future will realize the real-time medical intervention for pain by medical staffs. The EMR system can cooperate with the MNPDA to enable bedside nurses to implement care measures in accordance with an automatically generated nursing plan. The downstream health education system can further perform pain-knowledge education for newborns' family members so as to realize the traceability, standardization, and intelligence of the whole process of pain management.

Author Contributions: Conceptualization, X.C. (Xiaoying Cheng), H.Z.; methodology, H.Z. and X.C. (Xiaoying Cheng); software, H.Z. and Y.Z.; validation, F.L. and X.C. (Xiaofei Chen); formal analysis, X.C. (Xiaoying Cheng), F.L., X.C. (Xiaofei Chen), and H.Z.; investigation, L.M.; resources, S.C.; data curation, L.M.; writing—original draft preparation, X.C. (Xiaoying Cheng) and H.Z.; writing—review and editing, H.Z., Y.Z., Y.P. and S.C.; visualization, H.Z. and Y.Z.; supervision, S.C. and Y.P.; project administration, S.C. and Y.P.; funding acquisition, S.C. and Y.P. All authors have read and agreed to the published version of the manuscript.

Funding: This research was funded in part by the Zhejiang Provincial Natural Science Foundation of China under Grant No. LGF20H040008, and in part by the Zhejiang Provincial Health Commission's Science and Technology Program of Medicine and Health (2019PY045).

Institutional Review Board Statement: The study was approved by the Institutional Ethics Committee of The Children's Hospital of Zhejiang University (ethics number: 2018-IRB-051) on 31 July 2018.

Informed Consent Statement: Informed Consents that include consent for research publication were obtained from all subjects (guardians) involved in the study.

Data Availability Statement: The data are stored at the Children's Hospital, Zhejiang University School of Medicine, and will be available upon a reasonable request to the corresponding authors with acceptable ethical clearance.

Acknowledgments: The authors express their great appreciation to all the participants who joined in the experiment.

Conflicts of Interest: The authors declare no conflict of interest.

References

1. Kaur, H.; Mahajan, G. A comprehensive analysis of neonatal pain and measures to reduce pain. *J. Pediatric Crit. Care* **2019**, *6*, 43–48. [CrossRef]
2. Boyle, E.M.; Bradshaw, J.; Blake, K.I. Persistent pain in neonates: Challenges in assessment without the aid of a clinical tool. *Acta Paediatr.* **2018**, *107*, 63–67. [CrossRef] [PubMed]
3. Wan, Y. *The Occurrent Status and Influencing Factors of Neonatal Procedural Pain in Neonatal Intensive Care Unit*; Chinese Academy of Medical Sciences & Peking Union Medical College: Beijing, China, 2017.
4. Anand, K.J.; Eriksson, M.; Boyle, E.M.; Avila-Alvarez, A.; Andersen, R.D.; Sarafidis, K.; Polkki, T.; Matos, C.; Lago, P.; Papadouri, T.; et al. Assessment of continuous pain in newborns admitted to NICUs in 18 European countries. *Acta Paediatr.* **2017**, *106*, 1248–1259. [CrossRef]
5. Relland, L.M.; Gehred, A.; Maitre, N.L. Behavioral and physiological signs for pain assessment in preterm and term neonates during a nociception-specific response: A systematic review. *Pediatric Neurol.* **2019**, *90*, 13–23. [CrossRef] [PubMed]
6. Walker, S.M. Translational studies identify long-term impact of prior neonatal pain experience. *Pain* **2017**, *158*, S29–S42. [CrossRef]
7. Grunau, R.E.; Oberlander, T.; Holsti, L.; Whitfield, M.F. Bedside application of the neonatal facial coding system in pain assessment of premature infants. *Pain* **1998**, *76*, 277–286. [CrossRef]
8. Büttner, W.; Finke, W. Analysis of behavioural and physiological parameters for the assessment of postoperative analgesic demand in newborns, infants and young children: A comprehensive report on seven consecutive studies. *Pediatric Anesth.* **2000**, *90*, 13–23. [CrossRef]
9. Stevens, B.; Johnston, C.; Petryshen, P.; Taddio, A. Premature infant pain profile: Development and initial validation. *Clin. J. Pain* **1996**, *12*, 13–22. [CrossRef]
10. Lawrence, J.; Alcock, D.; McGrath, P.; Kay, J.; MacMurray, S.B.; Dulberg, C. The development of a tool to assess neonatal pain. *Neonatal Netw.* **1993**, *12*, 59–66. [CrossRef]
11. Cong, X.; McGrath, J.M.; Delaney, C.; Liang, S.; Vazquez, V.; Keating, L.; Chang, K.; Dejong, A. Neonatal nurses' perceptions of pain management: Survey of the United States and China. *Pain Manag. Nurs.* **2014**, *15*, 834–844. [CrossRef]
12. Guinsburg, R.; de Araújo Peres, C.; de Almeida, M.F.B.; Balda, R.D.C.X.; Berenguel, R.C.; Tonelotto, J.; Kopelman, B.I. Differences in pain expression between male and female newborn infants. *Pain* **2000**, *85*, 127–133. [CrossRef]
13. Zamzmi, G.; Kasturi, R.; Goldgof, D.; Zhi, R.; Ashmeade, T.; Sun, Y. A review of automated pain assessment in infants: Features, classification tasks, and databases. *IEEE Rev. Biomed. Eng.* **2017**, *11*, 77–96. [CrossRef] [PubMed]
14. Gholami, B.; Haddad, W.M.; Tannenbaum, A.R. Relevance vector machine learning for neonate pain intensity assessment using digital imaging. *IEEE Trans. Biomed. Eng.* **2010**, *57*, 1457–1466. [CrossRef]
15. Brahnam, S.; Nanni, L.; Sexton, R. Introduction to neonatal facial pain detection using common and advanced face classification techniques. In *Advanced Computational Intelligence Paradigms in Healthcare*; Springer: Berlin/Heidelberg, Germany, 2007; pp. 225–253. [CrossRef]
16. Lu, G.; Li, X.; Li, H. Research on recognition for facial expression of pain in neonates. *Acta Opt. Sin.* **2008**, *28*, 2109.
17. Brahnam, S.; Nanni, L.; McMurtrey, S.; Lumini, A.; Brattin, R.; Slack, M.; Barrier, T. Neonatal pain detection in videos using the iCOPEvid dataset and an ensemble of descriptors extracted from Gaussian of Local Descriptors. *Appl. Comput. Inform.* **2019**, *in press*. [CrossRef]
18. Egede, J.; Valstar, M.; Torres, M.T.; Sharkey, D. Automatic neonatal pain estimation: An acute pain in neonates database. In Proceedings of the 2019 8th International Conference on Affective Computing and Intelligent Interaction, Cambridge, UK, 3–6 September 2019. [CrossRef]
19. Zamzmi, G.; Paul, R.; Salekin, M.S.; Goldgof, D.; Kasturi, R.; Ho, T.; Sun, Y. Convolutional neural networks for neonatal pain assessment. *IEEE Trans. Biom. Behav. Identity Sci.* **2019**, *1*, 192–200. [CrossRef]
20. He, K.; Zhang, X.; Ren, S.; Sun, J. Deep residual learning for image recognition. In Proceedings of the IEEE Conference on Computer Vision and Pattern Recognition, Las Vegas, NV, USA, 27–30 June 2016. [CrossRef]
21. Huang, G.; Liu, Z.; van der Maaten, L.; Weinberger, K.Q. Densely connected convolutional networks. In Proceedings of the IEEE Conference on Computer Vision and Pattern Recognition, Honolulu, HI, USA, 22–25 July 2017. [CrossRef]
22. Sun, Y.; Hu, J.; Wang, W.; He, M.; de With, P.H.N. Camera-based discomfort detection using multi-channel attention 3D-CNN for hospitalized infants. *Quant. Imaging Med. Surg.* **2011**, *11*, 3059. [CrossRef]
23. Chen, S.; Luo, F.; Chen, X.; Yan, J.; Zhong, Y.; Pan, Y. A video database of neonatal facial expression based on painful clinical procedures. In Proceedings of the 2019 41st Annual International Conference of the IEEE Engineering in Medicine and Biology Society, Berlin, Germany, 23–27 July 2019. [CrossRef]
24. Huang, R.; Zhang, S.; Li, T.; He, R. Beyond face rotation: Global and local perception GAN for photorealistic and identity preserving frontal view synthesis. In Proceedings of the IEEE International Conference on Computer Vision, Venice, Italy, 22–29 October 2017. [CrossRef]
25. Wang, F.; Jiang, M.; Qian, C.; Yang, S.; Li, C.; Zhang, H.; Wang, X.; Tang, X. Residual attention network for image classification. In Proceedings of the IEEE Conference on Computer Vision and Pattern Recognition, Honolulu, HI, USA, 22–25 July 2017. [CrossRef]
26. Li, S.; Deng, W. Reliable crowdsourcing and deep locality-preserving learning for unconstrained facial expression recognition. *IEEE Trans. Image Process.* **2018**, *28*, 356–370. [CrossRef]

27. Witt, N.; Coynor, S.; Edwards, C.; Bradshaw, H. A guide to pain assessment and management in the neonate. *Curr. Emerg. Hosp. Med. Rep.* **2016**, *4*, 1–10. [CrossRef]
28. Grunau, R.; Craig, K. Pain expression in neonates: Facial action and cry. *Pain* **1987**, *28*, 395–410. [CrossRef]
29. Peters, J.; Koot, H.; Grunau, R.; de Boer, J.; van Druenen, M.; Tibboel, D.; Duivenvoorden, H. Neonatal facial coding system for assessing postoperative pain in infants: Item reduction is valid and feasible. *Clin. J. Pain* **2003**, *19*, 353–363. [CrossRef] [PubMed]
30. Zamzmi, G.; Pai, C.; Goldgof, D.; Kasturi, R.; Sun, Y.; Ashmeade, T. Automated pain assessment in neonates. In Proceedings of the 20th Scandinavian Conference on Image Analysis, Tromsø, Norway, 12–14 June 2017. [CrossRef]
31. Zamzmi, G.; Pai, C.; Goldgof, D.; Kasturi, R.; Ashmeade, T.; Sun, Y. A comprehensive and context-sensitive neonatal pain assessment using computer vision. *IEEE Trans. Affect. Comput.* **2019**, *13*, 28–45. [CrossRef]

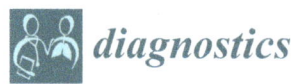 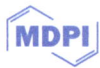

Article

Assessment of Sepsis Risk at Admission to the Emergency Department: Clinical Interpretable Prediction Model

Umran Aygun [1], Fatma Hilal Yagin [2,*], Burak Yagin [2,*], Seyma Yasar [2], Cemil Colak [2], Ahmet Selim Ozkan [3] and Luca Paolo Ardigò [4]

[1] Department of Anesthesiology and Reanimation, Malatya Yesilyurt Hasan Calık State Hospital, Malatya 44929, Turkey; umranaygun92@gmail.com
[2] Department of Biostatistics and Medical Informatics, Faculty of Medicine, Inonu University, Malatya 44280, Turkey; seyma.yasar@inonu.edu.tr (S.Y.); cemil.colak@inonu.edu.tr (C.C.)
[3] Department of Anesthesiology and Reanimation, Malatya Turgut Ozal University School of Medicine, Malatya 44210, Turkey; ahmet.ozkan@ozal.edu.tr
[4] Department of Teacher Education, NLA University College, 0166 Oslo, Norway; luca.ardigo@nla.no
* Correspondence: hilal.yagin@inonu.edu.tr (F.H.Y.); burak.yagin@inonu.edu.tr (B.Y.)

Citation: Aygun, U.; Yagin, F.H.; Yagin, B.; Yasar, S.; Colak, C.; Ozkan, A.S.; Ardigò, L.P. Assessment of Sepsis Risk at Admission to the Emergency Department: Clinical Interpretable Prediction Model. *Diagnostics* **2024**, *14*, 457. https://doi.org/10.3390/diagnostics14050457

Academic Editor: Zhongheng Zhang

Received: 23 January 2024
Revised: 18 February 2024
Accepted: 19 February 2024
Published: 20 February 2024

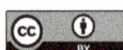

Copyright: © 2024 by the authors. Licensee MDPI, Basel, Switzerland. This article is an open access article distributed under the terms and conditions of the Creative Commons Attribution (CC BY) license (https://creativecommons.org/licenses/by/4.0/).

Abstract: This study aims to develop an interpretable prediction model based on explainable artificial intelligence to predict bacterial sepsis and discover important biomarkers. A total of 1572 adult patients, 560 of whom were sepsis positive and 1012 of whom were negative, who were admitted to the emergency department with suspicion of sepsis, were examined. We investigated the performance characteristics of sepsis biomarkers alone and in combination for confirmed sepsis diagnosis using Sepsis-3 criteria. Three different tree-based algorithms—Extreme Gradient Boosting (XGBoost), Light Gradient Boosting Machine (LightGBM), Adaptive Boosting (AdaBoost)—were used for sepsis prediction, and after examining comprehensive performance metrics, descriptions of the optimal model were obtained with the SHAP method. The XGBoost model achieved accuracy of 0.898 (0.868–0.929) and area under the ROC curve (AUC) of 0.940 (0.898–0.980) with a 95% confidence interval. The five biomarkers for predicting sepsis were age, respiratory rate, oxygen saturation, procalcitonin, and positive blood culture. SHAP results revealed that older age, higher respiratory rate, procalcitonin, neutrophil–lymphocyte count ratio, C-reactive protein, plaque, leukocyte particle concentration, as well as lower oxygen saturation, systolic blood pressure, and hemoglobin levels increased the risk of sepsis. As a result, the Explainable Artificial Intelligence (XAI)-based prediction model can guide clinicians in the early diagnosis and treatment of sepsis, providing more effective sepsis management and potentially reducing mortality rates and medical costs.

Keywords: sepsis; machine learning; explainable artificial intelligence; biomarker

1. Introduction

Sepsis is a complex syndrome characterized by a dysregulated host response to infection, leading to severe and potentially fatal organ dysfunction. The syndrome's lethality significantly surpasses that of simple infections, highlighting the imperative for swift recognition and intervention. Early stages of sepsis, even with minor organ dysfunction, are associated with an in-hospital mortality rate exceeding 10% [1,2], emphasizing the critical need for prompt and accurate identification of the syndrome [3]. Sepsis is caused by an imbalance between pro-inflammatory and anti-inflammatory mediators, resulting in a systemic inflammatory response syndrome (SIRS) that can impair the function of multiple organs, such as the lungs, kidneys, liver, heart, and brain. The severity of sepsis is classified according to the presence and number of organ failures, as well as the degree of hypotension and lactate elevation [1]. The diagnosis of sepsis is based on clinical criteria, such as fever, tachycardia, tachypnea, and altered mental status, as well as laboratory tests, such as blood cultures, inflammatory markers, and lactate levels [3]. The treatment of sepsis consists of early administration of appropriate antibiotics, fluid resuscitation, vasopressors, and supportive care for organ dysfunction. The timely initiation of these interventions can reduce the mortality and morbidity associated with sepsis [3,4].

Sepsis is a major challenge for healthcare systems in Turkey and worldwide, requiring prompt diagnosis, appropriate antimicrobial therapy, and supportive care to improve outcomes and reduce mortality. According to the World Health Organization (WHO) data, sepsis affects about 50 million people every year and 11 million of them lose their lives. In Turkey, the prevalence of sepsis varies roughly between 0.5% and 1% [5]. Despite the absence of a universally accepted gold standard for diagnosis, various definitions and scoring systems have been devised to aid in the rapid detection and diagnosis of sepsis. The Sequential Organ Failure Assessment (SOFA) score is a widely validated tool for assessing mortality risk and provides clear bedside criteria for identifying sepsis in adults [1]. Organ dysfunction is indicated by an acute change in the total SOFA score, specifically an increase of two or more points consequent to an infection. Typically, patients with no pre-existing organ dysfunction are presumed to have a baseline SOFA score of zero, and a score of two or higher correlates with a mortality risk of about 10% in a general hospital population with suspected infection. The potential for rapid deterioration even in cases of modest dysfunction underscores the urgency of timely and appropriate clinical responses [6].

For patients with suspected infection and the risk of prolonged intensive care unit (ICU) stays or adverse outcomes, the Quick Sequential Organ Failure Assessment (qSOFA) criteria can be used for early bedside evaluation [6]. These criteria include changes in mental status, systolic blood pressure of 100 mm Hg or less, or a respiratory rate of 22/min or more. However, the sensitivity of qSOFA for detecting early-stage sepsis in certain patient populations has been questioned, potentially delaying the initiation of necessary treatments [7]. Consequently, the 2021 Surviving Sepsis Campaign guidelines recommend against the exclusive use of qSOFA as a solitary screening tool for sepsis. In clinical practice, the integration of blood biomarkers may provide additional valuable information for identifying high-risk patients or those progressing toward organ failure, even when presenting with low SOFA scores [4]. From this clinical point, the SOFA scale is a clinical marker for sepsis prognosis [8]. Similarly, the Acute Physiology and Chronic Health Evaluation II (APACHE II) score exhibits efficacy in prognosticating the mortality risk associated with sepsis, with a positive correlation observed between score elevation and increased likelihood of death [9].

Recent advancements in Explainable Artificial Intelligence (XAI) have shown promising results in the early prediction of sepsis, a critical area in healthcare that demands timely and accurate decision-making. XAI models, by offering transparency in their decision processes, enable clinicians to understand and trust the predictions made by AI systems [10]. This is particularly vital in sepsis prediction, where the interpretability of AI models aids in identifying the onset of sepsis, potentially improving patient outcomes. Furthermore, XAI facilitates the identification of key clinical variables and their interactions, enhancing the ability of healthcare professionals to make informed decisions [11]. The integration of XAI in sepsis prediction not only augments the accuracy of diagnoses but also aligns with the ethical need for transparency and accountability in AI applications in healthcare [10]. Recognizing these benefits, the current study focuses on leveraging the capabilities of XAI to develop a more effective and reliable tool for healthcare professionals in the battle against sepsis. In addition, although there are many studies on machine learning-based sepsis classification in the literature, there are very few studies on classification with explainable artificial intelligence and candidate biomarkers [12–15]. This study would contribute to the literature in this respect. Therefore, the study aims to construct an XAI classification model for predicting the status of sepsis based on the candidate biomarker features.

2. Materials and Methods

2.1. Data Source

In this study, an open-access dataset of a prospective observational study on adult patients with and without sepsis was used. All patients aged 18 years and older (18–100) who presented to the emergency department with suspected sepsis were included [16]. A total of 1572 adult patients were studied; of these, 560 tested positive for sepsis, while 1012 tested negative. Using the Sepsis-3 criteria, we examined the diagnostic performance characteristics of sepsis biomarkers, both individually and in combination, for confirmed sepsis diagnosis. This study received ethical approval from the Inonu University Non-Interventional Clinical Research Institutional Review Board (decision no: 2023/5215). Informed consent was obtained from all subjects participating in the study.

2.2. Outcome Measures

The current study evaluated the presence and absence of sepsis as outcome measurements based on Sepsis-3 criteria. Sepsis was assessed as follows [16].

- Organ dysfunction was identified as an acute change in total SOFA score ≥ 2 points consequent to the infection.
- The baseline SOFA score was assumed to be zero in patients not known to have pre-existing organ dysfunction.
- The confirmed bacterial infection for Sepsis-3 was defined as a clinical infection, identification of relevant bacteria through culture, and a positive blood culture for bacteremia.

2.3. Biostatistical Analyses

Analytical (Shapiro–Wilk test) and visual (histogram and probability graphs) techniques were used to assess the quantitative characteristic eligibility for a normal distribution. The interquartile range (IQR) and median were used to describe the quantitative data since they were not normally distributed, and the Mann–Whitney U test was employed to compare the two groups. If a p-value was less than 0.05, it was deemed statistically significant. Cohen's D was used to calculate the effect size. The following thresholds were taken into account while determining the effect size: Cohen proposed that an impact size of d = 0.2 be categorized as "small", 0.5 as "medium", and 0.8 as "large" [17]. For qualitative measures, frequency (n) and percentage (%) values were computed, and the chi-square test was used to look at the associations between these features. The statistical analysis was carried out with IBM Corp.'s SPSS 28.0, located in Armonk, NY, USA.

2.4. ML Models and Validation

The methodology for assessing the predictive power of machine learning techniques for sepsis is described in this section. The random forest approach was used to approximate the missing values. Within the research, there was an issue of class imbalance in the distribution of sepsis (560 patients with sepsis and 1012 patients without sepsis). The class imbalance problem was resolved by applying the Synthetic Minority Oversampling Technique for Nominal and Continuous (SMOTE-NC). When dealing with real-world data, class imbalance is a prevalent issue that can be characterized as one in which the number of instances in the majority class is much more than the number of cases in the minority class. Balanced data are important because machine learning models might be biased towards the majority class, leading to problems with underfitting or overfitting. SMOTE-NC was applied only to the training set. The second phase was identifying the most important sepsis biomarkers using the ML-based Least Absolute Shrinkage and Selection Operator (LASSO) approach. A popular regularization and feature selection strategy in machine learning and linear regression is called LASSO. Its purpose is to keep regression models from overfitting by choosing a subset of the most pertinent characteristics from a wider range of features. Following preprocessing, the data were split into 80% training and 20% testing, with 10-fold cross-validation (CV) serving as the resampling technique throughout the training phase. This allowed the ML models to be validated. Three models were trained and evaluated using the tree-based AdaBoost, LightGBM, and XGBoost algorithms to find the best model for sepsis prediction. The optimal hyperparameters of each model were determined by Grid Search with 5-fold and 10 repeated k-Fold CV. Accuracy, sensitivity, specificity, F1 score, positive predictive value (PPV), and negative predictive value (NPV) were computed to evaluate and contrast the efficacy of the best ML model in predicting sepsis among various techniques.

2.5. Synthetic Minority Over-Sampling Technique (SMOTE)

The "Synthetic Minority Over-sampling Technique", or SMOTE for short, is a method used in data mining and ML to solve the issue of unbalanced datasets. One class (the minority class) contains substantially fewer examples than another (the majority class) in datasets that are unbalanced. As a result, ML models may perform poorly if they have a bias in favor of the majority class. SMOTE is a resampling method that generates artificial instances of the minority class in an effort to balance the distribution of classes. It functions by creating artificial samples that resemble instances of minority classes that already exist. SMOTE improves the dataset suitability for training ML models by reducing class imbalance and increasing the amount of samples from minority classes [18,19].

2.6. Extreme Gradient Boosting (XGBoost)

XGBoost is a powerful and versatile ML algorithm, renowned for its exceptional performance in various predictive modeling tasks. It falls under the category of gradient boosting algorithms, which sequentially combine a set of weak predictive models to create a strong ensemble model. The remarkable success of XGBoost can be attributed to several key innovations. First, it employs a novel regularization term that mitigates overfitting, enhancing model generalization. Furthermore, it optimizes computational efficiency by utilizing a data structure known as a "sparsity-aware block structure" and a technique called "column block compressed sparse column". These innovations enable XGBoost to efficiently handle large datasets. The algorithm also utilizes a weighted quantile sketch, improving accuracy when selecting splitting points during tree construction. Overall, XGBoost's combination of regularization, computational efficiency, and accurate splitting point selection has made it a popular choice for a wide range of machine-learning applications [20,21].

2.7. Light Gradient Boosting Machine (LightGBM)

LightGBM represents another cutting-edge gradient-boosting algorithm designed for efficient and high-performance ML tasks. It sets itself apart through its unique approach to tree construction, which differs from traditional depth-first or level-wise strategies. LightGBM utilizes a histogram-based approach, in which data are divided into histograms during tree construction, allowing for more efficient computation of gradient and Hessian values. This approach significantly reduces memory usage and speeds up the training process. LightGBM also introduces exclusive features such as "Gradient-based One-Side Sampling" and "Exclusive Feature Bundling", which further enhance training efficiency and enable the algorithm to tackle high-dimensional data effectively. Its ability to handle large datasets efficiently and its focus on minimizing memory consumption have made LightGBM a popular choice, particularly in real-time and large-scale ML applications [22,23].

2.8. Adaptive Boosting (AdaBoost)

AdaBoost is a classical ensemble learning technique that emphasizes adaptive model combinations to improve predictive accuracy. The central idea behind AdaBoost is to iteratively train a series of weak learners and assign them different weights based on their performance. In each iteration, AdaBoost assigns higher weights to the misclassified instances from the previous iteration, effectively forcing the algorithm to focus on the most challenging data points. By giving more weight to the errors, AdaBoost continually adapts and evolves its ensemble of weak learners, ultimately leading to a stronger, more accurate model. The final prediction is a weighted combination of the individual weak learner predictions, with higher-performing weak learners having more influence. AdaBoost has proven effective in boosting the performance of various base classifiers, making it a valuable tool in the ensemble learning toolbox [24,25].

2.9. Metrics Used to Evaluate the Performance of ML Models

Accuracy: Accuracy is a classification metric that measures the overall accuracy of a prediction model's decisions. This criterion is simple and intuitive, but may not be suitable for unbalanced data sets where one class is significantly superior to the other [26].

F1-Score: The F1-Score is a statistic that yields a single number by combining recall (sensitivity) and precision. When working with unbalanced datasets, it is helpful. The model's recall—its capacity to recognize all pertinent occurrences of the positive class—and precision—its capacity to prevent false positives—are both balanced by the F1-Score [27].

Sensitivity: This metric calculates the proportion of true positive samples that are predicted as positive by the ML model [26].

Specificity: Specificity measures the proportion of actual negative instances that are correctly predicted as negative by the model. It is the ratio of true negatives to the total number of actual negatives [26].

Negative Predictive Value (NPV): NPV measures the proportion of instances predicted as negative that are actually true negatives. It is the ratio of true negatives to the total number of instances predicted as negative [28].

Positive Predictive Value (PPV): PPV is a classification metric that measures the proportion of instances predicted as positive by a model that are actually true positive instances. In other words, PPV assesses the accuracy of the positive predictions made by a model. It is particularly relevant when the cost or consequences of making false positive predictions are significant [28].

Area Under the Receiver Operating Characteristic Curve (AUC): AUC is a metric that evaluates the ability of a classification model to distinguish between classes, particularly in binary classification problems. The ROC curve is a graphical representation of the true positive rate (sensitivity) against the false positive rate (1-specificity) at various threshold settings. AUC calculates the area under this curve, providing a single value that summarizes the model's ability to discriminate between positive and negative instances. A higher AUC value (closer to 1) indicates better discrimination and performance of the model [26,29].

Brier Score: The Brier Score measures the accuracy of probabilistic predictions made by a model. It is commonly used for assessing the calibration of predicted probabilities in binary or multi-class classification problems. The Brier Score is calculated as the mean squared difference between predicted probabilities and the actual outcomes. It penalizes both overconfidence (assigning high probability to the wrong class) and under confidence (assigning low probability to the correct class). The Brier Score ranges from 0 to 1, with 0 indicating perfect accuracy and 1 indicating the worst possible accuracy. Lower Brier Scores are preferable, indicating better-calibrated probability predictions [26,30].

3. Results

In the study, 1572 patients aged between 18 and 100 were examined. Of the patients, 44.3% were female and 55.7% were male. The median haemoglobin (g/L) of female patients was 126 and the median haemoglobin (g/L) of male patients was 135, while statistical tests showed that hemoglobin (g/L) levels were significantly higher in males than in females ($p < 0.001$). Age, systolic blood pressure (mmHg), respiratory rate (breaths/min), oxygen saturation (%), heart rate (beats/min), body temperature (°C), hemoglobin (g/L), leukocyte particle concentration ($\times 10^9$ cells/L), C-reactive protein(mg/L), procalcitonin (ng/mL), neutrophil–lymphocyte count ratio, lactate (mmol/L), intensive care unit, positive blood culture, and systemic inflammatory response syndrome are important biomarkers in sepsis following LASSO.

Table 1 provides a detailed summary of the descriptive statistics and effect size estimations for the sepsis biomarkers found after applying LASSO. The robustness of the feature selection procedure and the potential importance of these biomarkers in the setting of sepsis were reinforced when it was discovered that p values for every one of the chosen biomarkers were statistically significant with $p < 0.05$. On examining Table 1, it was seen that the group with sepsis had a considerably greater median age than the group without sepsis.

The sepsis group had substantially higher levels of respiratory rate (breaths/min), heart rate (beats/min), body temperature (°C), leukocyte particle concentration ($\times 10^9$ cells/L), C-reactive protein(mg/L), procalcitonin (ng/mL), neutrophil–lymphocyte count ratio, and plaque (mmol/L) ($p < 0.05$). Conversely, the sepsis group had substantially lower levels of hemoglobin (g/L), oxygen saturation (%), and systolic blood pressure (mmHg) ($p \leq 0.05$). Procalcitonin (ng/mL) had the largest significant effect size (ES: 0.0891) among the chosen biomarkers, according to our study. This implies that procalcitonin (ng/mL) functions as an effective sepsis-positive and sepsis-negative group discriminator and, as such, merits more research as a possible target for therapy or diagnostic biomarker.

Table 1. Descriptive statistics for the clinical biomarkers of sepsis.

Variable	Group				*p*-Value	ES
	Reference Values for No Sepsis	No Sepsis (*n* = 1012)	Reference Values for Sepsis	Sepsis (*n* = 560)		
Age (years)		68 (25)		76.5 (18)	<0.001	0.0669 (Small)
Systolic blood pressure (mmhg)	120–180	136 (31)	<90 or >140	130 (36)	<0.001	0.0115 (Small)
Respiratory rate (breaths/min)	12–20	22 (6.915)	>20 or <12	25.35 (8)	<0.001	0.0677 (Small)
Oxygen saturation (%)	95–100	96 (3)	<92	94 (6)	<0.001	0.0709 (Small)
Heart rate (beats/min)	60–100	95 (24.625)	>100 or <60	100 (26)	<0.001	0.00991 (Small)
Body temperature (°C)	36.5–37.5	37.8 (1.4)	<36 or >38	38 (1.5)	0.01	0.00418 (Small)
Haemoglobin (g/L)	13.5–17.5 (Male)	132 (24.812)	<13.5	128 (24)	0.001	0.00701 (Small)
Leukocyte particle concentration ($\times 10^9$ cells/L)	4–10	11.3 (6.3)	<4 or >12	13.1 (7.65)	<0.001	0.0307 (Small)
C-reactive protein(mg/L)	<5	91.5 (120.25)	>10	126 (148.25)	<0.001	0.0194 (Small)
Procalcitonin (ng/mL)	<0.5	0.13 (0.498)	>2.0	0.51 (3.88)	<0.001	0.0891 (Small)
Neutrophil–lymphocyte count ratio	<3.5	8 (9.45)	>10	13.013 (14.3)	<0.001	0.0755 (Small)
Lactate (mmol/L)	<2.0	1.6 (0.883)	>2.0	1.9 (1.253)	<0.001	0.039 (Small)

The values are reported by median (IQR); IQR: interquartile range; ES: effect size.

In Table 2, the optimum values of the parameters optimized by Grid Search for the three ML models are given.

Table 2. The optimal hyper-parameters of models determined by Grid Search.

Model	Optimal Hyper-Parameters
LightGBM	n_estimators = 1000, learning_rate = 0.1, colsample_bytree = 0.8, subsample = 0.8
AdaBoost	n_estimators = 100, learning_rate = 0.1
XGBoost	n_estimators = 1000, learning_rate = 0.1, max_depth = 2, subsample = 0.8

Three different ML models (AdaBoost, LightGBM, and XGBoost) were created using the important biomarkers of sepsis determined with the help of LASSO, and the prediction performances of these models were compared. Based on the findings of accuracy, F1 score, sensitivity, specificity, PPV, NPV, AUC, and Brier score, all the prediction models performed comparably. Optimum prediction was performed using the XGBoost model, one of the three tree-based ML classifiers. The performances of the models using the original data were lower than the models created after SMOTE-NC, and when the performance measures in the models using the original data were examined, it was observed that the results were biased and inconsistent. After SMOTE-NC, with a 95% confidence range, the XGBoost model produced accuracy of 0.898 (0.868–0.929) and an AUC of 0.940 (0.898–0.980).

Furthermore, the XGBoost model demonstrated exceptionally high specificity of 0.891 (0.837–0.932) and sensitivity of 0.905 (0.854–0.943). A lower false negative (FN) value is associated with a greater sensitivity rating. In comparative biological studies, mistakes including false positives and false negatives are frequent. This finding is significant since one of the primary objectives of this study was to reduce the number of false negatives, or missing sepsis patients (Table 3).

SHAP annotations were examined to interpret sepsis prediction results of the three tree-based models. With the help of SHAP, we were able to determine the levels of biomarkers important in predicting sepsis, identified by LASSO. The SHAP annotations of the optimal model XGBoost (Figure 1) and the LightGBM (Figure 2) model were more similar compared to the annotations for AdaBoost (Figure 3). According to the explanations of the XGBoost model, age, respiratory rate (breaths/minute), oxygen saturation (%), procalcitonin (ng/mL) and positive blood culture were determined as the five most important biomarkers in the early diagnosis of sepsis. In addition to old age there were higher respiratory rate (breaths/minute), procalcitonin (ng/mL), neutrophil–lymphocyte count ratio, C-reactive protein (mg/L), lactate (mmol/L), leukocyte particle concentration ($\times 10^9$ cells/L) It was determined that body temperature (°C) levels were associated with the risk of sepsis. Additionally, SHAP findings revealed that low oxygen saturation (%), systolic blood pressure (mmHg) and hemoglobin (g/L) levels increased the risk of sepsis (Figure 1).

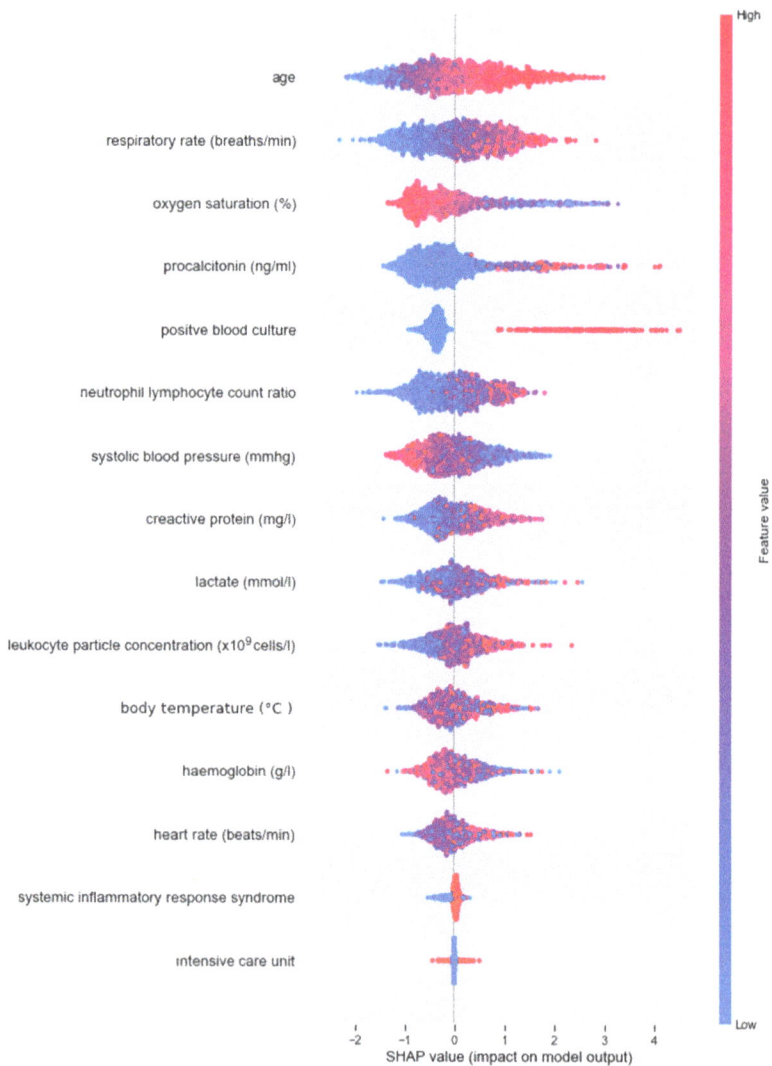

Figure 1. XGBoost model SHAP annotations; The importance of biomarkers is ranked by average (|SHAP value|); the graph's points are colored based on the normalized values of each patient's level of biomarker value. The feature value increases as it gets closer to pink and drops as it gets closer to blue. Sepsis is more likely when a feature's SHAP value is greater. The SHAP plot background for the optimal prediction model is drawn in grey.

Table 3. Results of ML models on original and SOMOTE-NC applied data in sepsis (Values in parentheses are 95% confidence interval (CI)).

Model/Metric		Accuracy	F1-Score	Sensitivity	Specificity	PPV	NPV	AUC	Brier Score
AdaBoost	Orijinal	0.732 (0.682–0.783)	0.813 (0.769–0.858)	0.92 (0.871–0.954)	0.407 (0.314–0.506)	0.729 (0.667–0.784)	0.746 (0.616–0.85)	0.782 (0.663–0.902)	0.121 (0.091–0.189)
	SMOTE-NC	0.869 (0.835–0.903)	0.871 (0.837–0.905)	0.882 (0.827–0.925)	0.856 (0.797–0.903)	0.859 (0.802–0.905)	0.879 (0.823–0.923)	0.917 (0.869–0.966)	0.027 (0.022–0.038)
LightGBM	Orijinal	0.746 (0.696–0.795)	0.824 (0.78–0.867)	0.936 (0.891–0.966)	0.417 (0.323–0.515)	0.735 (0.674–0.79)	0.789 (0.661–0.886)	0.799 (0.676–0.923)	0.104 (0.097–0.134)
	SMOTE-NC	0.888 (0.856–0.92)	0.89 (0.858–0.922)	0.895 (0.842–0.935)	0.88 (0.825–0.924)	0.885 (0.832–0.927)	0.89 (0.835–0.932)	0.931 (0.887–0.974)	0.025 (0.02–0.036)
XGBoost	Orijinal	0.766 (0.718–0.814)	0.834 (0.791–0.876)	0.925 (0.878–0.958)	0.491 (0.393–0.589)	0.759 (0.698–0.813)	0.791 (0.674–0.881)	0.815 (0.708–0.923)	0.080 (0.062–0.098)
	SMOTE-NC	0.898 (0.868–0.929)	0.901 (0.87–0.931)	0.905 (0.854–0.943)	0.891 (0.837–0.932)	0.896 (0.844–0.935)	0.901 (0.848–0.94)	0.94 (0.898–0.98)	0.018 (0.014–0.021)

AdaBoost: adaptive boosting; LightGBM: light gradient boosting; XGBoost: extreme gradient boosting; SMOTE-NC: Synthetic Minority Oversampling Technique for Nominal and Continuous; PPV: positive predictive value; NPV: negative predictive value; AUC: area under of the ROC curve; CI: confidence interval.

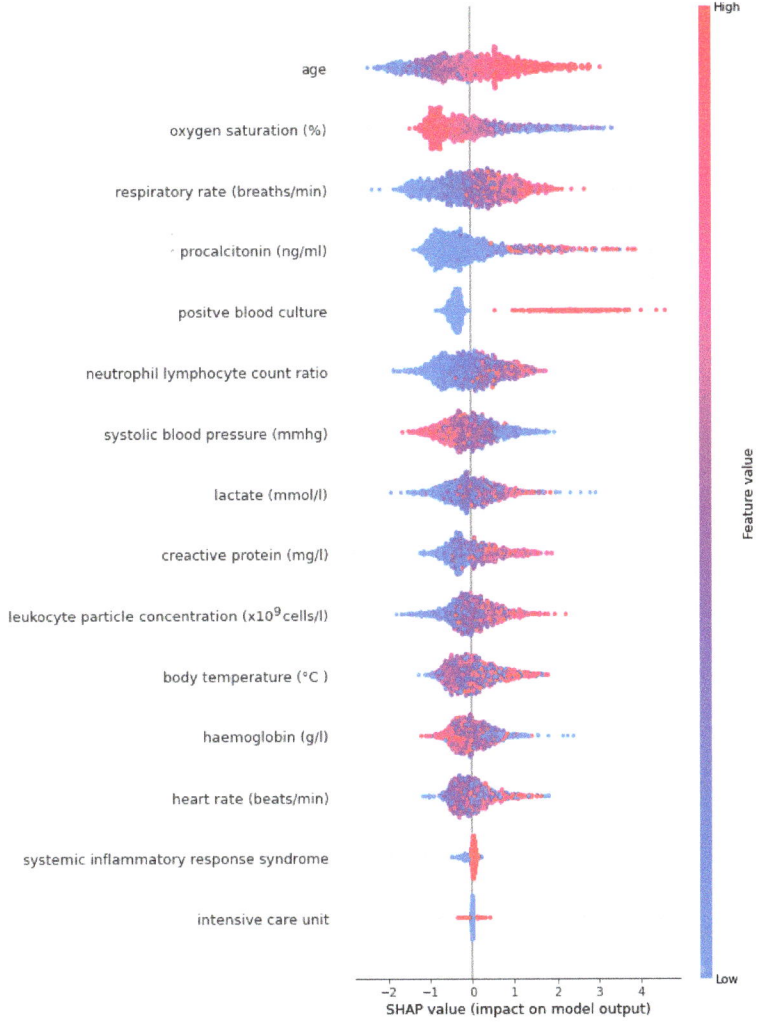

Figure 2. LightGBM model SHAP annotations.

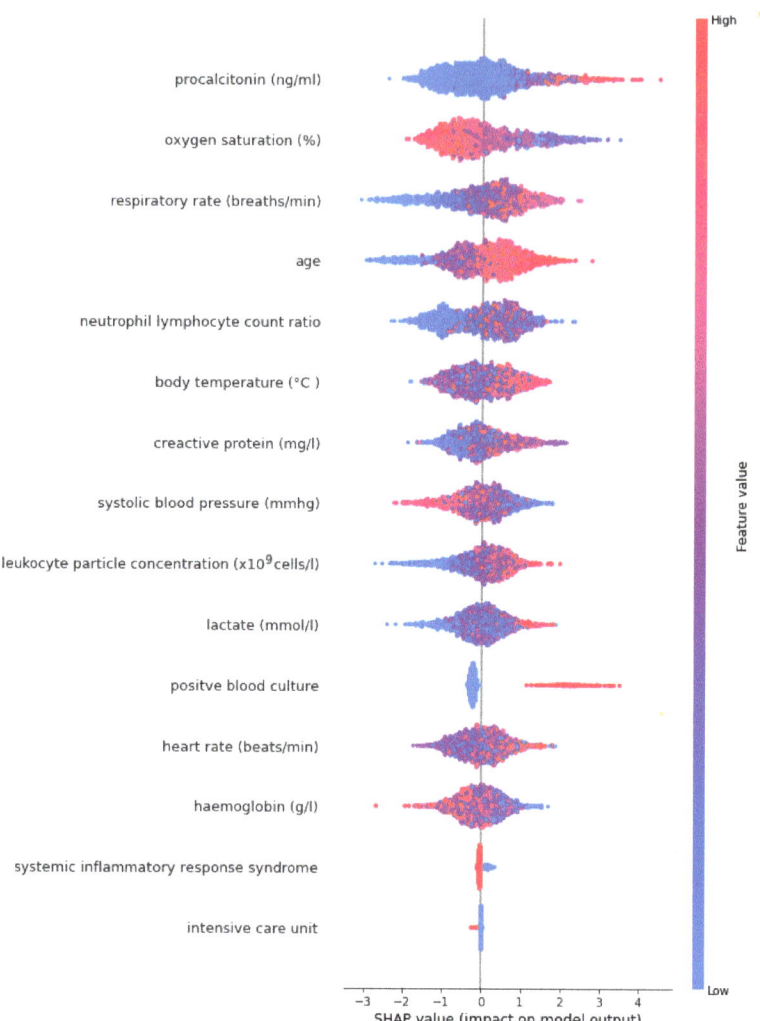

Figure 3. AdaBoost model SHAP annotations.

4. Discussion

Sepsis is a critical health condition triggered by an over-activation of the immune system to maintain its normal function, exceeding its capacity to fight widely disseminated infections. This pathophysiological state is characterized by an immune system response to prevent a local infection from having a systemic impact. Sepsis can lead to severe organ dysfunction and life-threatening complications caused by an excessive immune response. This complex process involves important factors that determine the clinical course of sepsis, affecting the ability to control infection and maintain a balanced inflammatory response [31,32]. Economically, sepsis has serious negative impacts due to high treatment costs, prolonged hospitalizations, and rehabilitation processes. An increase in sepsis cases puts financial pressure on health systems, strains hospital resources, and can push intensive care units to their limits. Globally and in Turkey, sepsis is challenged by expenditures and resource allocations that negatively impact economic growth. This emphasizes that sepsis is a significant burden on national economies as well as the health of individuals. In this context, the development of sepsis prevention strategies and effective treatment modalities is critical both to protect the health of individuals and to strengthen economic sustainability [33]. APACHE II and SOFA are two different clinical scales used to assess the severity and prognosis of intensive care unit patients. Both are designed to monitor and guide the treatment of patients in intensive care. The SOFA assesses the function of various organ systems and is used to identify patients with organ failure. The SOFA score is based on six different parameters that assess the function of the respiratory, cardiovascular, hepatic, coagulation, neurological, and renal systems. On the other hand, APACHE II is a scoring system based on the patient's physiologic status, chronic health status, and age. The APACHE II score is used to predict the patient's mortality risk and includes many parameters such as the oliguria system, cardiovascular system, neurologic status, and other physiologic measures. Sepsis is among the leading causes of infection-related deaths, such as COVID-19, and scoring systems such as SOFA and APACHE II are used to assess the severity and prognosis of the disease in patients who develop sepsis. Especially in patients with the severe form of COVID-19, these scoring systems can play an important role in directing intensive care resources and determining the treatment plan [34–36].

Anticipating sepsis can lower medical expenses and save lives by delaying the onset of multi-organ failure, decreasing admissions to critical care units, and enhancing patient outcomes. Therefore, early prediction of sepsis and initiation of treatment is vital to prevent mortality. Early identification of patients at high risk of sepsis with artificial intelligence (AI) algorithms can significantly improve health outcomes and treatment processes by enabling rapid intervention in intensive care units and halting disease progression. In this study, an artificial intelligence model (XGBoost, LightGBM, AdaBoost) was used to predict bacterial sepsis classified according to SOFA score. XGBoost has the highest performance metrics compared to the other two methods, with accuracy, F1-score, sensitivity, specificity, positive predictive value, negative predictive value, AUC, and Brier score values being 89.8%, 90.1%, 90.5%, 89.1%, 89.6%, 90.1%, 94.0%, and 0.018, respectively. According to the XGBoost model, the five possible biomarkers that can be used to predict sepsis are age, respiratory rate (breath/min), oxygen saturation (%), procalcitonin (ng/mL), and positive blood culture.

Age is an important factor that determines the resistance of individuals to infections. Advanced age is characterized by a series of changes that often lead to an age-related weakening of the immune system. Age-related immunosenescence involves a functional decline in immune cells, which can lead to a reduction in an effective defense mechanism against infections [37]. With advanced age, the increasing incidence of chronic diseases (especially diabetes, cardiovascular disease, and chronic renal failure) can reduce the body's defense capacity against bacterial infections. This can increase the risk of developing sepsis. With advanced age, the increasing incidence of chronic diseases (especially diabetes, cardiovascular disease, and chronic renal failure) can reduce the body's defense capacity against bacterial infections. This can increase the risk of developing sepsis [38]. On the other hand, the decline in the function of many organs such as the heart, lungs, and kidneys with increasing age can reduce the effectiveness in fighting infections. Affecting these organs can increase the severity of the sepsis process. Furthermore, in a systematic review of 17 articles, age was reported to be one of the most important predictors among 194 predictors [39].

Sepsis causes widespread inflammation, leading to increased metabolism and oxygen demand. This can result in elevated respiratory rate due to increased oxygen needs and tissue damage. Acidosis from lactic acid accumulation prompts faster breathing to remove excess acid. Lung damage or hypoxemia can occur, further increasing respiratory rate to compensate. Additionally, stress responses trigger hormonal release, boosting respiratory rate. Overall, the elevated respiratory rate in sepsis reflects efforts to combat infection, tissue repair, and oxygen demand, but it also indicates a serious condition requiring close clinical assessment, as lung damage and circulatory failure can impede oxygen exchange and utilization, leading to decreased oxygen saturation [40,41]. During sepsis, the metabolism of cells can increase, which can lead to acidosis. This can affect oxygen transport and lower oxygen saturation. Sepsis can often cause low blood pressure (hypotension). Low blood pressure can prevent enough blood from reaching the organs in the body, which can lower oxygen saturation. Therefore, it can be said that regular monitoring of oxygen saturation levels in a patient with sepsis and adjusting treatment, if necessary, will allow sepsis to be detected and prevented at an early stage.

Procalcitonin (PCT) is a host-directed biomarker used in the management of sepsis. PCT levels are used in many clinical situations, such as assessing the severity and extent of bacterial infections, differentiating sepsis from other inflammatory conditions, monitoring response to treatment, and managing antibiotic use. PCT levels can help in the early diagnosis of bacterial infections and in the differential diagnosis of sepsis from other inflammatory conditions. High PCT levels may indicate the presence of bacterial infections. Higher PCT levels can often indicate more serious bacterial infections. A further decline in PCT levels may indicate that the treatment is effective, and the infection is under control [42]. PCT levels can help manage the start and duration of antibiotic treatment. High PCT levels may indicate that bacterial infections persist, in which case antibiotic treatment can continue. However, low PCT levels may suggest that antibiotic treatment is unnecessary. PCT is considered a more specific marker, especially in bacterial infections. This may reduce the likelihood of PCT levels being confused with other conditions, such as viral infections [43,44]. Hence, PCT can be a timely, perfect, and effective diagnostic marker for sepsis brought on by bacterial infection [45].

There is a strong association between sepsis and positive blood cultures, and they play a critical role in the diagnosis of sepsis. Blood cultures are used to identify the causative microorganisms of an infection in the body. Positive blood cultures indicate that an infection in the body has spread into the bloodstream and bacteria have entered the blood. Positive blood cultures are also very useful in determining the severity of sepsis and how widespread the infection is. Different types and amounts of bacteria can affect the severity of sepsis. Positive blood cultures can also help to identify the source of focal infection [46–48].

Artificial intelligence studies, that contribute positively to the survival rates and treatment outcomes of patients by increasing the chances of early diagnosis and intervention in sepsis prediction, are frequently used in the literature [14,49,50]. However, in the current study, the performance criterion of the artificial intelligence model used to predict sepsis was significantly higher than the others. Therefore, XGBoost has a very high performance in predicting sepsis and the five proposed biomarkers will be very useful in the clinic for early diagnosis, treatment, and monitoring response to treatment.

5. Conclusions

The tree-based XGBoost algorithm proposed in this study can accurately distinguish and evaluate sepsis through selected biomarkers. A combination of XGBoost and XAI can provide a clear interpretation of the global risk estimate for sepsis and allow physicians to intuitively understand the impact of key biomarkers in the proposed model. As a result, research in which prediction models are used together with XAI is crucial, especially in medical applications, as it enhances the transparency and trustworthiness of the model predictions. It allows healthcare professionals to interpret and validate the model's decisions, ultimately aiding in the decision-making process.

Author Contributions: Conceptualization, U.A., F.H.Y. and B.Y.; Formal analysis, F.H.Y. and B.Y.; Investigation, S.Y. and C.C.; Methodology, U.A., F.H.Y. and B.Y.; Software, U.A. and F.H.Y.; Supervision, C.C. and L.P.A.; Validation, U.A., F.H.Y. and B.Y.; Writing—original draft, U.A., F.H.Y., B.Y., S.Y., C.C., A.S.O. and L.P.A.; Writing—review and editing, U.A., F.H.Y., B.Y., S.Y., C.C., A.S.O. and L.P.A. All authors have read and agreed to the published version of the manuscript.

Funding: This research received no external funding.

Institutional Review Board Statement: This study received ethical approval from the Inonu University Non-Interventional Clinical Research Institutional Review Board (decision no: 2023/5215). Informed consent was obtained from all subjects participating in the study.

Informed Consent Statement: Informed consent was obtained from all subjects involved in the study.

Data Availability Statement: In appropriate cases, it can be requested from the corresponding author.

Conflicts of Interest: The authors declare no conflicts of interest.

References

1. Singer, M.; Deutschman, C.S.; Seymour, C.W.; Shankar-Hari, M.; Annane, D.; Bauer, M.; Bellomo, R.; Bernard, G.R.; Chiche, J.-D.; Coopersmith, C.M.; et al. The third international consensus definitions for sepsis and septic shock (Sepsis-3). *JAMA* **2016**, *315*, 801–810. [CrossRef] [PubMed]
2. Shankar-Hari, M.; Phillips, G.S.; Levy, M.L.; Seymour, C.W.; Liu, V.X.; Deutschman, C.S.; Angus, D.C.; Rubenfeld, G.D.; Singer, M. Developing a new definition and assessing new clinical criteria for septic shock: For the Third International Consensus Definitions for Sepsis and Septic Shock (Sepsis-3). *JAMA* **2016**, *315*, 775–787. [CrossRef] [PubMed]
3. Seymour, C.W.; Gesten, F.; Prescott, H.C.; Friedrich, M.E.; Iwashyna, T.J.; Phillips, G.S.; Lemeshow, S.; Osborn, T.; Terry, K.M.; Levy, M.M. Time to treatment and mortality during mandated emergency care for sepsis. *N. Engl. J. Med.* **2017**, *376*, 2235–2244. [CrossRef] [PubMed]
4. Evans, L.; Rhodes, A.; Alhazzani, W.; Antonelli, M.; Coopersmith, C.M.; French, C.; Machado, F.R.; Mcintyre, L.; Ostermann, M.; Prescott, H.C.; et al. Surviving sepsis campaign: International guidelines for management of sepsis and septic shock 2021. *Intensive Care Med.* **2021**, *47*, 1181–1247. [CrossRef] [PubMed]
5. Baykara, N.; Akalın, H.; Arslantaş, M.K.; Hancı, V.; Çağlayan, Ç.; Kahveci, F.; Demirağ, K.; Baydemir, C.; Ünal, N. Epidemiology of sepsis in intensive care units in Turkey: A multicenter, point-prevalence study. *Crit. Care* **2018**, *22*, 1–14. [CrossRef]
6. Seymour, C.W.; Liu, V.X.; Iwashyna, T.J.; Brunkhorst, F.M.; Rea, T.D.; Scherag, A.; Rubenfeld, G.; Kahn, J.M.; Shankar-Hari, M.; Singer, M. Assessment of clinical criteria for sepsis: For the Third International Consensus Definitions for Sepsis and Septic Shock (Sepsis-3). *JAMA* **2016**, *315*, 762–774. [CrossRef]
7. Churpek, M.M.; Snyder, A.; Han, X.; Sokol, S.; Pettit, N.; Howell, M.D.; Edelson, D.P. Quick sepsis-related organ failure assessment, systemic inflammatory response syndrome, and early warning scores for detecting clinical deterioration in infected patients outside the intensive care unit. *Am. J. Respir. Crit. Care Med.* **2017**, *195*, 906–911. [CrossRef]
8. Jones, A.E.; Trzeciak, S.; Kline, J.A. The Sequential Organ Failure Assessment score for predicting outcome in patients with severe sepsis and evidence of hypoperfusion at the time of emergency department presentation. *Crit. Care Med.* **2009**, *37*, 1649. [CrossRef]
9. Abd-Elfattah, A.H.; Khaled, M.M.Y.; Ahmed, A.A.; Yahia, M.; Kotrob, A.M.E.-b.M. Comparison of Presepsin (CD14), Procalcitonin (PCT) and C-reactive protein (CRP) at different SOFA and APACHE II scores in sepsis patients. *Int. J. Health Sci.* **2022**, *6*, 3840–3864. [CrossRef]
10. Ribeiro, M.T.; Singh, S.; Guestrin, C. "Why should I trust you?" Explaining the predictions of any classifier. In Proceedings of the 22nd ACM SIGKDD International Conference on Knowledge Discovery and Data Mining, San Francisco, CA, USA, 13–17 August 2016; pp. 1135–1144.
11. Holzinger, A.; Biemann, C.; Pattichis, C.S.; Kell, D.B. What do we need to build explainable AI systems for the medical domain? *arXiv* **2017**, arXiv:1712.09923.
12. Jiang, Z.; Bo, L.; Xu, Z.; Song, Y.; Wang, J.; Wen, P.; Wan, X.; Yang, T.; Deng, X.; Bian, J. An explainable machine learning algorithm for risk factor analysis of in-hospital mortality in sepsis survivors with ICU readmission. *Comput. Methods Programs Biomed.* **2021**, *204*, 106040. [CrossRef]
13. Lemańska-Perek, A.; Krzyżanowska-Gołąb, D.; Kobylińska, K.; Biecek, P.; Skalec, T.; Tyszko, M.; Gozdzik, W.; Adamik, B. Explainable artificial intelligence helps in understanding the effect of fibronectin on survival of sepsis. *Cells* **2022**, *11*, 2433. [CrossRef]
14. Yang, M.; Liu, C.; Wang, X.; Li, Y.; Gao, H.; Liu, X.; Li, J. An explainable artificial intelligence predictor for early detection of sepsis. *Crit. Care Med.* **2020**, *48*, e1091–e1096. [CrossRef]
15. Guidotti, R.; Monreale, A.; Ruggieri, S.; Turini, F.; Giannotti, F.; Pedreschi, D. A survey of methods for explaining black box models. *ACM Comput. Surv. (CSUR)* **2018**, *51*, 1–42. [CrossRef]
16. Ljungström, L.; Pernestig, A.-K.; Jacobsson, G.; Andersson, R.; Usener, B.; Tilevik, D. Diagnostic accuracy of procalcitonin, neutrophil-lymphocyte count ratio, C-reactive protein, and lactate in patients with suspected bacterial sepsis. *PLoS ONE* **2017**, *12*, e0181704. [CrossRef]
17. Cohen, J. The effect size. In *Statistical Power Analysis for the Behavioral Sciences*; Academic Press: Cambridge, MA, USA, 1988; pp. 77–83.
18. Yi, H.; Jiang, Q.; Yan, X.; Wang, B. Imbalanced classification based on minority clustering synthetic minority oversampling technique with wind turbine fault detection application. *IEEE Trans. Ind. Inform.* **2020**, *17*, 5867–5875. [CrossRef]
19. Gozukara Bag, H.G.; Yagin, F.H.; Gormez, Y.; González, P.P.; Colak, C.; Gülü, M.; Badicu, G.; Ardigò, L.P. Estimation of obesity levels through the proposed predictive approach based on physical activity and nutritional habits. *Diagnostics* **2023**, *13*, 2949. [CrossRef] [PubMed]

20. Velthoen, J.; Dombry, C.; Cai, J.-J.; Engelke, S. Gradient boosting for extreme quantile regression. *Extremes* **2023**, *26*, 639–667. [CrossRef]
21. Yagin, B.; Yagin, F.H.; Colak, C.; Inceoglu, F.; Kadry, S.; Kim, J. Cancer Metastasis Prediction and Genomic Biomarker Identification through Machine Learning and eXplainable Artificial Intelligence in Breast Cancer Research. *Diagnostics* **2023**, *13*, 3314. [CrossRef]
22. Alzamzami, F.; Hoda, M.; El Saddik, A. Light gradient boosting machine for general sentiment classification on short texts: A comparative evaluation. *IEEE Access* **2020**, *8*, 101840–101858. [CrossRef]
23. Rufo, D.D.; Debelee, T.G.; Ibenthal, A.; Negera, W.G. Diagnosis of diabetes mellitus using gradient boosting machine (LightGBM). *Diagnostics* **2021**, *11*, 1714. [CrossRef]
24. Colakovic, I.; Karakatič, S. Adaptive Boosting Method for Mitigating Ethnicity and Age Group Unfairness. *SN Comput. Sci.* **2023**, *5*, 10. [CrossRef]
25. Guldogan, E.; Yagin, F.H.; Pinar, A.; Colak, C.; Kadry, S.; Kim, J. A proposed tree-based explainable artificial intelligence approach for the prediction of angina pectoris. *Sci. Rep.* **2023**, *13*, 22189. [CrossRef]
26. Halasz, G.; Sperti, M.; Villani, M.; Michelucci, U.; Agostoni, P.; Biagi, A.; Rossi, L.; Botti, A.; Mari, C.; Maccarini, M.; et al. A machine learning approach for mortality prediction in COVID-19 pneumonia: Development and evaluation of the Piacenza score. *J. Med. Internet Res.* **2021**, *23*, e29058. [CrossRef]
27. Chicco, D.; Jurman, G. The advantages of the Matthews correlation coefficient (MCC) over F1 score and accuracy in binary classification evaluation. *BMC Genom.* **2020**, *21*, 1–13. [CrossRef] [PubMed]
28. Jehi, L.; Ji, X.; Milinovich, A.; Erzurum, S.; Rubin, B.P.; Gordon, S.; Young, J.B.; Kattan, M.W. Individualizing risk prediction for positive coronavirus disease 2019 testing: Results from 11,672 patients. *Chest* **2020**, *158*, 1364–1375. [CrossRef] [PubMed]
29. Nahm, F.S. Receiver operating characteristic curve: Overview and practical use for clinicians. *Korean J. Anesthesiol.* **2022**, *75*, 25–36. [CrossRef] [PubMed]
30. Rufibach, K. Use of Brier score to assess binary predictions. *J. Clin. Epidemiol.* **2010**, *63*, 938–939. [CrossRef]
31. Wiersinga, W.J.; van der Poll, T. Immunopathophysiology of human sepsis. *EBioMedicine* **2022**, *86*, 104363. [CrossRef]
32. Jacobi, J. The pathophysiology of sepsis—2021 update: Part 2, organ dysfunction and assessment. *Am. J. Health-Syst. Pharm.* **2022**, *79*, 424–436. [CrossRef]
33. van den Berg, M.; van Beuningen, F.; Ter Maaten, J.; Bouma, H. Hospital-related costs of sepsis around the world: A systematic review exploring the economic burden of sepsis. *J. Crit. Care* **2022**, *71*, 154096. [CrossRef]
34. Huang, Y.; Jiang, S.; Li, W.; Fan, Y.; Leng, Y.; Gao, C. Establishment and effectiveness evaluation of a scoring system-RAAS (RDW, AGE, APACHE II, SOFA) for sepsis by a retrospective analysis. *J. Inflamm. Res.* **2022**, *15*, 465–474. [CrossRef]
35. Basile-Filho, A.; Lago, A.F.; Menegueti, M.G.; Nicolini, E.A.; de Brito Rodrigues, L.A.; Nunes, R.S.; Auxiliadora-Martins, M.; Ferez, M.A. The use of APACHE II, SOFA, SAPS 3, C-reactive protein/albumin ratio, and lactate to predict mortality of surgical critically ill patients: A retrospective cohort study. *Medicine* **2019**, *98*, e16204. [CrossRef]
36. Zou, X.; Li, S.; Fang, M.; Hu, M.; Bian, Y.; Ling, J.; Yu, S.; Jing, L.; Li, D.; Huang, J. Acute physiology and chronic health evaluation II score as a predictor of hospital mortality in patients of coronavirus disease 2019. *Crit. Care Med.* **2020**, *48*, e657. [CrossRef]
37. Nedeva, C. Inflammation and cell death of the innate and adaptive immune system during sepsis. *Biomolecules* **2021**, *11*, 1011. [CrossRef] [PubMed]
38. Bermejo-Martin, J.F.; Martín-Fernandez, M.; López-Mestanza, C.; Duque, P.; Almansa, R. Shared features of endothelial dysfunction between sepsis and its preceding risk factors (aging and chronic disease). *J. Clin. Med.* **2018**, *7*, 400. [CrossRef] [PubMed]
39. Goh, K.H.; Wang, L.; Yeow, A.Y.K.; Poh, H.; Li, K.; Yeow, J.J.L.; Tan, G.Y.H. Artificial intelligence in sepsis early prediction and diagnosis using unstructured data in healthcare. *Nat. Commun.* **2021**, *12*, 711. [CrossRef] [PubMed]
40. Lee, C.U.; Jo, Y.H.; Lee, J.H.; Kim, J.; Park, S.M.; Hwang, J.E.; Lee, D.K.; Park, I.; Jang, D.-H.; Lee, S.-M. The index of oxygenation to respiratory rate as a prognostic factor for mortality in Sepsis. *Am. J. Emerg. Med.* **2021**, *45*, 426–432. [CrossRef] [PubMed]
41. Roca, O.; Caralt, B.; Messika, J.; Samper, M.; Sztrymf, B.; Hernández, G.; García-de-Acilu, M.; Frat, J.-P.; Masclans, J.R.; Ricard, J.-D. An index combining respiratory rate and oxygenation to predict outcome of nasal high-flow therapy. *Am. J. Respir. Crit. Care Med.* **2019**, *199*, 1368–1376. [CrossRef] [PubMed]
42. Gregoriano, C.; Heilmann, E.; Molitor, A.; Schuetz, P. Role of procalcitonin use in the management of sepsis. *J. Thorac. Dis.* **2020**, *12*, S5–S15. [CrossRef] [PubMed]
43. Cleland, D.; Eranki, A. *Procalcitonin*; StatPearls: Treasure Island, FL, USA, 2023.
44. Hamade, B.; Huang, D.T. Procalcitonin: Where are we now? *Crit. Care Clin.* **2020**, *36*, 23–40. [CrossRef]
45. Luhulima, D.E.J.; Amelia, R. Procalcitonin as a Marker of Sepsis Due to Bacterial Infection. *J. Complement. Altern. Med. Res.* **2022**, *18*, 66–76. [CrossRef]
46. Cheng, M.P.; Stenstrom, R.; Paquette, K.; Stabler, S.N.; Akhter, M.; Davidson, A.C.; Gavric, M.; Lawandi, A.; Jinah, R.; Saeed, Z. Blood culture results before and after antimicrobial administration in patients with severe manifestations of sepsis: A diagnostic study. *Ann. Intern. Med.* **2019**, *171*, 547–554. [CrossRef]
47. Scheer, C.; Fuchs, C.; Gründling, M.; Vollmer, M.; Bast, J.; Bohnert, J.; Zimmermann, K.; Hahnenkamp, K.; Rehberg, S.; Kuhn, S.-O. Impact of antibiotic administration on blood culture positivity at the beginning of sepsis: A prospective clinical cohort study. *Clin. Microbiol. Infect.* **2019**, *25*, 326–331. [CrossRef]

48. Santella, B.; Folliero, V.; Pirofalo, G.M.; Serretiello, E.; Zannella, C.; Moccia, G.; Santoro, E.; Sanna, G.; Motta, O.; De Caro, F.; et al. Sepsis—A retrospective cohort study of bloodstream infections. *Antibiotics* **2020**, *9*, 851. [CrossRef]
49. Horng, S.; Sontag, D.A.; Halpern, Y.; Jernite, Y.; Shapiro, N.I.; Nathanson, L.A. Creating an automated trigger for sepsis clinical decision support at emergency department triage using machine learning. *PLoS ONE* **2017**, *12*, e0174708. [CrossRef] [PubMed]
50. Mollura, M.; Lehman, L.-W.H.; Mark, R.G.; Barbieri, R. A novel artificial intelligence based intensive care unit monitoring system: Using physiological waveforms to identify sepsis. *Philos. Trans. R. Soc. A* **2021**, *379*, 20200252. [CrossRef]

Disclaimer/Publisher's Note: The statements, opinions and data contained in all publications are solely those of the individual author(s) and contributor(s) and not of MDPI and/or the editor(s). MDPI and/or the editor(s) disclaim responsibility for any injury to people or property resulting from any ideas, methods, instructions or products referred to in the content.

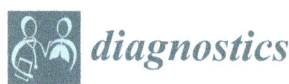

Article

Establishment of ICU Mortality Risk Prediction Models with Machine Learning Algorithm Using MIMIC-IV Database

Ke Pang [1,†], Liang Li [2,†], Wen Ouyang [1], Xing Liu [1] and Yongzhong Tang [1,*]

1. Department of Anesthesiology, Third Xiangya Hospital, Central South University, Changsha 410013, China; pangke97@gmail.com (K.P.); yangwenou@126.com (W.O.); xinxingmail@csu.edu.cn (X.L.)
2. Department of Gastrointestinal Surgery, Third Xiangya Hospital, Central South University, Changsha 410013, China; liliang97116@csu.edu.cn
* Correspondence: tangyongzhong@csu.edu.cn
† These authors contributed equally to this work.

Abstract: Objective: The mortality rate of critically ill patients in ICUs is relatively high. In order to evaluate patients' mortality risk, different scoring systems are used to help clinicians assess prognosis in ICUs, such as the Acute Physiology and Chronic Health Evaluation III (APACHE III) and the Logistic Organ Dysfunction Score (LODS). In this research, we aimed to establish and compare multiple machine learning models with physiology subscores of APACHE III—namely, the Acute Physiology Score III (APS III)—and LODS scoring systems in order to obtain better performance for ICU mortality prediction. **Methods:** A total number of 67,748 patients from the Medical Information Database for Intensive Care (MIMIC-IV) were enrolled, including 7055 deceased patients, and the same number of surviving patients were selected by the random downsampling technique, for a total of 14,110 patients included in the study. The enrolled patients were randomly divided into a training dataset (n = 9877) and a validation dataset (n = 4233). Fivefold cross-validation and grid search procedures were used to find and evaluate the best hyperparameters in different machine learning models. Taking the subscores of LODS and the physiology subscores that are part of the APACHE III scoring systems as input variables, four machine learning methods of XGBoost, logistic regression, support vector machine, and decision tree were used to establish ICU mortality prediction models, with AUCs as metrics. AUCs, specificity, sensitivity, positive predictive value, negative predictive value, and calibration curves were used to find the best model. **Results:** For the prediction of mortality risk in ICU patients, the AUC of the XGBoost model was 0.918 (95%CI, 0.915–0.922), and the AUCs of logistic regression, SVM, and decision tree were 0.872 (95%CI, 0.867–0.877), 0.872 (95%CI, 0.867–0.877), and 0.852 (95%CI, 0.847–0.857), respectively. The calibration curves of logistic regression and support vector machine performed better than the other two models in the ranges 0–40% and 70%–100%, respectively, while XGBoost performed better in the range of 40–70%. **Conclusions:** The mortality risk of ICU patients can be better predicted by the characteristics of the Acute Physiology Score III and the Logistic Organ Dysfunction Score with XGBoost in terms of ROC curve, sensitivity, and specificity. The XGBoost model could assist clinicians in judging in-hospital outcome of critically ill patients, especially in patients with a more uncertain survival outcome.

Keywords: machine learning; postoperative death; prediction model

Citation: Pang, K.; Li, L.; Ouyang, W.; Liu, X.; Tang, Y. Establishment of ICU Mortality Risk Prediction Models with Machine Learning Algorithm Using MIMIC-IV Database. *Diagnostics* **2022**, *12*, 1068. https://doi.org/10.3390/diagnostics12051068

Academic Editor: Zhongheng Zhang

Received: 18 March 2022
Accepted: 22 April 2022
Published: 24 April 2022

Publisher's Note: MDPI stays neutral with regard to jurisdictional claims in published maps and institutional affiliations.

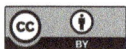

Copyright: © 2022 by the authors. Licensee MDPI, Basel, Switzerland. This article is an open access article distributed under the terms and conditions of the Creative Commons Attribution (CC BY) license (https://creativecommons.org/licenses/by/4.0/).

1. Introduction

As the number of critically ill patients is increasing, the demand for intensive care units (ICUs) has also substantially increased. Increasing demand for critical care has made capacity limitations commonplace in ICUs [1]. Critically ill patients admitted to ICUs are at a high risk of mortality [2]. Previous studies have indicated that the overall mortality rate was 20.5–43% among patients with an ICU stay, and the most common causes of death among patients in ICUs were sepsis, cardiac arrest, pneumonia, and cardiac arrhythmia [3].

Previous evidence has suggested that the severity and extent of disease upon admission to the ICU are strongly associated with ICU in-hospital mortality [4]. Therefore, the outcome of ICU patients predicted by multifactorial scores upon admission to the ICU is critical for long-term treatment and humanistic care [5]. At present, when patients are admitted to the ICU, they are scored with scales such as the Acute Physiology and Chronic Health Evaluation III (APACHE III) score, the Logistic Organ Dysfunction Score (LODS), and the Sequential Organ Failure Assessment (SOFA) [6,7]. Some scales, including SOFA, Systemic Inflammatory Response Syndrome (SIRS), and APACHE II, have been used to predict outcomes in critically ill patients and achieved adequate results [8,9].

Machine learning techniques have been widely used in clinics, ranging from diagnosis to predicting survival outcomes [10,11]. For ICU mortality prediction, the current prognosis models employ the logistic regression classifier or the single long short-term memory (LSTM) classifier [12] and single scoring system [13]. However, logistic regression constructs linear decision boundaries, and therefore, nonlinear problems may have relatively poor prediction results with logistic regression [14]. Previous research showed that an ensemble machine learning algorithm could have better prediction performance with Simplified Acute Physiology Score (SAPSII) and SOFA scores as input variables compared with logistic regression [15]. The XGBoost algorithm has been used to predict mortality based on the MIMIC-III database. A study used admission and laboratory variables to construct an XGBoost model to predict in-hospital mortality among patients with heart failure and achieved a high AUC of 0.84 [16]. Another study used the XGBoost algorithm to predict all-cause mortality based on the MIMIC-III database with some acute physiology variables and chronic conditions and achieved the highest AUC of 0.86 compared with other models [17].

It remains to be seen if we can achieve higher accuracy of survival outcome prediction by taking each score of both APS III and LODS scoring systems as the input features of nonlinear classifiers based on an ensemble machine learning algorithm. There were a few studies that used APS II or LODS to predict mortality in the ICU. A study on assessing the physiological instability of pediatric intensive care unit patients found that APS III could be sensitive to small changes in physiological status [18]. A previous study based on the MIMIC-III database used APS III data as input variables to construct a model to predict mortality among trauma patients with acute respiratory distress syndrome and found that the model achieved an AUC of 0.718 [19]. Another study used LODS to predict all-cause 30-day mortality and achieved an AUC of 0.733 among intensive care patients with sepsis based on the MIMIC-III database. As a result, we chose two kinds of scoring systems to construct models and achieve higher prediction performance [20]. There are few other research works that combine two scoring systems to predict mortality in ICUs.

We aimed to integrate the physiology subscores of APACHE III—namely, the APS III scoring system—and the LODS scoring system, and compare four different machine learning models (XGBoost [21], logistic regression, SVM, and decision tree) based on the data of 14,110 patients in the MIMIC-IV database [22] to predict the different performances of ICU patient mortality.

2. Methods

2.1. Data Source and Population

The study data were taken from the Medical Information Mart for Intensive Care (MIMIC)-IV database [22]. MIMIC-IV is a large, single-center database with more than 70,000 patients. For this study, we selected 67,748 adult patients with LODS scores and acute physiology subscores as part of APACHE III scores in the MIMIC-IV database and performed a retrospective review.

The inclusion criteria were patients admitted to the ICU for the first time who were older than 18 years. The first ICU admission was considered when a subject had multiple admissions to the ICU. The exclusion criteria were patients with admission to an ICU two or more times, patients younger than 18 years, and patients with the same hospital admission IDs. We did not exclude patients with any diseases, similar to the method used in previous studies [23]. Class imbalance is a major problem in ICU datasets, as the number of deceased patients (7055, 10.4%) is much lower than the number of living patients (60,693, 89.6%). Methods for dealing with datasets with class imbalance include resampling [24,25] and classifying cost functions [26]. Downsampling is a kind of resampling that entails decreasing the number of records in the majority class with more samples. We used random downsampling to randomly select the same number of positive samples as the negative samples from the original dataset of 60,693 patients [27]. After random downsampling, a total of 14,110 patients (7055 in-hospital deceased patients and 7055 surviving patients) were considered in the study. The sample size was sufficiently large, and no sample size calculation was undertaken. The flow chart of the study is shown in Figure 1. PostgreSQL was used to extract clinical information, including age, sex, weight, admission type, Logistic Organ Dysfunction Score (LODS), and Acute Physiology Score III (APS III) on the PostgreSQL database server (version 10).

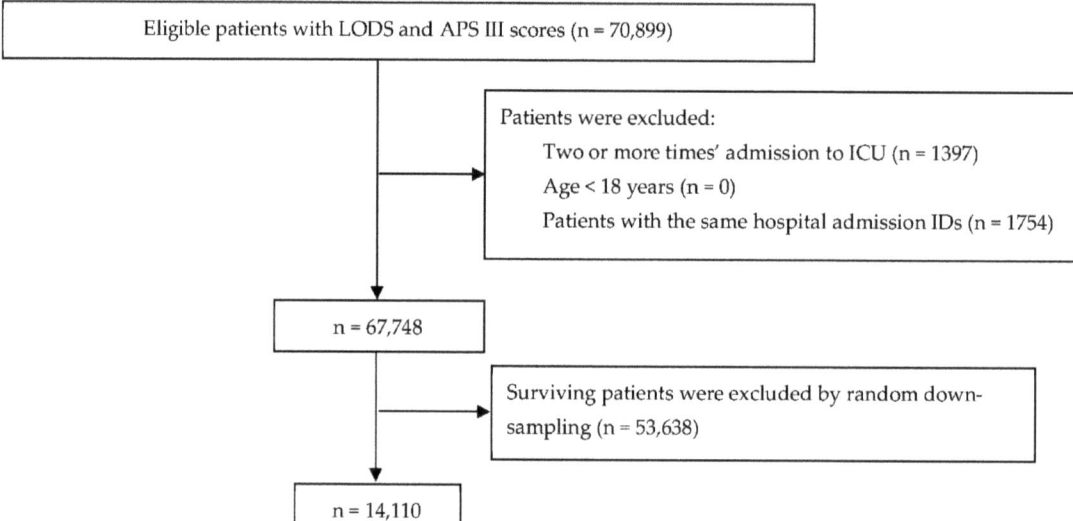

Figure 1. Flow chart.

2.2. Selection of Variables

The LODS score is based on six different scores, one each for the respiratory, cardiovascular, hepatic, coagulation, renal, and neurological systems. APS III scores include heart rate score, mean blood pressure score, temperature score, respiratory rate score, PaO2-aadO2 score, hematocrit score, white blood count score, serum creatinine score, urine output score, blood urea nitrogen score, sodium score, albumin score, bilirubin score, glucose score, acid base score, Glasgow Coma Scale score, and total APS III score.

2.3. Data Analysis and Model Construction

After employing the random downsampling technique to select surviving patients, the dataset was partitioned into the training set (70%) and the testing set (30%). After the completion of the feature engineering, the machine learning algorithms, including XGBoost, support vector machine (SVM), logistic regression (LR), and decision tree, were used to construct the models [28]. Receiver operating characteristic (ROC) curve analysis was considered as a metric to tune model parameters. Grid search and 5-fold cross-validation [29] were performed for hyperparameter optimization and the construction of prediction models. The AUCs, sensitivity, specificity, positive predictive rate, and negative predictive rate were calculated, and calibration curves [30] were plotted to evaluate the advantages or disadvantages of the models.

We performed statistical analyses using the *sklearn* machine learning package (0.24.2), xgboost package (1.5.0), and shap package (0.40.0) in Python 3.7.4 and R 4.1.0 programs. The normality of continuous variables was analyzed by the normality test. Continuous variables with normal distribution were expressed as mean ± standard deviations and continuous variables with non-normal distribution were expressed as median [IQR]. Categorical data are shown as numbers (percent). Group comparisons for continuous data with normal distribution were calculated with Student's t-test, while continuous data with non-normal distribution were calculated with the Kruskal–Wallis test, and categorical data were compared using χ^2 or Fisher's exact test with the tableone package in R 4.1.0. Effects with *p*-values smaller than 0.05 were considered significant.

3. Results

The pre- and post-sampling characteristics of the study subjects are presented in Table 1. The data show significant differences between surviving and in-hospital deceased patients in terms of admission type, weight, neurological score, cardiovascular score, renal score, pulmonary score, hematological score, hepatic score, total LODS score in the LODS scoring system, heart rate score, mean blood pressure score, temperature score, PaO_2-$aadO_2$ score, white blood count score, serum creatinine score, urine output score, blood urea nitrogen score, blood sodium score, albumin score, bilirubin score, glucose score, acid base score, Glasgow Coma Scale score, and total APS III score in the APS III scoring system ($p < 0.001$). However, there were no statistical differences between surviving and in-hospital deceased patients in respiratory rate score, hematocrit score, and gender.

Table 1. Baseline data of participants.

Variable (Score)	Dataset before Downsampling			Dataset after Downsampling		
	Survived (60,693)	Dead (7055)	p	Survived (7055)	Dead (7055)	p
Female [1]	26,774 (44.1)	3235 (45.9)	0.006	3193 (45.3)	3235 (45.9)	0.488
Age [3]	64.37 ± 17.10	71.44 ± 15.23	<0.001	64.25 ± 17.32	71.44 ± 15.23	<0.001
Weight [3]	81.48 ± 26.00	77.34 ± 23.89	<0.001	81.08 ± 26.33	77.34 ± 23.89	<0.001
Emergency [1]	43,724 (72.0)	6016 (85.3)	<0.001	5102 (72.3)	6016 (85.3)	<0.001
LODS [2]	3.00 [2.00, 5.00]	8.00 [5.00, 11.00]	<0.001	3.00 [2.00, 6.00]	8.00 [5.00, 11.00]	<0.001
Neurologic [2]	0.00 [0.00, 1.00]	1.00 [0.00, 3.00]	<0.001	0.00 [0.00, 1.00]	1.00 [0.00, 3.00]	<0.001
Cardiovascular [2]	0.00 [0.00, 1.00]	1.00 [0.00, 1.00]	<0.001	0.00 [0.00, 1.00]	1.00 [0.00, 1.00]	<0.001
Renal [2]	1.00 [1.00, 3.00]	3.00 [1.00, 5.00]	<0.001	1.00 [1.00, 3.00]	3.00 [1.00, 5.00]	<0.001
Pulmonary [2]	0.00 [0.00, 1.00]	1.00 [0.00, 3.00]	<0.001	0.00 [0.00, 1.00]	1.00 [0.00, 3.00]	<0.001
Hematologic [2]	0.00 [0.00, 0.00]	0.00 [0.00, 0.00]	<0.001	0.00 [0.00, 0.00]	0.00 [0.00, 0.00]	<0.001
Hepatic [2]	0.00 [0.00, 1.00]	1.00 [0.00, 1.00]	<0.001	0.00 [0.00, 1.00]	1.00 [0.00, 1.00]	<0.001
APS III [2]	39.00 [29.00, 52.00]	73.00 [53.00, 95.00]	<0.001	39.00 [29.00, 52.00]	73.00 [53.00, 95.00]	<0.001
Heart rate [2]	1.00 [0.00, 5.00]	5.00 [0.00, 7.00]	<0.001	1.00 [0.00, 5.00]	5.00 [0.00, 7.00]	<0.001
Mean pressure [2]	9.00 [7.00, 15.00]	15.00 [7.00, 15.00]	<0.001	9.00 [7.00, 15.00]	15.00 [7.00, 15.00]	<0.001
Temperature [2]	0.00 [0.00, 0.00]	0.00 [0.00, 2.00]	<0.001	0.00 [0.00, 0.00]	0.00 [0.00, 2.00]	<0.001
Respiratory rate [2]	6.00 [6.00, 8.00]	6.00 [6.00, 8.00]	<0.001	6.00 [6.00, 8.00]	6.00 [6.00, 8.00]	0.001
PaO_2-$aadO_2$ [2]	0.00 [0.00, 0.00]	0.00 [0.00, 0.00]	<0.001	0.00 [0.00, 0.00]	0.00 [0.00, 0.00]	<0.001
Hematocrit [2]	3.00 [3.00, 3.00]	3.00 [3.00, 3.00]	0.670	3.00 [3.00, 3.00]	3.00 [3.00, 3.00]	0.735
White blood count [2]	0.00 [0.00, 0.00]	0.00 [0.00, 1.00]	<0.001	0.00 [0.00, 0.00]	0.00 [0.00, 1.00]	<0.001
Creatinine [2]	0.00 [0.00, 3.00]	4.00 [0.00, 7.00]	<0.001	0.00 [0.00, 4.00]	4.00 [0.00, 7.00]	<0.001
Urine output [2]	4.00 [0.00, 5.00]	5.00 [4.00, 8.00]	<0.001	4.00 [0.00, 5.00]	5.00 [4.00, 8.00]	<0.001

Table 1. Cont.

Variable (Score)	Dataset before Downsampling			Dataset after Downsampling		
	Survived (60,693)	Dead (7055)	p	Survived (7055)	Dead (7055)	p
Blood urea nitrogen [2]	2.00 [0.00, 7.00]	7.00 [7.00, 11.00]	<0.001	2.00 [0.00, 7.00]	7.00 [7.00, 11.00]	<0.001
Blood sodium [2]	0.00 [0.00, 0.00]	0.00 [0.00, 2.00]	<0.001	0.00 [0.00, 0.00]	0.00 [0.00, 2.00]	<0.001
Albumin [2]	0.00 [0.00, 0.00]	0.00 [0.00, 0.00]	<0.001	0.00 [0.00, 0.00]	0.00 [0.00, 0.00]	<0.001
Bilirubin [2]	0.00 [0.00, 0.00]	0.00 [0.00, 0.00]	<0.001	0.00 [0.00, 0.00]	0.00 [0.00, 0.00]	<0.001
Glucose [2]	0.00 [0.00, 3.00]	0.00 [0.00, 3.00]	<0.001	0.00 [0.00, 3.00]	0.00 [0.00, 3.00]	<0.001
Acid base [2]	0.00 [0.00, 2.00]	3.00 [0.00, 9.00]	<0.001	0.00 [0.00, 2.00]	3.00 [0.00, 9.00]	<0.001
Glasgow Coma Scale [2]	0.00 [0.00, 3.00]	3.00 [0.00, 29.00]	<0.001	0.00 [0.00, 3.00]	3.00 [0.00, 29.00]	<0.001
Hypertension [1]	38,236 (63.0)	4608 (65.3)	<0.001	4399 (62.4)	4608 (65.3)	<0.001
Ischemic heart disease [1]	20,317 (33.5)	2568 (36.4)	<0.001	2307 (32.7)	2568 (36.4)	<0.001
Diabetes [1]	18,001 (29.7)	2135 (30.3)	0.301	2053 (29.1)	2135 (30.3)	0.136
Chronic pulmonary disease [1]	15,248 (25.1)	1916 (27.2)	<0.001	1721 (24.4)	1916 (27.2)	<0.001
Cerebrovascular disease [1]	8919 (14.7)	1630 (23.1)	<0.001	1072 (15.2)	1630 (23.1)	<0.001

Data are number of subjects (percentage) or median [IQR]. [1] Chi-square test or Fisher's exact test was used to compare the percentage between participants between surviving and deceased patients. [2] Kruskal–Wallis test was used to compare the median [IQR] between surviving and deceased patients. [3] Student's t-test was used to compare the mean ± standard deviations between surviving and deceased patients.

For the prediction of mortality in ICU patients (Figure 2), the AUC of the XGBoost model was 0.918 (95%CI, 0.915–0.922). The AUCs of logistic regression, SVM, and decision tree were 0.872 (95%CI, 0.867–0.877), 0.872 (95%CI, 0.867–0.877), and 0.852 (95%CI, 0.847–0.857), respectively (Table 2). XGBoost showed better accuracy, sensitivity, specialty, positive predictive value, and negative predictive value compared with SVM, logistic regression, and decision tree. The calibration curves of logistic regression and SVM performed better than the other two models in the low and high probability range (0–40% and 70–100%), while the calibration curve of XGBoost performed better in the medium probability range of 40–70% (Figure 3). The XGBoost feature importance plot shows that apart from total LODS score, total APS III score, weight, and age, the three most important characteristics in predicting ICU mortality were Glasgow Coma Scale score, respiratory rate score, and acid base score (Figure 4). The SHAP bee swarm plot shows the SHAP value importance of all features in the XGBoost model (Supplementary Figure S2), and the results show that in the plot, the Glasgow Coma Scale score, acid base score, and urine output score were the three most important features in predicting mortality [31]. The hyperparameters of the models are shown in Supplementary Table S1.

Table 2. AUC, accuracy, sensitivity, specialty, positive predictive value, and negative predictive value of different models.

Models	ROC (95%CI)	Accuracy	SEN	SPE	PPV	NPV
XGBOOST	0.918 (0.915–0.922)	0.834	0.822	0.846	0.842	0.826
SVM	0.872 (0.867–0.877)	0.789	0.773	0.805	0.799	0.780
Logistic regression	0.872 (0.867–0.877)	0.787	0.756	0.818	0.806	0.771
Decision Tree	0.852 (0.847–0.857)	0.776	0.727	0.825	0.806	0.752

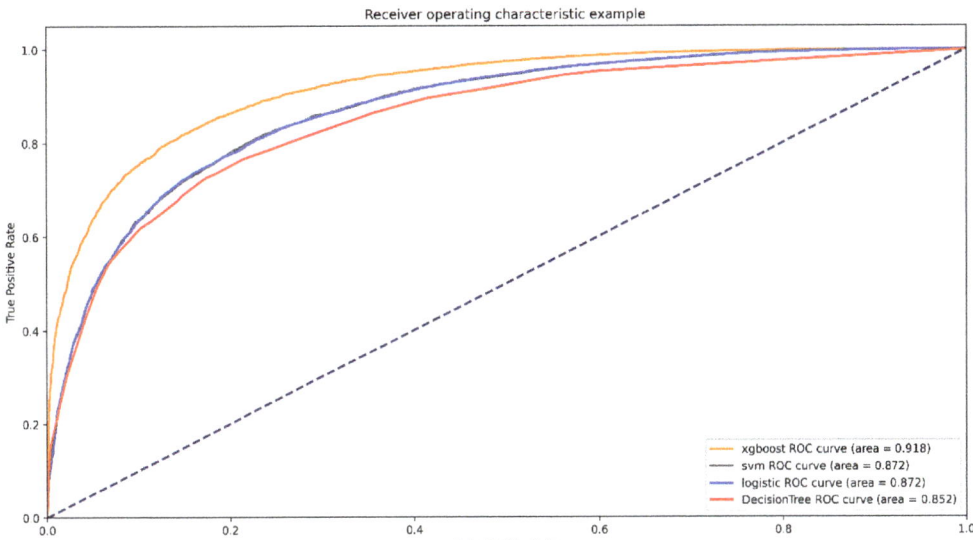

Figure 2. ROCs of different models.

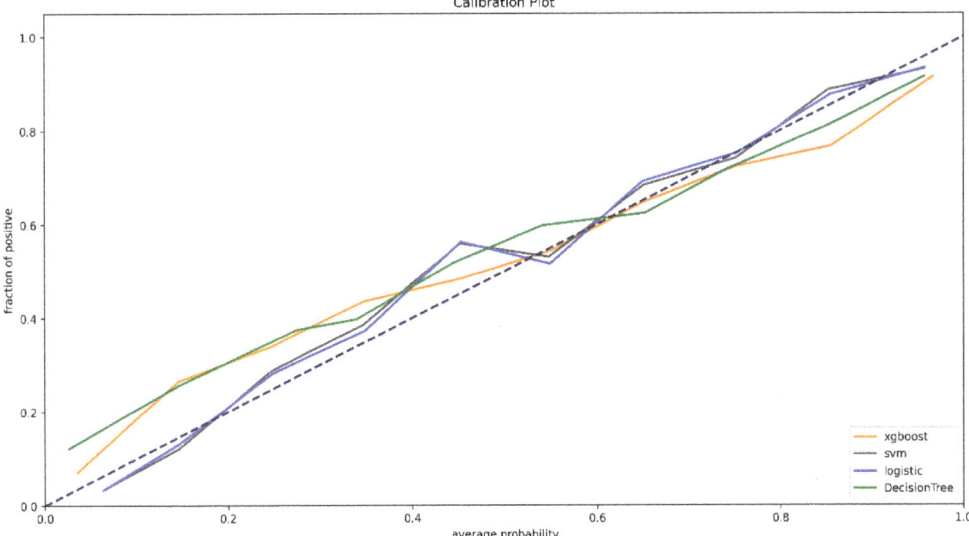

Figure 3. Calibration curve.

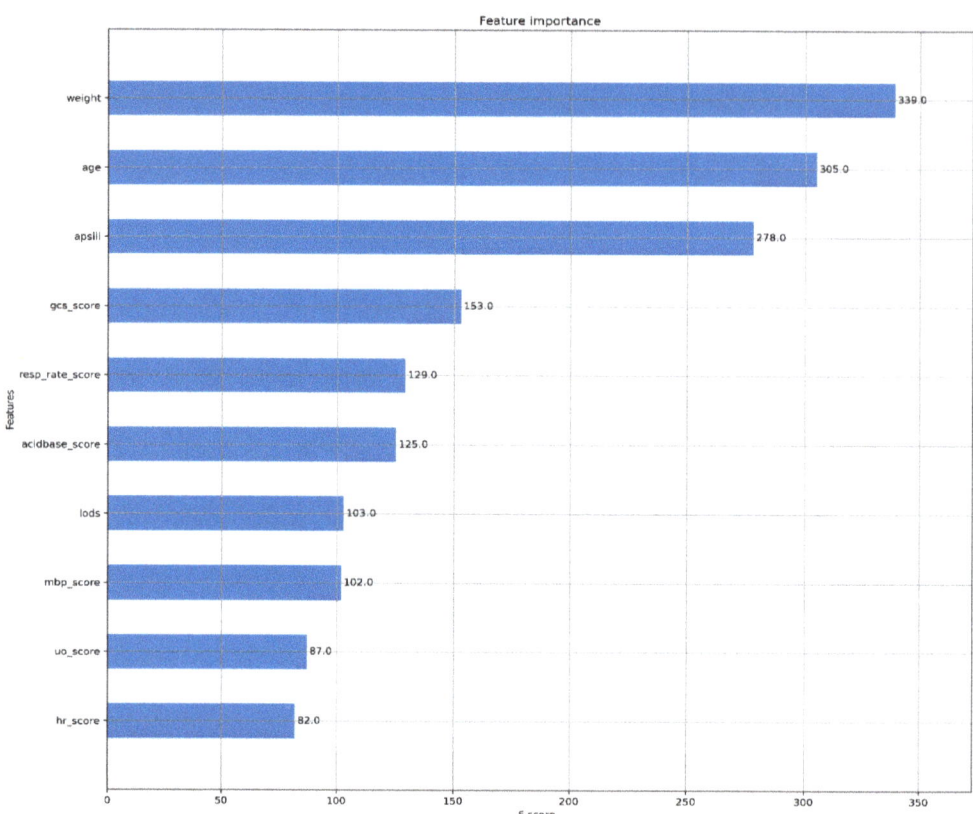

Figure 4. Feature importance plot of XGBoost.

4. Discussion

Critical illness in the ICU is associated with in-hospital mortality and substantial economic burden. The in-hospital mortality in ICUs accounts for 20–50% of all in-hospital deaths [32,33], and the ICU accounts for 22% of the aggregate costs [34] for all hospitalizations, or nearly USD 81.3 billion in 2005 [35]. Early aggressive therapy can retard progression and control disease. However, it is difficult for clinicians to predict which patients will worsen and to evaluate the risk of not treating patients or if they will respond to specific therapy. As a result, better prediction models are needed to predict the mortality risk of critically ill patients in the ICU. Several prognostic scoring systems in ICUs have been developed to predict the outcome of patients. The advantages of such scoring systems are that they are easy to measure and interpret and are less prone to measurement and calculation errors. In this study, we used two prognostic scoring systems (LODS and APS III, the physiology subscore part of the APACHE III scoring system) as input variables, as more variables could provide better prediction performance [36,37]. The Logistic Organ Dysfunction Score (LODS) system is a common and important scoring system. LODS scores are used to assess six organ or system states and record the worst score within 24 h after admission to the hospital. The organ scoring system assesses for dysfunction of neurological, cardiovascular, renal, pulmonary, hematological, and hepatic systems [38]. As a weighted system, LODS is summed by six subscores, ranging from 0 to 5, and each subscore represents an organ or system's function or state. However, for the respiratory and hematological systems, the highest score is 3 points, and for the hepatic system, the highest is 1 point. Since its development in 1996 [39], it has been widely used for assessing mortality in ICUs. The Acute Physiology and Chronic Health Evaluation system was introduced in the early 1980s and has experienced three major revisions [40]. Although the APACHE II model is old, and new scoring systems have been developed using more recent cohorts and better features, APACHE II is still widely used in clinical practice [41]. The APACHE III scoring system was developed in 1991. Compared to the APACHE II scoring system, APACHE III performs better in terms of correct classification and the AUCs [42]. The APACHE III scores several factors, including clinical complications, vital signs, and partial blood biochemical examination results [43]. A higher score of LODS or APACHE III is associated with high mortality in the ICU. Although some studies took APACHE III as features to establish machine learning models, there is little literature on using LODS or APS III data as partial input variables at present.

Our study aimed to compare the predictive power mortality between four different machine learning models using subscores of LODS and APS III in predicting in-hospital mortality of ICU patients. In the dataset, the mortality rate of ICU patients was 10.4%. Of the four models, XGBoost showed the best performance in predicting mortality, followed by SVM, logistic regression, and decision tree. Moreover, calibration curves were plotted to evaluate the clinical usefulness of different mortality ranges. The results showed that in the uncertain medium mortality risk range (40–70%), XGBoost was more valuable than logistic regression and SVM models.

As the most widely used model, logistic regression has been used to diagnose diseases and predict outcomes. A study based on a Spanish ICU database revealed that a logistic regression model could achieve an AUC of 0.82 with APACHE III data as input variables, which showed prediction ability to some extent [36]. Another study based on an American ICU database found that using APACHE IV data as input variables could achieve high prediction results [44]. Previous studies found that logistic regression and artificial neural network (ANN) had similar performance when the sample size was adequate [45]. Although logistic regression could not provide a nonlinear decision boundary, it still achieved suitable prediction results. However, more studies revealed that, compared with logistic regression, ANN demonstrated a better degree of discrimination in complex clinical situations [46]. And another research revealed that using ANN to predict early hospital mortality in acute pancreatitis in MIMIC-III could achieve higher prediction performance compared with logistic regression [47]. This may be because ANNs have an inherently flexible nature that suits more complicated interactions between the clinical input variables. In comparison, logistic regression lacks modeling for complex interactions in clinical issues. Some studies found that logistic regression had a relatively worse performance in AUCs, prediction accuracy, or other metrics [36]. Meanwhile, there is research revealing a better discrimination in predicting ICU mortality using XGBoost and gradient-boosted decision trees (GBDT) models compared to SVM [48]. However, a better performance using SVM classification to predict mortality risk for ICU patients with sepsis compared with logistic regression has also been shown [49]. That might be because, depending on the particular dataset or subject population, nonlinear classifiers (XGBoost and SVM) could obtain better predictive performance compared with linear classifiers (logistic regression), which means researchers need to take practical issues into account and select the optimal model.

Some previous studies used vital signs and laboratory variables available in conventional clinical scoring systems as input features to predict mortality based on the MIMIC-III, MIMIC-IV, and eICU databases with recurrent neural networks and achieved similar prediction performance [31]. Another study used partial vital signs and Glasgow Coma Scale scores at different time points after admission to the hospital as input features to predict mortality based on the MIMIC-III database with a convolutional neural network-based prediction model for multivariate time series [50]. The above studies used SHAP or heatmaps to interpret the importance or contribution of the models. However, the studies used a single scoring system as input variables. In contrast, our study selected all subscores of LODS and APS III scoring systems as input variables, as they were completed within the first 24 h of admission to ICU [51], and we used SHAP to explore the features' importance following the method employed in previous studies. Additionally, we used the calibration curve to find the best prediction range of different models. Previous studies showed that constructing models based on SVM, neural network, and logistic regression with SOFA scores as input variables to predict ICU mortality all performed well [23]. A study using APACHE III as variables to construct an XGBoost model based on the MIMIC-III database showed that XGBoost could perform better in accuracy, sensitivity, specificity, and AUC [52], and the comparisons between XGBoost and other models (including logistic regression and multilayer perceptron models) were statistically significant. Our research drew a similar conclusion, as XGBoost had advantages in accuracy, AUCs, and discrimination ability compared with SVM, logistic regression, and decision tree. However, among the population with high mortality probability (more than 70%) and low mortality probability (less than 40%), the calibration of SVM and logistic regression was better than XGBoost, while among the population with medium mortality probability (40–70%), XGBoost had advantages in calibration and discrimination compared with SVM and logistic regression. As a result, in terms of ROC curve, sensitivity, and specificity, for patients whose prognosis is difficult to predict by clinical experience, XGBoost performs better.

Although the importance of variables in XGBoost is shown in Figure 4, the recognition of variables' importance and mortality in the ICU could not be completely explained. However, the reason why the variables of weight, age, and APS III total score had high importance was because the values of the three variables were relatively large compared with other scores. The three variables of the Glasgow Coma Scale score, respiratory rate score, and acid base score were the most important variables. The SHAP bee swarm plot shown in Supplementary Figure S2 showed a similar result, that the Glasgow Coma Scale score, respiratory rate score, and acid base score were the three most important variables. As a result, special attention should be paid to these physiological indices. This result is consistent with previous studies. A study by Daniel found that the Glasgow Coma Scale score dominates in predicting 30-day mortality in a mixed ICU with admission Sequential Organ Failure Assessment scores as input variables [53]. Another study revealed that the Glasgow Coma Scale was more suitable for early in-hospital death assessment among patients with acute head injury [54]. A study by Piotr found that in multivariate analysis, the Glasgow Coma Scale score was the most important variable in critically ill surgical and nonsurgical patients [55]. There are few studies about respiratory rate predicting value for mortality. A multicenter study developed a machine learning analysis with age, heart rate, and respiratory rate as input features and found that the two most important prediction factors were respiratory rate and heart rate [56]. Considering acid base, a study by Anja found that in the ICU, some acid base imbalance factors (including lactate, base excess, and pH) were all suitable predictors of mortality [57].

Compared with previous related studies, our study introduced each score in the APS III and LODS scales to predict mortality in the ICU based on a newly released database and achieve better prediction performance and used calibration curves to judge the best prediction range of different patients with different mortality risk. In the SHAP plots of value importance and feature importance of XGBoost, we explained the most influential physiological conditions for survival. Clinicians can judge patients' mortality probability by whether the patients were at high or low mortality risk.

The strengths of this study rest on several aspects. First, we used the updated MIMIC-IV database with complex and comprehensive information. Second, relatively novel machine learning methods were used to replace the traditional logistic regression, and the results showed better performance of XGBoost methods than the conventional logistic regression model. Third, better statistical methods were used to replace traditional methods, such as 5-fold cross-validation to evaluate the model, and the results showed that XGBoost had better performance. Fourth, we plotted calibration curves and found that patients with different mortality risks could be assessed with different machine learning models. In our study based on the MIMIC-IV database, the relatively certain in-hospital outcome of patients with high or low mortality probability (0–40% and 70–100%) could be predicted with a logistic regression model or SVM, while the relatively uncertain survival outcome of patients with medium mortality probability (40–70%) could be predicted with XGBoost. Fifth, we used the SHAP bee swarm to explain the importance of all input features. Additional different machine learning models should be developed, aiming to predict the outcomes of critically ill patients with different scores.

However, there were also limitations in the present study. First, it was a single-center retrospective study. Thus, further prospective multicenter studies are needed to validate the current results. Second, this observational study used the random downsampling technique to select surviving patients, which might result in some information loss and potential bias. A better sampling technique or more datasets in order to obtain balanced datasets can achieve better performance [58].

5. Conclusions

Compared with models with a single scoring system to predict mortality, our models of data analysis provide strong evidence for the accuracy of predicting mortality in the ICU with the APS III–LODS-based scoring system. In conclusion, this study showed that a machine learning method based on XGBoost could perform better than conventional logistic regression and support vector machine models. The Glasgow Coma Scale, acid base score, urine output, and respiratory rate should be considered in order to improve clinical prognosis. The XGBoost model could assist clinicians in judging in-hospital outcome of critically ill patients, especially in patients with a more uncertain survival outcome.

Supplementary Materials: The following supporting information can be downloaded at: https://www.mdpi.com/article/10.3390/diagnostics12051068/s1, Figure S1: ROC curves of training dataset (A) and testing dataset (B); Figure S2: SHAP values importance of all features in the Xgboost model; Table S1: Hyperparameter values of models.

Author Contributions: W.O. and Y.T. designed the study. K.P. organized data. K.P. and L.L. analyzed data and wrote the first draft of the manuscript. X.L. revised the manuscript. All authors have read and agreed to the published version of the manuscript.

Funding: This work was supported by the National Key R&D Program of China (Grant Number 2018YFC2001800) and the Project of Health and Health Commission of Hunan Province (Grant Number 20201802).

Institutional Review Board Statement: This study was carried out in accordance with the recommendations and approval (R21178) of the Institutional Review Board of the Third Xiangya Hospital of Central South University, which abides by the Declaration of Helsinki and is registered at the Chinese Clinical Trial Registry (ChiCTR2200055703, website: http://www.chictr.org.cn (accessed on 16 January 2022)).

Informed Consent Statement: Patient consent was waived because the study was an analysis of a third-party anonymized publicly available database.

Data Availability Statement: Restrictions apply to the availability of these data. Data were obtained from MIMIC-IV and are available at https://physionet.org/content/mimiciv/1.0/ (accessed on 1 October 2021) with the permission of PhysioNet.

Acknowledgments: We are deeply grateful to all persons who participated in this study. To all people who made efforts for this study, we would equally like to thank their collaboration.

Conflicts of Interest: The authors declare no conflict of interest.

References

1. Terwiesch, C.; Diwas, K.C.; Kahn, J.M. Working with capacity limitations: Operations management in critical care. *Crit. Care* **2011**, *15*, 308. [CrossRef]
2. Lin, W.-T.; Chen, W.-L.; Chao, C.-M.; Lai, C.-C. The outcomes and prognostic factors of the patients with unplanned intensive care unit readmissions. *Medicine* **2018**, *97*, e11124. [CrossRef] [PubMed]
3. Akkoç, I.; Yücetaş, E.; İşitemiz, İ.; Toptaş, M.; Tas, A.; Sen, O.; Ozgur, F.; Erguven, H. Mortality Rate In Intensive Care Units of Tertiary Health Institutions and Identifying Risk Factors: Analysis of 3945 Patients. *Bezmialem Sci.* **2017**, *5*, 116–120. [CrossRef]

4. Mayr, V.D.; Dünser, M.W.; Greil, V.; Jochberger, S.; Luckner, G.; Ulmer, H.; Friesenecker, B.E.; Takala, J.; Hasibeder, W.R. Causes of death and determinants of outcome in critically ill patients. *Crit. Care* **2006**, *10*, R154. [CrossRef]
5. Huber, W.; Rauch, J.; Saugel, B.; Mair, S.; Messer, M.; Lahmer, T.; Schultheiss, C.; Luppa, P.; Schmid, R.J.C.C. Prognostic value of neutrophil gelatinase-associated lipocalin and transpulmonary thermodilution-derived parameters within 48 hours after admission. *Crit. Care* **2013**, *17*, 1–200. [CrossRef]
6. Sekulic, A.D.; Trpkovic, S.V.; Pavlovic, A.P.; Marinkovic, O.M.; Ilic, A.N. Scoring systems in assessing survival of critically ill ICU patients. *Med. Sci. Monit. Int. Med. J. Exp. Clin. Res.* **2015**, *21*, 2621. [CrossRef] [PubMed]
7. Wu, S.-C.; Chou, S.-E.; Liu, H.-T.; Hsieh, T.-M.; Su, W.-T.; Chien, P.-C.; Hsieh, C.-H. Performance of Prognostic Scoring Systems in Trauma Patients in the Intensive Care Unit of a Trauma Center. *Int. J. Environ. Res. Public Health* **2020**, *17*, 7226. [CrossRef]
8. Ferreira, F.L.; Bota, D.P.; Bross, A.; Mélot, C.; Vincent, J.L. Serial evaluation of the SOFA score to predict outcome in critically ill patients. *JAMA* **2001**, *286*, 1754–1758. [CrossRef] [PubMed]
9. Basile-Filho, A.; Lago, A.F.; Menegueti, M.G.; Nicolini, E.A.; Rodrigues, L.A.d.B.; Nunes, R.S.; Auxiliadora-Martins, M.; Ferez, M.A. The use of APACHE II, SOFA, SAPS 3, C-reactive protein/albumin ratio, and lactate to predict mortality of surgical critically ill patients: A retrospective cohort study. *Medicine* **2019**, *98*, e16204. [CrossRef]
10. Goldstein, B.A.; Navar, A.M.; Carter, R.E. Moving beyond regression techniques in cardiovascular risk prediction: Applying machine learning to address analytic challenges. *Eur. Heart J.* **2017**, *38*, 1805–1814. [CrossRef] [PubMed]
11. Szlosek, D.A.; Ferrett, J. Using Machine Learning and Natural Language Processing Algorithms to Automate the Evaluation of Clinical Decision Support in Electronic Medical Record Systems. *EGEMS* **2016**, *4*, 1222. [CrossRef] [PubMed]
12. Ge, W.; Huh, J.-W.; Park, Y.R.; Lee, J.-H.; Kim, Y.-H.; Turchin, A. An Interpretable ICU Mortality Prediction Model Based on Logistic Regression and Recurrent Neural Networks with LSTM units. *AMIA Annu. Symp. Proc.* **2018**, *2018*, 460–469. [PubMed]
13. Raith, E.P.; Udy, A.A.; Bailey, M.; McGloughlin, S.; MacIsaac, C.; Bellomo, R.; Pilcher, D.V. Prognostic Accuracy of the SOFA Score, SIRS Criteria, and qSOFA Score for In-Hospital Mortality Among Adults With Suspected Infection Admitted to the Intensive Care Unit. *JAMA* **2017**, *317*, 290–300. [CrossRef]
14. Kulin, M.; Fortuna, C.; De Poorter, E.; Deschrijver, D.; Moerman, I. Data-Driven Design of Intelligent Wireless Networks: An Overview and Tutorial. *Sensors* **2016**, *16*, 790. [CrossRef]
15. Pirracchio, R.; Petersen, M.L.; Carone, M.; Rigon, M.R.; Chevret, S.; van der Laan, M.J. Mortality prediction in intensive care units with the Super ICU Learner Algorithm (SICULA): A population-based study. *Lancet Respir. Med.* **2015**, *3*, 42–52. [CrossRef]
16. Li, F.; Xin, H.; Zhang, J.; Fu, M.; Zhou, J.; Lian, Z. Prediction model of in-hospital mortality in intensive care unit patients with heart failure: Machine learning-based, retrospective analysis of the MIMIC-III database. *BMJ Open* **2021**, *11*, e044779. [CrossRef] [PubMed]
17. Luo, Y.; Wang, Z.; Wang, C. Improvement of APACHE II score system for disease severity based on XGBoost algorithm. *BMC Med. Inform. Decis. Mak.* **2021**, *21*, 237. [CrossRef] [PubMed]
18. Pollack, M.M.; Patel, K.M.; Ruttimann, U.E. The Pediatric Risk of Mortality III–Acute Physiology Score (PRISM III-APS): A method of assessing physiologic instability for pediatric intensive care unit patients. *J. Pediatr.* **1997**, *131*, 575–581. [CrossRef]
19. Tang, R.; Wang, H.; Peng, J.; Wang, D. A trauma-related survival predictive model of acute respiratory distress syndrome. *J. Clin. Lab. Anal.* **2021**, *35*, e24006. [CrossRef] [PubMed]
20. Hu, T.; Lv, H.; Jiang, Y. The association between four scoring systems and 30-day mortality among intensive care patients with sepsis: A cohort study. *Sci. Rep.* **2021**, *11*, 11214. [CrossRef] [PubMed]
21. Chen, T.; Guestrin, C. Xgboost: A scalable tree boosting system. In Proceedings of the 22nd Acm Sigkdd International Conference on Knowledge Discovery and Data Mining, San Francisco, CA, USA, 13–17 August 2016; pp. 785–794.
22. Johnson, A.; Bulgarelli, P.L.; Pollard, T.; Horng, S.; Celi, L.A.; Mark, R. MIMIC-IV (version 1.0). 2021. *PhysioNet* **2021**. [CrossRef]
23. Aperstein, Y.; Cohen, L.; Bendavid, I.; Cohen, J.; Grozovsky, E.; Rotem, T.; Singer, P. Improved ICU mortality prediction based on SOFA scores and gastrointestinal parameters. *PLoS ONE* **2019**, *14*, e0222599. [CrossRef] [PubMed]
24. Berry, M.J.A.; Linoff, G.S. *Data Mining Techniques: For. Marketing, Sales, and Customer Relationship Management*; John Wiley & Sons, Inc.: Hoboken, NJ, USA, 2004.
25. Bader-El-Den, M. Self-adaptive heterogeneous random forest. In Proceedings of the 2014 IEEE/ACS 11th International Conference on Computer Systems and Applications (AICCSA), Doha, Qatar, 10–13 November 2014; pp. 640–646.
26. Bader-El-Den, M.; Teitei, E.; Adda, M. Hierarchical classification for dealing with the Class imbalance problem. In Proceedings of the 2016 International Joint Conference on Neural Networks (IJCNN), Vancouver, BC, Canada, 24–29 July 2016; pp. 3584–3591.
27. He, H.; Ma, Y. *Imbalanced Learning: Foundations, Algorithms, and Applications*; Wiley: Hoboken, NJ, USA, 2013.
28. Zhang, Z.; Chen, L.; Xu, P.; Hong, Y.J.L. Predictive analytics with ensemble modeling in laparoscopic surgery: A technical note. *Laparosc. Endosc. Robot. Surg.* **2022**, *5*, 25–34. [CrossRef]
29. Li, C.; Zhang, Z.; Ren, Y.; Nie, H.; Lei, Y.; Qiu, H.; Xu, Z.; Pu, X. Machine learning based early mortality prediction in the emergency department. *Int. J. Med. Inform.* **2021**, *155*, 104570. [CrossRef]
30. Zhu, Y.; Zhang, J.; Wang, G.; Yao, R.; Ren, C.; Chen, G.; Jin, X.; Guo, J.; Liu, S.; Zheng, H.; et al. Machine Learning Prediction Models for Mechanically Ventilated Patients: Analyses of the MIMIC-III Database. *Front. Med.* **2021**, *8*, 662340. [CrossRef] [PubMed]
31. Pattalung, T.N.; Ingviya, T.; Chaichulee, S. Feature Explanations in Recurrent Neural Networks for Predicting Risk of Mortality in Intensive Care Patients. *J. Pers. Med.* **2021**, *11*, 934. [CrossRef]

32. Teres, D.; Lemeshow, S. The APACHE III prognostic system. *Chest* **1992**, *102*, 1919–1920. [CrossRef]
33. Beck, D.H.; Taylor, B.L.; Millar, B.; Smith, G.B. Prediction of outcome from intensive care: A prospective cohort study comparing Acute Physiology and Chronic Health Evaluation II and III prognostic systems in a United Kingdom intensive care unit. *Crit. Care Med.* **1997**, *25*, 9–15. [CrossRef]
34. Halpern, N.A.; Pastores, S.M. Critical care medicine in the United States 2000–2005: An analysis of bed numbers, occupancy rates, payer mix, and costs. *Crit. Care Med.* **2010**, *38*, 65–71. [CrossRef]
35. Halpern, N.A.; Bettes, L.; Greenstein, R. Federal and nationwide intensive care units and healthcare costs: 1986–1992. *Crit. Care Med.* **1994**, *22*, 2001–2007.
36. Rivera-Fernández, R.; Vázquez-Mata, G.; Bravo, M.; Aguayo-Hoyos, E.; Zimmerman, J.; Wagner, D.; Knaus, W. The Apache III prognostic system: Customized mortality predictions for Spanish ICU patients. *Intensive Care Med.* **1998**, *24*, 574–581. [CrossRef] [PubMed]
37. Timsit, J.-F.; Fosse, J.-P.; Troché, G.; De Lassence, A.; Alberti, C.; Garrouste-Orgeas, M.; Bornstain, C.; Adrie, C.; Cheval, C.; Chevret, S. Calibration and discrimination by daily Logistic Organ Dysfunction scoring comparatively with daily Sequential Organ Failure Assessment scoring for predicting hospital mortality in critically ill patients. *Crit. Care Med.* **2002**, *30*, 2003–2013. [CrossRef] [PubMed]
38. Jang, H.N.; Park, H.J.; Cho, H.S.; Bae, E.; Lee, T.W.; Chang, S.-H.; Park, D.J. The logistic organ dysfunction system score predicts the prognosis of patients with alcoholic ketoacidosis. *Ren. Fail.* **2018**, *40*, 693–699. [CrossRef] [PubMed]
39. Le Gall, J.R.; Klar, J.; Lemeshow, S.; Saulnier, F.; Alberti, C.; Artigas, A.; Teres, D. The Logistic Organ Dysfunction system. A new way to assess organ dysfunction in the intensive care unit. ICU Scoring Group. *JAMA* **1996**, *276*, 802–810. [CrossRef] [PubMed]
40. Metnitz, P.G.H.; Moreno, R.P.; Almeida, E.; Jordan, B.; Bauer, P.; Campos, R.A.; Iapichino, G.; Edbrooke, D.; Capuzzo, M.; Le Gall, J.-R. SAPS 3—From evaluation of the patient to evaluation of the intensive care unit. Part 1: Objectives, methods and cohort description. *Intensive Care Med.* **2005**, *31*, 1336–1344. [CrossRef]
41. Ho, K.M.; Dobb, G.J.; Knuiman, M.; Finn, J.; Lee, K.Y.; Webb, S.A.R. A comparison of admission and worst 24-hour Acute Physiology and Chronic Health Evaluation II scores in predicting hospital mortality: A retrospective cohort study. *Crit. Care* **2006**, *10*, R4. [CrossRef]
42. Markgraf, R.; Deutschinoff, G.; Pientka, L.; Scholten, T. Comparison of acute physiology and chronic health evaluations II and III and simplified acute physiology score II: A prospective cohort study evaluating these methods to predict outcome in a German interdisciplinary intensive care unit. *Crit. Care Med.* **2000**, *28*, 26–33. [CrossRef]
43. Knaus, W.A.; Wagner, D.P.; Draper, E.A.; Zimmerman, J.E.; Bergner, M.; Bastos, P.G.; Sirio, C.A.; Murphy, D.J.; Lotring, T.; Damiano, A. The APACHE III prognostic system. Risk prediction of hospital mortality for critically ill hospitalized adults. *Chest* **1991**, *100*, 1619–1636. [CrossRef]
44. Zimmerman, J.E.; Kramer, A.A.; McNair, D.S.; Malila, F.M. Acute Physiology and Chronic Health Evaluation (APACHE) IV: Hospital mortality assessment for today's critically ill patients. *Crit. Care Med.* **2006**, *34*, 1297–1310. [CrossRef]
45. Clermont, G.; Angus, D.C.; DiRusso, S.M.; Griffin, M.; Linde-Zwirble, W.T. Predicting hospital mortality for patients in the intensive care unit: A comparison of artificial neural networks with logistic regression models. *Crit. Care Med.* **2001**, *29*, 291–296. [CrossRef]
46. Dybowski, R.; Weller, P.; Chang, R.; Gant, V. Prediction of outcome in critically ill patients using artificial neural network synthesised by genetic algorithm. *Lancet* **1996**, *347*, 1146–1150. [CrossRef]
47. Ding, N.; Guo, C.; Li, C.; Zhou, Y.; Chai, X. An Artificial Neural Networks Model for Early Predicting In-Hospital Mortality in Acute Pancreatitis in MIMIC-III. *Biomed. Res. Int.* **2021**, *2021*, 6638919. [CrossRef] [PubMed]
48. Zhai, Q.; Lin, Z.; Ge, H.; Liang, Y.; Li, N.; Ma, Q.; Ye, C. Using machine learning tools to predict outcomes for emergency department intensive care unit patients. *Sci. Rep.* **2020**, *10*, 20919. [CrossRef] [PubMed]
49. Ribas, V.J.; López, J.C.; Ruiz-Sanmartin, A.; Ruiz-Rodríguez, J.C.; Rello, J.; Wojdel, A.; Vellido, A. Severe sepsis mortality prediction with relevance vector machines. *Annu. Int. Conf. IEEE Eng. Med. Biol. Soc.* **2011**, *2011*, 100–103. [CrossRef]
50. Viton, F.; Elbattah, M.; Guérin, J.-L.; Dequen, G. Heatmaps for visual explainability of cnn-based predictions for multivariate time series with application to healthcare. In Proceedings of the 2020 IEEE International Conference on Healthcare Informatics (ICHI), Oldenburg, Germany, 30 November–3 December 2020; pp. 1–8.
51. George, N.; Moseley, E.; Eber, R.; Siu, J.; Samuel, M.; Yam, J.; Huang, K.; Celi, L.A.; Lindvall, C. Deep learning to predict long-term mortality in patients requiring 7 days of mechanical ventilation. *PLoS ONE* **2021**, *16*, e0253443. [CrossRef]
52. Allen, A.; Mataraso, S.; Siefkas, A.; Burdick, H.; Braden, G.; Dellinger, R.P.; McCoy, A.; Pellegrini, E.; Hoffman, J.; Green-Saxena, A.; et al. A Racially Unbiased, Machine Learning Approach to Prediction of Mortality: Algorithm Development Study. *JMIR Public Health Surveill.* **2020**, *6*, e22400. [CrossRef]
53. Knox, D.B.; Lanspa, M.J.; Pratt, C.M.; Kuttler, K.G.; Jones, J.P.; Brown, S.M. Glasgow Coma Scale score dominates the association between admission Sequential Organ Failure Assessment score and 30-day mortality in a mixed intensive care unit population. *J. Crit. Care* **2014**, *29*, 780–785. [CrossRef]
54. Cho, D.Y.; Wang, Y.C. Comparison of the APACHE III, APACHE II and Glasgow Coma Scale in acute head injury for prediction of mortality and functional outcome. *Intensive Care Med.* **1997**, *23*, 77–84. [CrossRef]
55. Fuchs, P.A.; Czech, I.J.; Krzych, Ł.J. Mortality Prediction Using SOFA Score in Critically Ill Surgical and Non-Surgical Patients: Which Parameter Is the Most Valuable? *Medicina* **2020**, *56*, 273. [CrossRef]

56. Akel, M.A.; Carey, K.A.; Winslow, C.J.; Churpek, M.M.; Edelson, D.P. Less is more: Detecting clinical deterioration in the hospital with machine learning using only age, heart rate, and respiratory rate. *Resuscitation* **2021**, *168*, 6–10. [CrossRef]
57. Schork, A.; Moll, K.; Haap, M.; Riessen, R.; Wagner, R. Course of lactate, pH and base excess for prediction of mortality in medical intensive care patients. *PLoS ONE* **2021**, *16*, e0261564. [CrossRef] [PubMed]
58. Branco, P.; Torgo, L.; Ribeiro, R.P. A Survey of Predictive Modeling on Imbalanced Domains. *ACM Comput. Surv. (CSUR)* **2016**, *49*, 31. [CrossRef]

MDPI
St. Alban-Anlage 66
4052 Basel
Switzerland
www.mdpi.com

Diagnostics Editorial Office
E-mail: diagnostics@mdpi.com
www.mdpi.com/journal/diagnostics

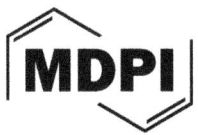

Disclaimer/Publisher's Note: The statements, opinions and data contained in all publications are solely those of the individual author(s) and contributor(s) and not of MDPI and/or the editor(s). MDPI and/or the editor(s) disclaim responsibility for any injury to people or property resulting from any ideas, methods, instructions or products referred to in the content.

www.ingramcontent.com/pod-product-compliance
Lightning Source LLC
LaVergne TN
LVHW070611100526
838202LV00012B/624